Pediatric Allergy

Second Edition

MEDICAL OUTLINE SERIES

R. Michael Sly, M.D.
Director of Allergy and Immunology
Children's Hospital National Medical Center;
Professor of Child Health and Development
George Washington University School of
Medicine and Health Sciences
Washington, D.C.

illustrated by

Don Alvarado

 Medical Examination Publishing Co., Inc.
an Excerpta Medica company

SIMULTANEOUSLY PUBLISHED IN:

| Europe | : | HANS HUBER PUBLISHERS |
| | | Bern, Switzerland |

| Japan | : | IGAKU-SHOIN Ltd. |
| | | Tokyo, Japan |

Mexico,	:	EDITORIAL EL MANUAL MODERNO
Central America, and		Mexico City, Mexico
South America		
(except Brazil)		

notice

The editor(s) and/or author(s) and the publisher of this book have made
every effort to ensure that all therapeutic modalities that are recommended are in accordance with accepted standards at the time of
publication.

The drugs specified within this book may not have specific approval by
the Food and Drug Administration in regard to the indications and
dosages that are recommended by the editor(s) and/or author(s). The
manufacturer's package insert is the best source of current prescribing
information.

Preface

Numerous recent advances in the immunology, physiology, biochemistry, and pharmacology of atopic diseases have clarified the pathogenesis of these disorders, facilitated accurate diagnosis, and permitted the development of rational, safe, and effective programs of therapy. The clinician is called upon for a synthesis of the best of the old with the new for optimal patient care.

This book was written to supply practicing physicians and students with a concise reference on current diagnosis and treatment of atopic respiratory and cutaneous diseases, systemic anaphylaxis, and drug allergy in children. Much of the clinical and laboratory research of recent years has necessitated extensive revision of the first edition. Although the most extensive changes describe the immunopathology of atopy, the treatment of asthma, and insect sting allergy, every chapter has been revised.

Extensive bibliographies follow each chapter to facilitate more detailed exploration of subjects of special interest to the reader. The magnitude of my debt to the many authors who have preceded me will be evident from the length of these lists of references.

R. Michael Sly, M.D.

This book is dedicated to

my wife, Ann, and daughters, Terri and Cindy—
without their understanding patience
it could not have been written;

and to

the authors whose names appear among the references—
without their observations and insight there
would have been nothing to write.

Contents

Continuing Medical Education Credits

As an organization accredited for Continuing Medical Education, Temple University School of Medicine has designated this continuing medical educational activity as meeting the criteria for 10 credit hours in Category I for educational materials for the Physician's Recognition Award of AMA, provided it has been completed according to instructions.

The purpose of this activity is to give information which the physician can apply to practice. By means of the self-assessment test the participant can evaluate the effectiveness of the educational experience.

Suggestions concerning the educational aspects of the program are encouraged and should be directed to:

Albert J. Finestone, M.D.
Associate Dean, Continuing Medical Education
Office for Continuing Medical Education
Temple University School of Medicine
3400 North Broad Street
Philadelphia, PA 19140

CHAPTER I | ALLERGY AND ATOPY

ALLERGY

While seeking a means of affording protection against the toxic effects of an extract prepared from actinaria tentacles Charles Richet observed that injection after 2-3 weeks of a second dose into dogs which had survived the initial injection was followed within a few seconds by panting, prostration, diarrhea, and hematemesis. The reaction was often fatal within 25 minutes. Since this seemed the opposite of protection (phylaxis), he coined the word "anaphylaxis" in 1902.[1]

The term "allergy" was introduced in 1906 by Clemens von Pirquet, a pediatrician.[2] He had observed deaths in animals following administration of small amounts of tetanus toxin when hyperimmunity had previously been induced by injection of the toxin and had also noticed the change in the reaction to tuberculin which followed tuberculosis.

"...the tuberculous patient (behaves) towards tuberculin, the person injected with serum towards serum, in a different manner from him who has not previously been in contact with such an agent. Yet he is not insensitive to it. We can only say of him that his power to react has undergone a change".[2]

He concluded that there was a close relationship between immunity and increased sensitivity and defined allergy as an acquired specific alteration in an animal's capacity to react following contact with a foreign substance. More recently the term "allergy" has been restricted to clinical hypersensitivity, and it is no longer used to include immunity.

In current usage "allergy" is usually applied to a response mediated by an immunologic mechanism, and it has been recommended that its definition restrict its usage to such responses.[3] Thus, allergy can usually be defined as a specific, acquired alteration in reactivity mediated by an immunologic mechanism which results in an untoward physiological response. Physical allergy is one of the very few exceptions, since these responses are not usually mediated by immunologic mechanisms.

1

CLASSIFICATION OF HYPERSENSITIVITY REACTIONS

Within 20 years after the introduction of the term "allergy", it was evident that allergic reactions could be classified into at least two groups: immediate hypersensitivity, including anaphylaxis, and delayed hypersensitivity, including the tuberculin reaction which von Pirquet had observed. With immediate hypersensitivity the peak of the reaction is reached within minutes or a few hours, and reactivity can be transferred from hypersensitive to normal subjects by serum containing the specific antibody. With delayed hypersensitivity the peak of the reaction is reached only after 12 hours or more, and delayed hypersensitivity can be transferred only by lymphoid cells or leukocyte extracts. Arthus reactions and serum sickness are further examples of immediate hypersensitivity.

More recently Gell and Coombs proposed a further classification of allergic reactions based upon "the circumstances of the initial reaction between allergen (or antigen) and antibody or specifically modified cells... subgrouping subsequently on other secondary phenomena" (Fig. 1.1).[4]

TYPE I REACTION
(ANAPHYLACTIC REACTION)

This response followed reaction between antigen and antibody fixed to the surface of mast cells or basophils. This causes the release of chemical mediators (See Chapter 2), and the pharmacological actions of these agents are responsible for the clinical manifestations. The cytotropic antibodies (antibodies which can become fixed to cell surfaces) which participate in this reaction are usually of the immunoglobulin E (IgE) class.

Type I reactions can be subclassified into generalized anaphylactic reactions and local anaphylactic reactions. Generalized anaphylaxis is the systemic reaction characterized by flushing, urticaria, anxiety, coughing, dyspnea, wheezing, cyanosis, vomiting and shock which may follow the antigen-antibody reaction. Local anaphylactic reactions include allergic rhinitis, allergic asthma, and some forms of urticaria.

TYPE II REACTION
(CYTOLYTIC OR CYTOTOXIC REACTION)

In a Type II reaction antibody usually of the IgG or IgM class reacts with an antigenic component of a cell or with an antigen or hapten which has become intimately associated with the cell. The target cell is destroyed by polymorphonuclear

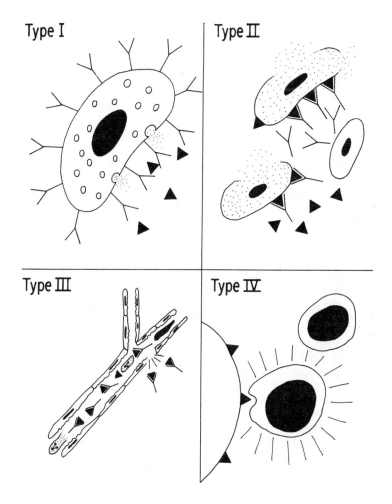

Fig. 1-1.   Four types of allergic reaction which may cause tissue injury (modified from Coombs and Gell). [4]

leukocytes or macrophages through opsonic adherence (mediated by the Fc portion of the antibody molecule) or by immune adherence (mediated by the antigen-antibody-C3b complex). Antibody-dependent cell-mediated toxicity is a mechanism through which the target cell is destroyed without participation of complement by neutrophils, monocytes, or small lymphocytes lacking surface markers of B or T cells, known as K cells.

Examples of Type II reactions include transfusion reactions due to blood group incompatibility resulting in hemolysis, hemolytic disease of the newborn due to Rh incompatibility or A or B incompatibility, some forms of drug hypersensitivity such as penicillin-induced hemolytic anemia, and the glomerulonephritis and alveolitis of Goodpasture's syndrome.

TYPE III REACTION (ARTHUS TYPE REACTION, TOXIC COMPLEX REACTION)

A reaction of this type results from the formation of soluble antigen-antibody complexes. In moderate antigen excess systemic reactions may occur, while complex formation in antibody excess usually is followed by reactions localized to the site of introduction of antigen.

The reaction between antigen and precipitating antibody (IgG or IgM) results in deposition of microprecipitates in and around small blood vessels following complement activation. Polymorphonuclear leukocytes, attracted by chemotactic factors associated with C5, 6, and 7, phagocytize the complexes. Some of the polymorphonuclear leukocytes are destroyed, releasing proteolytic enzymes which cause tissue damage. Platelet aggregation may occur, causing formation of microthrombi, which can cause local ischemia.

Local injection of the antigen into tissues when antibody is circulating in the blood results in an Arthus type reaction. It has been suggested that local reactions which may follow frequent immunization with tetanus toxoid may be Arthus-type reactions.[5]

When large amounts of antigen are circulating, serum sickness can result from formation of antigen-antibody complexes as antibody is produced.

Other diseases ascribed to Type III reactions include hypersensitivity pneumonitis (extrinsic allergic alveolitis) and some forms of glomerulonephritis, including the nephritis of systemic lupus erythematosus. There is also evidence suggesting at least partial mediation of hypersensitivity pneumonitis through a Type IV reaction.[6]

TYPE IV REACTION (DELAYED OR CELL MEDIATED HYPERSENSITIVITY)

As indicated previously, delayed hypersensitivity can be transferred to a normal subject by lymphoid cells or leukocyte extracts, but not by serum. The reaction becomes maximal only after 12 hours, usually at 24-72 hours.

Although Type IV reactions are not yet fully understood, available evidence indicates that contact of thymus-dependent lymphocytes with antigen is followed by blast transformation and sensitization of the lymphocyte. Further interaction of sensitized lymphocytes with antigen is followed by release from the lymphocytes of lymphokines, biologically active factors mostly defined by their activity (Table 1.1). Migration inhibitory factor, one of the lymphokines, may induce activation of macrophages (increased cell size; increased numbers of mitochondria, lysosomal granules, and vesicles; increased phagocytosis). Cytolysis of the target cell may then occur through the action of other lymphokines. Cytolysis of the Type IV reaction is not complement dependent, unlike that of the Type II reaction. Immunologic memory for Type IV reactions is retained by small lymphocytes.

Examples of Type IV reactions include contact dermatitis, tuberculin allergy, autoimmunity, homograft rejection, and immunologic response to cancer cells.

ATOPY

The recognized relationships between hay fever and allergic asthma caused Coca to introduce the term "atopy", a word derived by Perry from the Greek, meaning strange disease.[7] He defined atopy as that form of hypersensitivity which was peculiar to humans, acquired spontaneously, and influenced by heredity. This atopic state was characterized by an immediate whealing reaction and circulating reaginic antibody (Type I reaction). Because of similarities and the clinical association between atopic respiratory disease and allergic eczema it was soon referred to as atopic dermatitis.[8] Gastrointestinal allergy and some forms of urticaria are also considered atopic diseases.

Allergic rhinitis and asthma are now known to occur in dogs, and reaginic antibody formation has been induced by injection of antigen into human subjects.[9] Furthermore, discordance with respect to atopic diseases reported in what were considered to be identical twins has raised questions about the mode of inheritance.[10,11] Nevertheless, atopy has retained its usefulness as a term which seems to characterize most of the subjects to whom it is applied appropriately.

HEREDITY

An influence of heredity upon the development of atopic diseases was suspected as early as 1650 when Sennertus reportedly recognized that asthma could be familial.[12] Numerous

TABLE 1.1   POSSIBLE EFFECTORS OF
             DELAYED HYPERSENSITIVITY

LYMPHOKINE	ACTIVITY
Migration Inhibitory Factor (MIF) or Macrophage Activating Factor	Inhibition of macrophage migration Stimulation of macrophage phagocytic capacity, metabolism, membrane activity, and killing of microorganisms
Macrophage Aggregation Factor	(Probably identical with MIF)
Macrophage Chemotactic Factor	Macrophage chemotaxis
Neutrophil Chemotactic Factor	Neutrophil chemotaxis
Lymphotoxic Factors	Killing target cells
Cloning Inhibition Factor	Reversible inhibition of cloning of target cells
Proliferation Inhibition Factor	Inhibition of growth of human cell lines
Inhibitor of DNA Synthesis	Inhibition of DNA synthesis
Mitogenic Factors (Blastogenic Factors	Blast transformation of non-sensitive lymphocytes
Skin Reactive Factor	Induction of erythema, induration, and mobilization of mononuclear cells and polymorphonuclear leukocytes in guinea pig skin
Transfer Factor	Transfer of activity to uncommitted lymphocytes
Platelet aggregating factor	Platelet aggregation
Interferon	Inhibition of virus replication
Antibody	Reaction with antigen

subsequent studies have confirmed an increased incidence of atopy in the siblings and parents of subjects with atopic diseases, but the results of different studies are difficult to compare and figures cannot be quoted with great confidence because of differences in the definition and diagnosis of specific diseases, lack of agreement concerning criteria for classification of some conditions as atopic, and variations in assessing the significance of atopy in distant relatives.

Cooke and Vander Veer reported in 1916 positive family histories in 48% of 504 subjects with "sensitization" (hay fever, asthma, eczema, gastrointestinal allergy, urticaria), compared with 14.5% in 76 normal subjects.[13] Positive family history was defined to include siblings, parents, aunts and uncles, and grandparents, but excluded cousins. Their data indicated that what was inherited was an atopic tendency rather than one of the specific diseases or allergy to a specific allergen. Inheritance was from the paternal side of the family as frequently as the maternal side, implicating genetic factors rather than transplacental transmission of sensitization. Age of onset of symptoms of an atopic disease as determined by history was earlier with bilateral "inheritance" than unilateral "inheritance" or in those with negative family histories for atopy.

Spain and Cooke later found a positive family history in 58% of 462 subjects when only hay fever and asthma were included, compared with a frequency of 7% in 115 normal subjects.[14] The age of onset of symptoms was again found to be related to the extent of the hereditary influence, but subsequent studies have failed to confirm such an association.[15] After adjustments for the ages of their subjects, the authors estimated that 71.6% of the children with bilateral family histories of hay fever or asthma could expect to develop one of these conditions while 56.1% of those with unilateral family histories would.

Although these early studies were subject to the limitations of any study dependent largely upon historical data compounded further by what was then a very limited knowledge of allergy, the conclusions have largely been confirmed by subsequent studies reporting family histories of "allergy" in 40-70% of children with asthma and 35-80% of subjects with hay fever.[12, 16]

Others have also reported that a bilateral family history of atopy carries an increased risk for the development of atopic diseases as compared with a unilateral family history.[16]

Schwartz concluded from the incidence of various possibly atopic diseases in a group of 191 asthmatic subjects compared with 200 controls that vasomotor rhinitis, hay fever, and atopic dermatitis were genetically related to asthma, while gastrointestinal allergy and urticaria were not definitely related.[17]

Although there has been general agreement that atopy is hereditary, the mode of inheritance remains undetermined. Some have suggested inheritance as a Mendelian dominant, [13] but this cannot account for the large number of atopic subjects without any family history of atopy. A recessive mode of inheritance, on the other hand, would fail to explain the frequent occurrence of unaffected children when both parents are atopic. Wiener et al., proposed that transmission might be as an incomplete recessive trait. [18] Subjects homozygous for the normal gene would be normal; those homozygous for the allergic gene might be those who developed atopic disease by 10 years of age. It was suggested that approximately 18% of heterozygotes developed atopy at some time after 10 years of age, depending upon environmental conditions. Subsequently most others have agreed that inheritance of atopy is probably mediated through such a mechanism [16, 17] (estimates of penetrance have varied) or through more than one pair of genes. [16, 19] Tips has proposed three separate pairs of alleles for asthma, hay fever, and atopic dermatitis, respectively. [19]

Studies of identical twins have not supplied conclusive evidence regarding the question of heredity, partly because of a lack of proof that many of the twins were monozygotic. Nevertheless it is of interest that of 44 pairs of twins considered identical, in which at least one of each pair had an allergic disease, at least 4 pairs were discordant with respect to the presence of allergic disease. [20] Bowen reported that of 59 pairs of "monozygotic" twins, in 52 "the allergic condition existed in only one twin to the degree that medical aid was sought." [10] Criteria for the diagnosis of "the allergic condition" were not supplied, however, and monozygosity was established only by examination of obstetrical records to determine that a single placenta had been recognized, an unreliable criterion for monozygosity. Discordance with respect to atopy has also been reported in other apparently identical twins, however, [11] although a much higher rate of concordance with respect to atopy has generally been reported among "monozygotic" twins than among dizygotic twins. In the three reports where monozygosity was well established [21-23] some evidence of concordance with respect to atopy was reported although in one case one twin was much more severely affected than the other. [23]

Serum IgE concentrations have been reported to agree much more closely in monozygotic twins than in dizygotic twins, [24] but sufficiently great differences were found in some pairs of monozygotic twins to emphasize the likelihood of dependence upon nongenetic as well as probably genetic factors.

Immune response genes linked to the major histocompatibility (H) system of inbred mice are known to control specific IgE antibody responses, but their total IgE production is not H-linked. It is inferred that immune response genes linked to the major histocompatibility complex in humans may also exist (Fig. 1.2).

This inference has been supported by a significant association between hay fever due to hypersensitivity to the antigen E component of ragweed pollen and the HLA-A1, 8 haplotype in one family, and by similar associations with six other haplotypes in each of six other families (W-28, x; HLA-A-10, Da; HLA-A3, 7; HLA-A3, 5; HLA-A2, x; and HLA-A-2, W14).[26] Highly significant associations have also been found between HLA-B7 and hypersensitivity to the Ra5 component of short ragweed pollen, and between HLA-B8 and A1, B8 and hypersensitivity to the group I allergen of rye grass pollen.[27, 28] Among patients with total IgE concentrations in the serum of less than 130 units/ml, a highly significant association has been found between HLA-A2 and Ra3 hypersensitivity.[29]

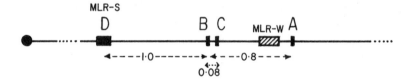

Fig. 1-2. Genetic map of a portion of the short arm of chromosome 6, showing the human major histocompatibility complex, HLA, with the relationships of the serologically defined (SD) loci, A, B, and C, and the lymphocyte-defined (LD) regions, D (or MLR-S) and MLR-w, which control mixed lymphocyte reactions. Map distances are expressed as percentage frequency of recombination. (From Marsh, D. G., used by permission[25])

PREVALENCE

Attempts to determine the prevalence of allergic diseases have also been limited by differences in definition and methods of diagnosis. Most have depended upon completion of questionnaires by subjects whose ability to supply accurate data has varied. Variations with the geographic location and mobility of the population also seem likely and are confirmed to some extent by data from the Health Interview Survey of 1970 of the United States Bureau of the Census (Figs. 1.3, 1.4).[30] Most of

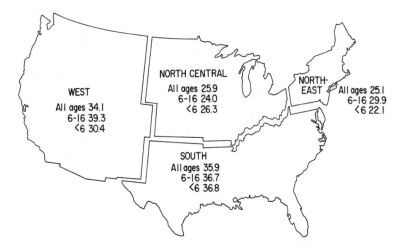

Fig. 1-3. Prevalence of asthma with or without hay fever per 1,000 population as determined from data from the Health Interview Survey of 1970 of the United States Bureau of the Census.[30]

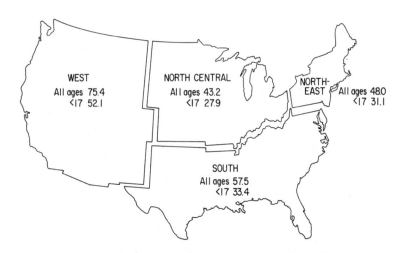

Fig. 1-4. Prevalence of hay fever without asthma per 1,000 population as determined from data from the Health Interview Survey of 1970 of the United States Bureau of the Census.[30]

these variables have probably caused an underestimation of the incidence of allergic diseases.

Nevertheless most recent studies have suggested that at least 20-25% of children in the United States have or have had allergic rhinitis, asthma and/or atopic dermatitis by 18 years of age. [31,32] The frequency of seasonal hay fever has been reported to be 21% among 12th grade students[31] or college freshmen;[32] nonseasonal allergic rhinitis, 5%; and asthma 3-5%. Study of a community in Michigan, however, disclosed that 10.7% of boys 10-15 years old had had probable asthma and another 4.4% had "suspect asthma".[33] The frequency among girls of this age was 7.6% and 3.6%, respectively. Data from the National Health Examination Survey of 1963-65 confirmed the frequent observation of an increased prevalence of a history of asthma in boys (6.5%) as compared with girls (2.9%) for ages 6-11 years. [34]

Atopic dermatitis (past or present) has been reported at a frequency of 1.6% (questionnaire, 12th grade students)[31] to 4.3% (diagnosis by pediatrician in 1753 children examined periodically from birth until 1/2-7 years of age). [35]

The National Health Survey of 1959-61, based upon household interviews, disclosed that "hay fever, asthma, and other allergies accounted for 32.8% of chronic conditions in children".[36] Despite the estimate of prevalence of allergy at only 7.4%, low compared to more recent data, asthma accounted for 22.9% of days reported lost from school because of chronic conditions in children. Thus, allergy is the commonest chronic illness in children, and asthma accounts for more time lost from school than any other single chronic disease except other respiratory diseases.

REFERENCES

1. Portier, P., and Richet, C.: De l'action anaphylactique de certains venins. C R Soc Biol 54:170, 1902.
2. Pirquet, C. von: Allergie, Munchen med. Wchshr 53:1457, 1906 (Translated by C. Prausnitz and quoted by Gell, P. G. H., and Coombs, R. R. A.), eds.: Clinical Aspects of Immunology, F. A. Davis Co., Philadelphia, 1963, p 807.
3. Minden, P., and Farr, R. S.: The management of allergic disorders in children. Ped Clin N A 16:305, 1969.
4. Coombs, R. R. A., and Gell, P. G. H.: The classification of allergic reactions underlying disease in Gell, P. G. H. and Coombs, R. R. A., eds.: Clinical Aspects of Immunology, F. A. Davis Co., Philadelphia, 1963, p 317.
5. Edsall, G., Elliot, M. W., Peebles, T. C., Levine, L., and Eldred, M. C.: Excessive use of tetanus toxoid boosters. JAMA 202:17, 1967.
6. Lake, W. W., Salvaggio, J. E., and Buechner, H. A.: "Infiltrative 'Hypersensitivity' Lung Disease" in Frazier, C. A., ed: Annual Review of Allergy 1973, Med Exam Pub Co., Inc., Garden City, N. Y., 1974.
7. Coca, A. F., and Cooke, R. A.: On the classification of the phenomena of hypersensitiveness. J Imm 8:163, 1923.
8. Coca, A. F. and Sulzberger, M. B.: Yearbook of Dermatology and Syphilology, Year Book Pub., Chicago, 1933, p 59.
9. Feinberg, A. R., Becker, R. J., Slavin, R. G., and Feinberg, S. M.: Induction of immediate and delayed skin reactivity with emulsion of purified ragweed antigen. J All 38:236, 1966.
10. Bowen, R.: Allergy in identical twins. J All 24:236, 1953.
11. Rajka, G.: Prurigo Besnier (atopic dermatitis) with special reference to the role of allergic factors. 1. The influence of atopic hereditary factors. Acta Dermat-Vener 40:285, 1960.
12. Vaughan, W. T., and Black, J. H.: Practice of Allergy, 3rd ed., C. V. Mosby Co., St. Louis, 1954.
13. Cooke, R. A., and Vander Veer, A., Jr.: Human Sensitization. J Imm 1:201, 1916.
14. Spain, W. C., and Cooke, R. A.: Studies in specific hypersensitiveness XI. The familial occurrence of hay fever and bronchial asthma. J Imm 9:521, 1924.
15. Ratner, B., and Silberman, D. E.: Critical analysis of the hereditary concept of allergy. J All 24:371, 1953.
16. VanArsdel, P. P., Jr., and Motulsky, A. G.: Frequency and heritability of asthma and allergic rhinitis in college students. Acta Genet Stat Med 9:101, 1959.

17. Schwartz, M.: Heredity in Bronchial Asthma. Acta Allergol (Suppl 2), 1952.
18. Wiener, A. S., Zieve, I. and Fries, J. H.: The inheritance of allergic disease. Ann Eugen 7:141, 1936.
19. Tips, R. L.: A study of the inheritance of atopic hypersensitivity in man. Am J Hum Gen 6:328, 1954.
20. Spaich, D., and Ostertag, M.: Untersuchungen uber allergische Erkrankungen bei Zwillingen. Ztschr menschl Vererb u Konstitutionslehre 19:731, 1936.
21. Wiener, S.: Desensitization for asthma in identical twins. Med J Austr 1:1004, 1967.
22. Sly, R. M., and Heimlich, E. M.: Identical twins with short stature, elevated IgA, and Asthma. Ann All 25:578, 1967.
23. Falliers, C. J., de A. Cardoso, R. R., Bane, H. N., Coffey, R., and Middleton, E., Jr.: Discordant allergic manifestations in monozygotic twins: Genetic identity versus clinical, physiologic, and biochemical differences. J All 47:207, 1971.
24. Bazaral, M., Orgel, H. A., and Hamburger, R. N.: Genetics of IgE and allergy: Serum IgE levels in twins. J All Clin Imm 54:288, 1974.
25. Marsh, D. G.: "Allergy: a model for studying the genetics of human immune response", in Johansson, S. G. O., and Strandberg, K. (eds): Molecular and Biological Aspects of the Acute Allergic Reaction, Plenum Press, New York, 1976, p 23.
26. Levine, B. B., Stember, R. H., and Fotino, M.: Ragweed hay fever: Genetic control and linkage to HLA haplotypes. Science 178:1201, 1972.
27. Marsh, D. G., Bias, W. B., Santilli, J., Schacter, B., and Goodfriend, L.: Ragweed allergen Ra5: A new tool in understanding the genetics and immunochemistry of immune response in man. Immunochemistry 12:539, 1975.
28. Marsh, D. G., and Bias, W. B.: Basal serum IgE levels and HLA antigen frequencies in allergic subjects. II Studies in populations sensitive to rye grass group I and ragweed antigen E and of postulated immune response loci in the HLA region. Immunogenetics 5:235, 1977.
29. Marsh, D. G., and Bias, W. B.: "The genetics of atopic allergy", in Samter, M. (Ed): Immunological Diseases, 3rd Ed., Little, Brown, & Co., Boston, 1978, p 819.
30. Wilder, C. S.: Prevalence of selected chronic respiratory conditions, U. S., 1970. U. S. Vital and Health Statistics, Series 10, No. 84, September, 1973.

31. Freeman, G. L. , and Johnson, S. : Allergic diseases in adolescents. Am J Dis Child 107:549, 1964.
32. Hay, G. W. , and Settipane, G. A. : Bronchial asthma, allergic rhinitis, and allergy skin tests among college students. J All 44:323, 1969.
33. Broder, I. , Higgins, M. W. , Mathews, K. P. , and Keller, J. B. : Epidemiology of asthma and allergic rhinitis in a total community, Tecumseh, Michigan, J All Clin Imm 53:127, 1974.
34. Roberts, J. : Examination and health history findings among children and youths, 6-17 years. U. S. Vital and Health Statistics, Series 11, No. 129, U. S. Dept. Health, Education, and Welfare, November, 1973.
35. Halpern, S. R. , Sellars, W. A. , Johnson, R. B. , Anderson, D. W. , Saperstein, S. , and Reisch, J. S. : Development of childhood allergy in infants fed breast, soy, or cow milk. J All Clin Imm 51:139, 1973.
36. Schiffer, C. G. , and Hunt, E. P. : Illness Among Children. U. S. Dept. Health, Education, and Welfare, 1963.

REAGIN

The presence of a sensitizing factor in the sera of atopic subjects was suggested in 1919 by the report of Ramirez of the occurrence of asthma due to exposure to horses in a previously nonallergic man following transfusion with blood from an asthmatic with hypersensitivity to horse dander.[1]

In 1920 Prausnitz and Kustner demonstrated that the skin reactivity associated with Kustner's allergy to fish could be transferred by serum to the skin of nonallergic subjects.[2] Intradermal injection of fish extract at sites which had received intradermal injections of Kustner's serum the previous day was followed within 15 minutes by the appearance of a wheal and erythema at each site. Since then, similar passive transfer or P-K reactions have frequently been used to demonstrate or to detect the presence of specific immediate hypersensitivity.

Coca and Grove introduced the term 'atopic reagin' to designate the "specifically reacting substances in the serum of atopic individuals".[3] The Ishizakas found that reagin activity was usually due to a specific class of immunoglobulins, IgE,[4] observations confirmed by Johansson and Bennich after discovery of a patient with IgE myeloma.[5]

The IgE molecule consists of four polypeptide chains, two heavy chains and two light chains, bound together by disulfide bonds and noncovalent forces to form a bivalent antibody molecule with two antigen combining sites. Thus, its structure resembles the basic structure of immunoglobulins of the other four classes, but its heavy chains are unique. Differences in the heavy chains of the five classes of immunoglobulins confer differences in their physiochemical, metabolic, and biologic properties. (Tables 2.1, 2.2 and 2.3).

Immunoglobulin G is the major serum antibody globulin, including the protective antibodies against most bacterial and viral infections. Antibodies to castor allergen have been found to be restricted to the IgG4 subclass in some patients with cas-

TABLE 2.1 PHYSICOCHEMICAL PROPERTIES OF IMMUNOGLOBULINS

	IgG	IgA	Secretory IgA	IgM	IgD	IgE
Heavy Chains	γ	α	α	μ	δ	ε
Light Chains	κ or λ	κ or λ	κ or λ	κ or λ	κ or λ	κ or λ
Monomer Units	1	1	2	5	1	1
Electrophoretic Mobility	γ_2 ($\gamma_2 - \alpha_2$)	$\gamma_1 - \alpha_1$ (β)	$\gamma_1 - \alpha_1$ (β)	γ_1 ($\gamma_1 - \alpha_1$)	γ_1 ($\gamma_1 - \beta$)	β ($\gamma_1 - \beta$)
Sedimentation Coefficient	6.7s	7-15s	11.4-11.7s (7-19s)	19s	7s	8s
Molecular Weight	150,000	160,000-318,000	370,000	900,000	175,000	190,000
Carbohydrate	2.9%	5-7%	(SC 9.5%)	11.8%	14.8%	12%
Heat Lability	$\pm$	+		++	++++	+++
Genetic Factors	Gm, Inv	Am, Inv	Am, Inv	Inv	Inv	Inv

TABLE 2.2   METABOLIC PROPERTIES OF IMMUNOGLOBULINS

	IgG	IgG1	IgG2	IgG3	IgG4	IgA	IgA1	IgA2	IgM	IgD	IgE
Normal Adult Serum Concentration (mg/dl)	1200	500-1200	200-600	50-100	20-100	200	50-200	0-20	50-150	0-40	0-0.13
(I.U./ml)	138					120			58-173	0-280	1-550
Biologic half-life (days)	23	23	23	9	23	6	6	6	5	2.8	2.3 (9-14 in skin)
Distribution (% intravascular)	45					45	most	little	80	75	50
Total body pool (mg/Kg)	1150					230			49	1.5	0.04
Synthetic rate (mg/Kg/day)	35					25			7	0.4	0.02
Placental transfer	+	+	+	+	+	-	-	-	-	-	-
% Body content catabolized each day	3					12			14	35	89

TABLE 2.3 BIOLOGIC PROPERTIES OF IMMUNOGLOBULINS

	IgG	IgG1	IgG2	IgG3	IgG4	IgA1	IgA2	IgM	IgD	IgE
Complement Activation (classical pathway)	+	‡	+	‡	-	-	-	+	-	-
(alternate)	-	-	-	-	-	+	+	-	+−	+−
Agglutination	+					-	-	‡	-	-
Opsonization	+					-	-	‡	-	-
Virus Neutralization	+					-	+	+	-	-
Hemolysis	+					-	-	‡	-	-
Fixation to mast cells or basophils		-	-	-	+	-	-	-	-	‡
Blocking of IgE binding		-	-	-	+	-	-	-	-	
Cytophilic binding to macrophages and polymorphonuclear leukocytes	+					-	-	-	-	-
Present in body secretions	+					+	‡	+−	-	+−

tor bean hypersensitivity, and IgG4 antibodies to grass pollen have been found in some patients with pollenosis. [6,7] Elevated serum IgG4 concentrations have been reported in some patients with atopic dermatitis and some with cystic fibrosis. [8,9] There is also evidence that specific IgG4 antibody induced by immunotherapy may act as a blocking antibody. [10]

Immunoglobulin M is a polymer consisting of five monomers held together by disulfide bonds and a J chain, a relatively small polypeptide chain high in sulfhydryl content. Primary immunization is usually characterized initially by production of IgM followed within two weeks by production of larger amounts of IgG. Production of IgG usually predominates in the secondary response.

Serum IgA globulin contains isoagglutinins and antibodies against some bacteria and viruses. Serum IgA consists mostly of 7s molecules composed of two heavy chains and two light chains, but small amounts of molecular aggregates are also present in serum.

Secretory IgA consists predominantly of monomers joined by J chains to form dimers, each bound to a "secretory piece" or "secretory component," resulting in a molecular weight of 370,000. Secretory IgA is much more resistant to proteolysis than serum IgA or other immunoglobulins. Although small amounts of the other immunoglobulins can be found in external body secretions such as tears, colostrum, saliva, and nasal secretions, secretory IgA usually predominates and has been found to have antibody activity against many bacteria and viruses.

The secretory component is present in the secretions of patients with IgA deficiency. Isolated deficiency of secretory component has been reported in a boy with virtual absence of IgA in secretions, normal serum concentrations of IgA, and chronic intestinal candidiasis. [11]

Immunoglobulin D has also been demonstrated to have antibody activity, and sera from some subjects allergic to penicillin have been found to contain IgD globulins specific for the benzyl-penicilloyl antigenic determinant. [12] Three subjects with hypersensitivity to cow's milk have been found to have IgD antibodies directed against bovine gamma globulin. [13]

Immunoglobulin D, IgM, or both have been found on the surfaces of most peripheral B lymphocytes, and IgD may help determine the response of the B lymphocyte to antigen. [14]

Immunoglobulin E has been detected in low concentrations ($<$10 U/ml, median 2 U/ml) in cord sera from normal newborn infants, [15] and synthesis by fetal lung and liver has been detected at 11 weeks. [16] Most recent data indicate that there is normally a gradual increase in serum concentration of IgE until normal adult concentrations are reached at 7-10 years of age. [17]

Abnormal increases in total serum IgE concentrations have been reported in association with atopic dermatitis, hay fever, and allergic asthma, ascariasis, visceral larva migrans, and other helminthic parasitic infestations, and Wiskott-Aldrich Syndrome, a sex linked recessive disorder characterized by eczema, thrombocytopenia, and increased susceptibility to infections with increased serum concentrations of IgA and defective delayed hypersensitivity. Other conditions reported associated with increased serum concentrations of IgE include pemphigoid, chronic acral dermatitis, food allergy, allergic bronchopulmonary aspergillosis, pulmonary hemosiderosis, celiac disease, Laennec's cirrhosis, multiple myeloma patients without "M" peaks, isolated IgA deficiency, thymic alymphoplasia, (Nezelof Syndrome or DiGeorge Syndrome), gonorrhea, trichomoniasis, primary syphilis, infectious mononucleosis and other viral infections, and cystic fibrosis. Extremely high serum concentrations of IgE have been associated with a syndrome characterized by recurrent cutaneous, pulmonary and joint abscesses, growth retardation, coarse facies, chronic dermatitis, eosinophilia, and impairment of delayed hypersensitivity and antibody formation.[18] Extreme hyperimmunoglobulinemia E, eosinophilia, and increased numbers of circulating lymphocytes bearing surface IgE have also been described in a man without any evident morbidity except mild pruritus.[19]

Serum concentrations of IgE have been reported to be very low in subjects with primary generalized deficiency of immunoglobulin production.

Immunoglobulin E-forming plasma cells have been found in greatest profusion in tonsils and adenoids.[20] Lesser numbers have been found in bronchial and peritoneal lymph nodes, and respiratory and gastrointestinal mucosa, and very few IgE forming plasma cells have been found in the spleen and subcutaneous lymph nodes. Immunoglobulins of all five classes have been demonstrated in external secretions such as saliva, nasal secretions, tracheobronchial secretions, colostrum and intestinal secretions. Only secretory IgA has been found to differ in structure from its serum counterpart, and only secretory IgA and IgE have been found in secretions of normal subjects at concentrations higher relative to those of IgG than in the serum. Concentrations of IgE in some specimens of colostrum have been reported more than 20 times as great as the serum concentrations.[21] However, increased vascular permeability resulting from IgE-mediated hypersensitivity reactions may permit serum antibody also to participate in local immunity.

The presence of IgE in some secretions and a report of correlation between sinopulmonary infections and the combination of IgA deficiency and IgE deficiency in some subjects with ataxia-telangiectasia[22] suggested a protective function of IgE in secretions. Subsequent study of subjects with IgA deficiency who did not have ataxia-telangiectasia disclosed no relationship between serum IgE levels and susceptibility to infection,[23] however, and absence of serum IgE has been reported in apparently healthy subjects.

Increased concentrations of IgE in nasal washings have been reported in asthmatic children as compared with normal controls[24] although some asthmatics without elevated concentrations of IgE in nasal washings or sputum have also been found. Nasal washings from some but not most patients allergic to ragweed have been found to contain IgE antiragweed antibodies.[25]

Concentrations of IgE in both serum and nasal secretions have been reported to increase during pollen seasons in most patients with allergic rhinitis or asthma due to pollen hypersensitivity.[26]

Very high concentrations of IgE have been reported in nasal polyp fluid, ranging from 203-8638 ng/ml.[27]

REGULATION OF IgE

Although the possible function of IgE in normal subjects remains uncertain beyond its protective effect against parasitic infestation, its activity in the Type I anaphylactic reaction is well established.

Studies of experimental animals indicated that complex cellular interactions regulate the production of IgE (Fig. 2.1). When the allergen is a hapten-carrier conjugate, the carrier interacts with T lymphocytes, while the hapten interacts with B lymphocytes. A hapten is a substance that is not of itself immunogenic (capable of stimulating antibody formation or a cellular immune response), but when linked to a carrier molecule it becomes immunogenic. Haptens are antigenic (capable of reacting with antibody or sensitized lymphocytes).

Presentation of allergen by macrophages favors induction of helper T cells, that interact not only with the carrier portion of the allergen but also with "cell interaction molecules" on the surface of the macrophage.[28] Induction of antigen-specific suppressor T cells may occur, but nonspecific suppressor T cells have also been found, and a strain-specific, antigen-nonspecific substance that suppresses IgE production has been found in mouse serum.[28] Interaction of the haptenic determinants of the allergen with B lymphocytes results in a redistribution of immunoglobulin on the surface of the lymphocyte into a cap, and subsequent endocytosis of the surface immunoglobulin. Inter-

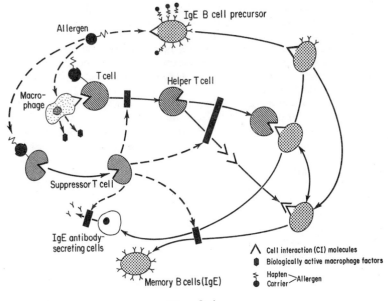

Fig. 2-1.

action of such B cell precursors, with helper T cells or soluble factors released from helper T cells, facilitates differentiation into IgE antibody-secreting plasma cells or memory B cells.

Suppressor T cells may interfere with activation of helper T cells, with interaction of helper T cells with B lymphocytes, with differentiation of B lymphocytes to mature, IgE antibody-producing or memory cells, or with secretion of IgE antibody by mature effector cells.

IMMUNOLOGIC RELEASE OF CHEMICAL MEDIATORS

Molecules of IgE have an affinity for the surfaces of circulating basophils or their tissue counterparts, mast cells. The Fc portion of this homocytotropic antibody molecule becomes attached to the cell surface, leaving the Fab portions free to react with antigen. The number of IgE receptor sites on the cell surface has been estimated to vary from 6,000 to 600,000, although the number of receptor sites on the cells of atopic subjects does not necessarily exceed that of normal subjects. The number of receptors does correlate closely with the serum IgE level, indicating either a genetic association or determination of receptor number by IgE concentration.[29] Binding of IgE molecules to these receptors is reversible, and affinity between IgE and receptors may differ from person to person. Correlation has been found between serum IgE concentration and the number of molecules bound to basophils, but receptor saturation has been reported at IgE concentrations of 400 ng/ml.[30] An inverse relationship was found between the number of IgE molecules bound to each cell and optimum concentration of anti-IgE for maximum histamine release from the cells.[29] Likewise, cell reactivity (maximum percent histamine release attainable) has been found dependent upon the number of antigen-specific IgE molecules on each basophil.[31] As few as 2500 molecules of ragweed antigen E-specific IgE have been found sufficient for a cellular reactivity of 50%.

The binding of IgE to mast cells is strong enough that the half-life of IgE in skin is 9-14 days, much longer than its half-life in plasma (See Table 2.2).[32] Reaction between IgE bound to basophils and anti-IgE is followed by a migration of both bound and free IgE receptors to one pole of the cell.[33]

Homocytotropic, skin sensitizing antibodies of the IgG class are found in experimental animals, and in rats such antibodies compete with IgE for the same receptors,[34] but IgG homocytotropic antibodies have been reported only very rarely in humans.[35]

BIOCHEMICAL EVENTS

Available evidence indicates that the initial event in the Type I allergic reaction is reaction between antigen and two adjacent IgE molecules bound to the surface of the sensitized mast cell. Consequent interaction between the IgE receptors may induce the series of intracellular biochemical reactions resulting in degranulation of the cell and secretion of biologically active chemical mediators through the microtubule system at least in the basophil. In their functional, aggregated form, microtubules are long, tubular, intracellular structures approximately 200 Å in diameter. When disaggregated they form smaller subunits with a molecular weight of 110,000. Colchicine binds to these subunits, preventing reaggregation and interfering with microtubule function, and colchicine has been shown to block IgE-mediated histamine release.[36] Deuterium oxide on the other hand facilitates the aggregation of microtubules and enhances histamine release.[37] Fusion of perigranular membranes with the cell membrane is followed by mediator release from mast cells.

That which is known about the sequence of biochemical events suggests that the antigen-antibody reaction is followed by activation of a serine esterase from its precursor form to a state in which activity can be inhibited by diisopropyl fluorophosphate (DFP) (Fig. 2.2). The activation of this serine es-

Immunologic Release of Chemical Mediators

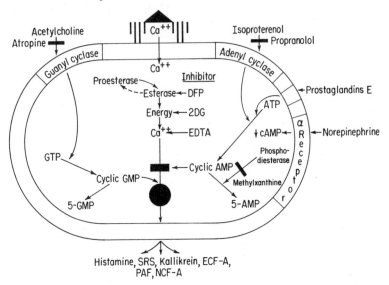

Fig. 2-2. Biochemical events and pharmacologic modification of immunologic release of chemical mediators (modified from Kaliner and Austen).[38]

terase is dependent upon the presence of extracellular calcium ions. A further autocatalytic feedback activation of the esterase can occur in the absence of inhibitor. Activation of the serine esterase is followed by an energy-requiring step which utilizes glycolysis or oxidative phosphorylation and can be inhibited by 2-deoxyglucose (2-DG). This is followed by a step requiring the intracellular presence of calcium ions and subject to inhibition by ethylenediaminetetraacetate (EDTA). The next step can be inhibited by cyclic 3,5-adenosine monophosphate (cyclic AMP). Finally this sequence of reactions results in the secretion of the chemical mediators.[38]

PHARMACOLOGIC MODIFICATION OF MEDIATOR RELEASE

Modification of the immunologic release of chemical mediators through intervention in this pathway has been most extensively investigated through study of the effects of cyclic AMP. An inverse relationship between tissue levels of cyclic AMP and the amount of histamine and slow reacting substance of anaphylaxis (SRS-A) released has been demonstrated. [39] Increased concentrations of cyclic AMP cause inhibition of mediator release.

β-adrenergic stimulating agents such as isoproterenol interact with membrane-bound adenyl cyclase to catalyze the formation of cyclic AMP from adenosine triphosphate (ATP). This effect can be prevented with a β-adrenergic blocking agent such as propranolol. The intracellular concentration of cyclic AMP can also be increased by inhibition of the specific phosphodiesterase responsible for its hydrolysis to adenosine monophosphate (AMP). Aminophylline and other methyl xanthines inhibit this reaction (see Fig. 2. 2). As would be anticipated, isoproterenol and aminophylline have been found to be synergistic in both increasing intracellular concentrations of cyclic AMP and inhibiting mediator release.

Prostaglandins E_1 and E_2 can also increase intracellular concentration of cyclic AMP and inhibit mediator release. [40] At lower concentrations prostaglandins E_1 and F_2 α decrease intracellular concentrations of cyclic AMP and enhance mediator release.

Use of α-adrenergic stimulating agents such as phenylephrine or epinephrine in combination with a β-blocking agent to prevent concomitant β-stimulation causes a decrease in the intracellular concentration of cyclic AMP and enhancement of mediator release, [39] possibly through stimulation of membrane adenosine triphosphatase. [41]

Histamine itself has been found to cause an increase in cyclic AMP levels in leukocyte preparations and to inhibit antigen-induced, IgE mediated histamine release, but such an inhibitory effect does not occur in the human lung mast cell. [43] These effects of histamine are not antagonized by H1 antihistamines but can be blocked by H2 antihistamines such as burimamide and metiamide. [44]

The H1 antihistamines have also been found to inhibit antigen-induced histamine release when present in relatively high contrations. [44] Phenothiazine antihistamines and other tricyclic antidepressant drugs were especially potent. At even higher concentrations they caused histamine release. These effects were not mediated through changes in cyclic AMP levels.

Cholinergic stimulation with acetylcholine or carbamylcholine enhances antigen-induced mediator release from sensitized tissues without changing cyclic AMP concentrations. [40] This effect can be prevented with atropine, a cholinergic blocking agent. Apparently cholinergic stimulation results in an increase in the intracellular concentration of cyclic guanosine monophosphate (cyclic GMP) through interaction with guanylate cyclase. [39] Thus, adrenergic stimulation and cholinergic stimulation have opposite effects upon the release of mediators.

Cyclic nucleotides not only inhibit or enhance secretion of preformed chemical mediators but can also modify the amount of SRS-A generated after immunologic activation.[45] Incubation of passively sensitized human lung fragments with cyclic AMP prevented SRS-A generation following antigenic challenge, while preincubation with cyclic GMP increased the amount of SRS-A generated.

Cromolyn sodium (disodium cromoglycate) and diethylcarbamazine have also been shown to inhibit antigen-induced mediator release from human lung fragments through mechanisms not yet fully defined.[46] The effect of cromolyn is probably largely due to prevention of movement of calcium ions into the cell.

NATURAL REGULATION OF THE ALLERGIC REACTION

The intensity and extent of the allergic reaction are influenced by the intensity of the initial stimulation of the mast cell, variations in the concentrations of cyclic AMP and cyclic GMP, the rate of inactivation of the chemical mediators released by the mast cell, and possibly by availability of mediator receptors and responsiveness of target cells. Increases in the number of IgE molecules bound to mast cells and in the amount of antigen available for interaction favor mediator release, while more limited activation of the mast cell can cause formation of SRS-A without release of mediators.[47]

Endogenous hydrocortisone may increase the number of beta-adrenergic receptors, and endogenous catecholamines may act upon these receptors to stimulate cyclic AMP formation, inhibiting further mediator release.[48] Prostaglandins E_1 and E_2 also influence cyclic AMP concentrations, and released histamine itself has been seen to cause increases in cyclic AMP in basophils.

Eosinophils are attracted to the site of the allergic reaction by ECF-A, which can then deactivate the eosinophils, preventing their further migration away from the site of the reaction. At some concentrations histamine is also chemotactic for eosinophils.

Arylsulfatase B, found in eosinophil granules, and the major basic protein of eosinophils both inactivate SRS-A. Eosinophils also contain histaminase, that inactivates histamines. Further release of histamine from mast cells can be inhibited by the increase in cyclic AMP, which can be caused by E prostaglandins released from eosinophils. Platelet-activating factor can be inactivated by phospholipase D, which is also found in eosinophils. Thus, the eosinophil has the capacity for limiting the allergic reaction.

CHEMICAL MEDIATORS

The chemical mediators of the Type I anaphylactic reaction (immediate hypersensitivity) are agents whose formation or release follows the antigen-antibody reaction and whose actions cause the clinical manifestations of the allergic reaction. They can be classified as primary mediators found in mast cells and secondary mediators formed or released as a result of action of primary mediators. The mediators of established importance in immediate hypersensitivity in humans (histamine, slow reacting substance of anaphylaxis, and eosinophil chemotactic factor of anaphylaxis) and some of possible significance are listed with some of their properties in Table 2.4.

HISTAMINE

Histamine, β-imidazolylethylamine (Fig. 2.3) is formed by decarboxylation of histidine by histidine decarboxylase.

It is found preformed in the metachromatically staining granules of mast cells where it is bound in a heparin-protein-

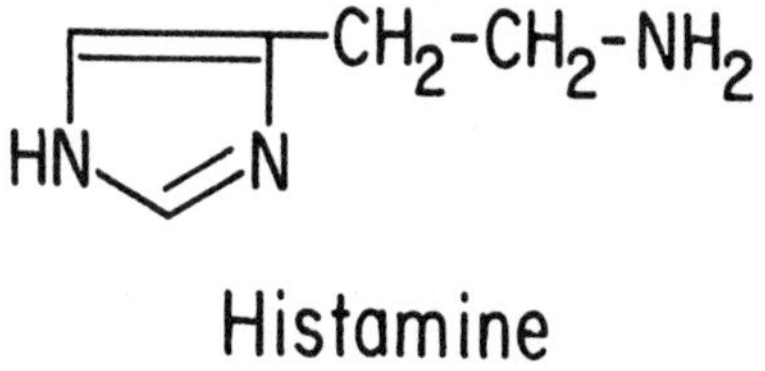

Fig. 2-3. Chemical structure of histamine.

Histamine

histamine complex. Histamine associated with mast cells is especially plentiful in human lung. Histamine is also found in substantial amounts in human epidermis, the central nervous system and the gastrointestinal mucosa where it is not necessarily associated with mast cells. The most important pathway through which histamine is metabolized involves ring N-methylation catalyzed by histamine-N-methyltransferase. The product, methylhistamine, is mostly converted by monoamine oxidase to methyl imidazole acetic acid.

The other important pathway of histamine metabolism consists of oxidative deamination by histaminase or diamine oxidase to produce imidazole acetic acid and its riboside. Histamine metabolites have little or no pharmacological activity and are excreted in the urine.

TABLE 2.4 CHEMICAL MEDIATORS OF IMMEDIATE HYPERSENSITIVITY

PRIMARY MEDIATORS	RECOGNIZED IMPORTANCE IN HUMANS	CHEMICAL STRUCTURE AND CHARACTERISTICS	ACTIONS	ANTAGONISTS OR INHIBITORS	ASSAY
Histamine	+	β-Imidazolylethylamine MW=111	H1: Itching, contraction of smooth muscle, increased vascular permeability, arteriolar dilatation (H1 & H2), stimulation of lacrimal, nasal, and bronchial secretions. H2: Gastric acid secretion, inhibition of histamine release from basophils, Eosinophil chemotaxis	H1: Ethanolamines Ethylenediamines Alkylamines Piperazines Phenothiazines H2: Burimamide Metiamide Cimetidine (Inactivated by histaminase)	Contraction of guinea pig ileum, Fluorometric, Enzymatic conversion of histamine to radioactive methylhistamine.
Slow-reacting substance of anaphylaxis (SRS-A)	+	Leukotriene C MW=400	Bronchoconstriction Increased vascular permeability	Inactivated by arylsulfatases A and B	Contraction of guinea pig ileum in presence of antihistamine and atropine
Eosinophil chemotactic factor of anaphylaxis (ECF-A)	+	Acidic tetrapeptides: val-gly-ser-glu ala-gly-ser-glu possibly others MW=360-390	Eosinophil (and neutrophil) chemotaxis followed by diminished chemotactic responsiveness (deactivation)		Attraction of eosinophils across millipore membrane

Neutrophil chemotactic factor of anaphylaxis (NCF-A)	−	Protein MW >750,000	Neutrophil (and eosinophil) chemotaxis followed by deactivation		Attraction of neutrophils
Basophil kallikrein of anaphylaxis (BK-A)	±	Tosyl-L-arginine methyl esterase	Formation of bradykinin from kininogen		Radioimmunoassay
Superoxide	−	O_2^-	Microbicidal activity	Superoxide dismutase	Chemiluminescence, cytochrome c reduction
Superoxide dismutase	−		Inactivation of superoxide		Inhib. of NBT or cytochrome c reduction
Platelet activating factor (PAF)	±	Mixture of phospholipids and free fatty acids (?) MW=400-1,000	Platelet aggregation Release of vasoactive amines from platelets	Inactivated by phospholipase D	Release of vasoactive amines from platelets
Heparin	−	Macromolecular acidic proteoglycan MW=750,000 approximately	Alteration of coagulation		Antithrombin activation or metachromasis

Table 2.4 (cont'd.)

SECONDARY MEDIATORS					
Bradykinin	±	Nonapeptide MW=1060	Bronchoconstriction, vasodilation, increased capillary permeability, perspiration, salivation, pain	Inactivated by carboxypeptidase, chymotrypsin	Bioassay: estrus rat uterus, cat jejunum, guinea pig ileum
Serotonin	−	3-(β-aminoethyl)-5-hydroxyindole MW=176	Bronchoconstriction in asthmatics, vasoconstriction or vasodilation, increase in small intestinal motility, pain.	Cyproheptadine Methysergide	Fluorometric
Prostaglandins	±	Unsaturated hydroxy aliphatic acids with cyclopentane rings MW=350 approximately	PGE: Bronchodilation, contraction of other smooth muscle, diverse vascular effects PGF: Bronchoconstriction	Indomethacin Mefenamic acid Flufenamic acid Phenylbutazone Aspirin Polyphloretin phosphate	Contraction of isolated smooth muscle (gerbil colon, rat colon, guinea pig colon, chick rectum, rat stomach)

Stress, epinephrine, and endotoxins have been found to increase histidine decarboxylase activity in various mouse tissues lacking many mast cells. [49] Antigen challenge of IgE-sensitized human peripheral leukocytes also causes increased histidine decarboxylase activity as well as an increase in cellular histamine. [50]

Release of histamine has been demonstrated in vitro following antigenic challenge of lung tissue and bronchi obtained from asthmatics, [51] but relatively high concentrations of histamine are necessary to induce contraction of human bronchial smooth muscle in vitro.

Some lack of specificity of antihistamines in the treatment of atopic diseases and the lack of correlation between their antihistaminic potency and antiallergic potency have also raised questions concerning the importance of histamine as a mediator.

Study of isolated stomach preparations has established that histamine can have indirect effects mediated through stimulation of nervous tissue. Reflex bronchoconstriction due to stimulation of cough receptors by histamine has been suggested by the observation that the bronchoconstriction induced by injection of small doses of histamine into the bronchial arteries of dogs could be abolished by bilateral cervical vagotomy or pretreatment with atropine. [52]

Although the specific mechanisms through which histamine acts remain unknown, its various actions seem to be mediated by at least two different types of receptors (see Table 2.4), each type inhibited by a specific group of antihistamines. [53] Thus, histamine's action on smooth muscle is subject to competitive inhibition by ethanolamines, ethylenediamines, and the other antihistamines frequently prescribed for the treatment of atopic diseases, while the stimulation of gastric secretion by histamine is inhibited instead by burimamide or metiamide. The hypotensive effect of intravenous doses of histamine can be prevented by simultaneous administration of mepyramine and burimamide, but not by either alone; thus this response results from stimulation of both H1 and H2 receptors. [54] There is also evidence that both H1 and H2 antagonists are necessary for most effective inhibition of the various effects of cardiac anaphylaxis in the isolated guinea pig heart. [55]

SLOW REACTING SUBSTANCE OF ANAPHYLAXIS (SRS-A)

SRS-A is the salt of an acid, hydrophilic substance which adsorbs readily to lipids and has a molecular weight of 400. It was first recognized as a substance liberated from perfused lungs of guinea pigs or cats following treatment with cobra venom and was distinguished from histamine and acetylcholine by the slower and more prolonged contraction of guinea pig ileum which it produced. [56] It was subsequently recognized in the perfusate of sensitized lungs (experimental animals and humans) challenged in vitro with specific allergen, and its activity upon guinea pig ileum was not affected by antihistamine. [51]

Physicochemical properties of SRS-A recovered from a variety of species have been very similar suggesting very close relationship if not structural identity.

Anaphylactic challenge of sensitized human lung fragments is followed by immediate cellular formation of SRS-A, which is then released 30-60 seconds later. [45] Since histamine and ECF-A are already formed and stored, awaiting antigenic challenge of the cell, their peak release precedes that of SRS-A. In vitro most SRS-A is formed within the first 5 minutes after antigenic challenge of sensitized tissue, but it is still detectable 1 hour later. [57]

SRS-A is a very potent bronchoconstrictor, and since guinea pig gut can both form and respond to SRS-A, it may also be an important mediator of food allergy. [57]

Enzymatic inactivation of SRS-A by an arylsulfatase found in eosinophils suggests that this may be another mechanism for limiting the results of the anaphylactic reaction. [58] At least one SRS has been identified as leukotriene C, a product of the action of lipooxygenase on arachidonic acid. [91]

EOSINOPHIL CHEMOTACTIC FACTOR OF ANAPHYLAXIS (ECF-A)

ECF-A consists of at least two acidic tetrapeptides. Its release was first demonstrated following antigenic challenge of sensitized guinea pig lung. Subsequently release from passively sensitized human lung fragments following antigenic challenge was also found. [59] Like histamine, ECF-A is found preformed in mast cell granules from which it can be released following antigenic challenge of sensitized cells. [60]

Neutrophils are also attracted to some extent by ECF-A, but the predominant activity is upon eosinophils. Histamine and kallikrein also have weak chemotactic activity for eosinophils.

NEUTROPHIL CHEMOTACTIC FACTOR OF ANAPHYLAXIS (NCF-A)

NCF-A is an incompletely characterized substance found preformed in human basophils and released from human lung fragments following IgE-dependent activation. [61]

BASOPHIL KALLIKREIN
OF ANAPHYLAXIS (BK-A)

Kallikrein is a term applied to any kinin-forming enzyme. A preformed kallikrein associated with basophil granules, tosyl-L-arginine methyl esterase, is released following antigenic challenge of sensitized human leukocytes.[62]

SUPEROXIDE AND
SUPEROXIDE DISMUTASE

Immunologic and nonimmunologic stimulation of mast cells has been found to cause release of superoxide (O_2^-) and superoxide dismutase from mast cell granules.[63] The possible role of superoxide in Type I reactions is unknown, but it is essential to the microbicidal activity of phagocytes.

BRADYKININ

Bradykinin (kallidin I) is a linear nonapeptide with a molecular weight of 1060. It is one of a group of kinins which resemble each other closely in chemical structure (Fig. 2.4) and pharmacological activity.[64]

Prekallikrein, kallikrein inhibitors, and kininogen are all found in the α 2-globulin fraction of plasma.[57]

Figure 2.5 indicates some of the complex interrelationships of the complement system and coagulation system through which kinins can be formed. Prekallikrein can be converted to kallikrein by Hageman factor, Hageman factor fragments, and by an activator released from tissue (including platelets).[57,65]

Kinins are among the most potent vasodilators known. They actively increase vascular permeability and cause constriction of certain smooth muscle. Inhalation of bradykinin has been found to induce bronchoconstriction in asthmatics but not in normal human subjects.

Bradykinin's role as a mediator of anaphylaxis has been less well established in humans than in experimental animals, but increased levels of bradykinin have been demonstrated in the nasal secretions of allergic subjects following challenge with ragweed,[66] kinins have been demonstrated in the perfusate of human skin following antigenic challenge,[67] and increased kinin levels have been measured in blood during acute asthmatic attacks.[68]

Kinins are rapidly degraded in blood (half life less than 1 minute) by carboxypeptidases and other kininases to inactive peptide fragments. Acetylsalicylic acid has been found to block kinin-induced bronchoconstriction in the guinea pig, but no safe, effective inhibitor is available yet for use in humans.

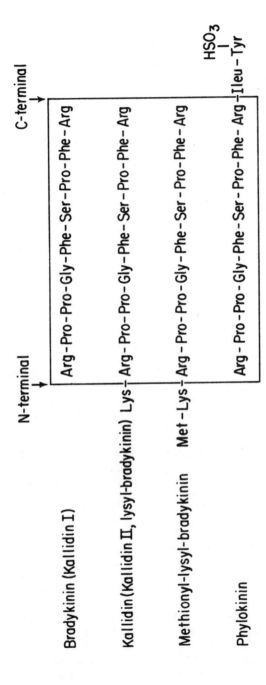

Fig. 2-4. Amino acid composition of some kinins.

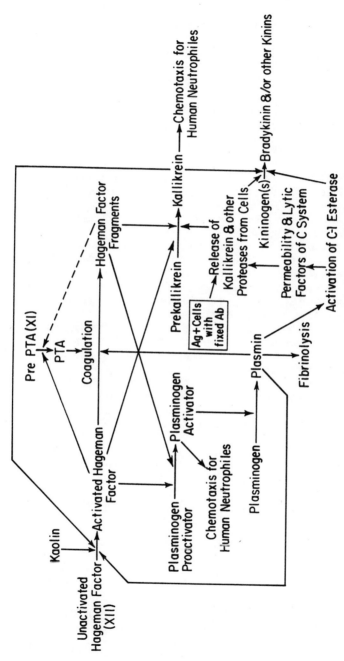

Fig. 2-5. Pathways of kinin formation.

PLATELET ACTIVATING FACTOR

Release of a platelet activating factor from IgE sensitized rabbit basophils has been found to follow antigenic challenge. This factor causes aggregation of rabbit platelets and release of their histamine and serotonin. Antigenic release of a similar factor from sensitized human leukocytes (possibly basophils) has also been demonstrated.[69]

SEROTONIN (5-HYDROXYTRYPTAMINE) (5-HT)

Serotonin, 3-(β-aminoethyl)-5-hydroxyindole (Fig. 2-6), is synthesized from dietary tryptophan. It is estimated that in humans 90% of 5-HT is found in the intestine, mostly in enterochromaffin cells. Much of the rest is found in brain and platelets, where it is stored in platelet granules. It is found in rat mast cells but not in human mast cells. 5-HT is mostly metabolized to 5-hydroxyindoleacetic acid which is excreted in the urine with other metabolites.

The pharmacological actions of 5-HT are variable depending upon the species and other circumstances. It is an active bronchoconstrictor in many experimental animals, but not usually in humans except for asthmatics. It can cause either vasoconstriction or vasodilation and stimulates small intestinal motility. Although it is very active in increasing capillary permeability in rodents. this effect does not occur in humans.

Although 5-HT has been implicated as a mediator of anaphylaxis in experimental animals[70] there is no conclusive evidence of such an effect in humans. There is now evidence, however, that it is released from human platelets by anaphylactic antigen-antibody reactions.[69]

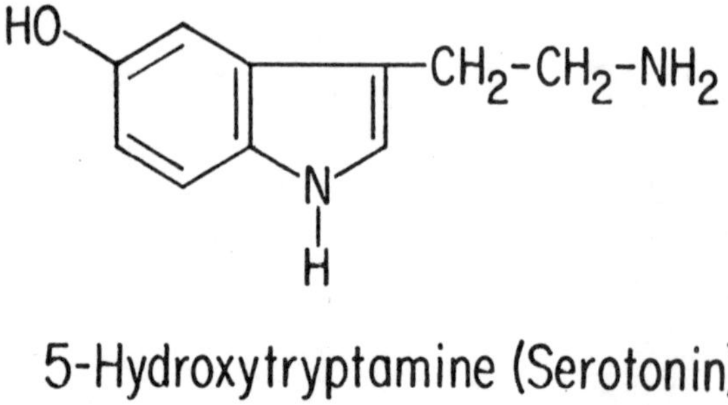

5-Hydroxytryptamine (Serotonin)

Fig. 2-6. Chemical structure of 5-hydroxytryptamine (serotonin).

PROSTAGLANDINS

The prostaglandins are a group of 20-carbon unsaturated hydroxyaliphatic acids (Fig. 2.7). Phospholipases found in association with cell membranes and lysosomes can split the fatty acid precursors of prostaglandins from lecithins, which are also common constituents of cell membranes. Consequently prostaglandin production is likely whenever cells are destroyed or damaged with resulting phospholipase activation. [57]

PGE_1 and E_2 are the most potent of the prostaglandins in activation of adenyl cyclase, an effect which is not blocked by propranolol. Thus, as would be anticipated, they inhibit antigen-induced histamine release from sensitized human basophils. [71]

PGE_1, PGE_2, and $PGF_2\alpha$ have been found in the perfusate of IgE sensitized human lung tissue following antigenic challenge, [72] and their appearance, like that of histamine and SRS-A, can be suppressed by cromolyn sodium. [73] Prostaglandins, however, were also found after agitation of lung tissue and

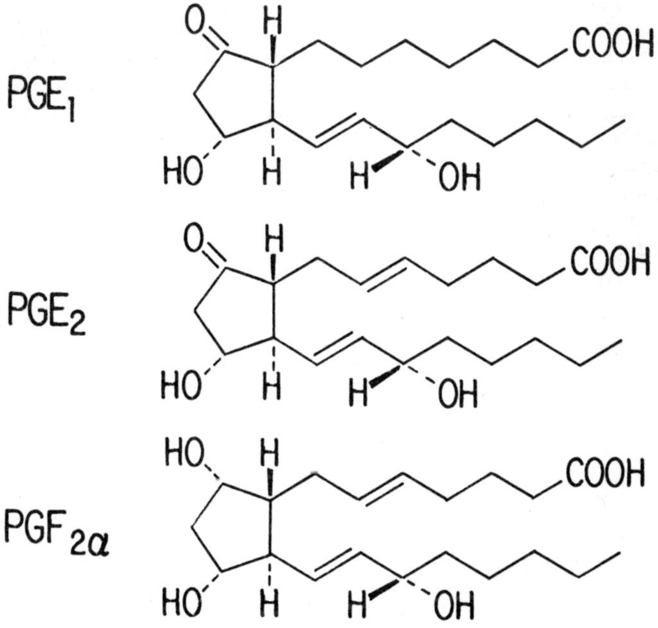

Fig. 2-7. Chemical structure of some prostaglandins.

their appearance after either agitation or antigen-induced mediator release was suppressed by indomethacin, an inhibitor of prostaglandin synthesis. This suggested that prostaglandin formation or release may have been secondary to the release of the primary mediators.

PGE_1 and E_2 cause bronchodilation, but $PGF_2 \alpha$ causes bronchoconstriction which is especially extreme in asthmatic subjects.[74] Asthmatic subjects were 8000 times more sensitive to inhaled $PGF_2 \alpha$ than normal subjects; it is a more potent bronchoconstrictor than any other known substance occurring naturally in the body.

Plasma PGF concentrations were not found to be elevated significantly in eight asthmatics as compared with normal controls.[75] In fact, PGE and PGE/F ratios were increased in the asthmatics, suggesting a possible regulatory function for PGE. However, increased plasma concentrations of a metabolite of $PGF_2 \alpha$ have been reported to follow allergen-induced asthmatic attacks.[76] A positive correlation between the release of histamine and that of $PGF_2 \alpha$ following antigen challenge of previously sensitized human lung fragments, has been reported.[77] Inhibition of such release by diphenhydramine suggests mediation by histamine through H1 receptors.[78] Some prostaglandins increase pulmonary vascular resistance while others decrease it, suggesting a role in the control of local blood flow. PGE_1 causes dilatation of both arteries and veins, but PGE_2 has no significant effect upon arteries and causes venous constriction.

PGE_1, PGE_2, and $PGF_2 \alpha$ are almost completely inactivated by one passage through the pulmonary circulation at least in experimental animals, apparently due to the action of 15-hydroxyprostaglandin dehydrogenase.[79] Prostaglandin synthesis can be inhibited by aspirin and sodium salicylate as well as indomethacin.

HEPARIN

The heparin found in mast cell granules is largely responsible for their metachromasia. The molecular weight is much greater than that of commercially available heparin. Although release of heparin follows challenge of rat peritoneal mast cells with anti-IgE, heparin is not of demonstrated importance as a mediator of Type I reactions in humans.

β ADRENERGIC THEORY

The observation that injection of <u>Bordetella pertussis</u> organisms into certain strains of mice and rats induced a state resembling human atopy (increased sensitivity to histamine, serotonin, bradykinin, and respiratory irritants; enhanced antibody formation; eosinophilia) with reduced sensitivity to catecholamines and that these abnormalities were due to a partial blockade of the beta-adrenergic receptors led Szentivanyi to propose that a partial beta-adrenergic blockade might be responsible for the increased irritability of the tracheobronchial tree characteristic of human asthma. [80] Some of the clinical evidence to support this includes abnormal metabolic and physiological responses to catecholamines consistent with a partial blockade of beta-adrenergic receptors in atopic subjects (Table 2.5).

Increased sensitivity to methacholine-induced bronchospasm has been shown to follow intravenous injection of the beta-adrenergic blocking agent, propranolol, in asthmatics but not in normal subjects, [81] however; and induction of beta-adrenergic blockade in normal subjects has failed to make them susceptible to the exercise induced bronchospasm which is typical of asthmatics. [82] Beta-adrenergic blockade alone seemed insufficient to cause these features of asthma in the normal subjects. Furthermore, evidence that pretreatment of normal subjects with ephedrine can alter metabolic and cardiovascular responses to epinephrine to resemble those reported as evidence of partial beta-adrenergic blockade in asthmatics suggests the possibility that some of these abnormalities may have been the result of treatment rather than a cause of the asthma, and similar receptor desensitization to isoproterenol has been found in lymphocytes of asthmatic and normal subjects. [83-85] However, evidence of partial beta-adrenergic blockade has been found in some patients who have not been treated previously with sympathomimetics. [86] Decreased binding of tritiated dihydroalprenolol, a beta-adrenergic antagonist, by lymphocytes of asthmatics has been reported to be independent of therapy with adrenergic agents, and lymphocytes of the patients with the most severe airway obstruction demonstrated the least binding. [87, 88]

Measurement of the capacity of phenylephrine to cause cutaneous vascular constriction and pupillary dilatation has disclosed alpha-adrenergic hyperresponsiveness in asthmatic adults as compared with normal controls and subjects with allergic rhinitis only. [92] Much smaller doses caused vascular constriction and pupillary dilatation in the asthmatics than in the control subjects.

There is evidence to suggest the possibility of interconversion of alpha- and beta-adrenergic receptors. [93] Alpha-adrenergic hyperresponsiveness might then be expected in patients with reduced beta-adrenergic responsiveness, but evidence of partial beta-adrenergic blockade has been found in patients with allergic rhinitis as well as those with asthma.

TABLE 2.5   EVIDENCE FOR PARTIAL BETA-
ADRENERGIC BLOCKADE IN ATOPY

Less than normal vasodilation induced by isoproterenol infusion in asthmatics

Less than normal hyperglycemia induced by isoproterenol infusion or epinephrine infusion or injection of asthmatics

Less than normal increase in blood lactate induced by epinephrine injection

Less than normal eosinopenia induced by epinephrine injection in asthmatics

Less than normal platelet aggregation induced by epinephrine in asthmatics

Less than normal increase in urinary cyclic AMP induced by epinephrine injection

Less than normal increase in leukocyte and lymphocyte cyclic AMP induced by norepinephrine, epinephrine and isoproterenol in asthmatics

Less than normal leukocyte and lymphocyte cyclic AMP concentrations in asthmatics

Fewer than normal beta-adrenergic receptor sites on lymphocytes of asthmatics

Less than normal inhibition by isoproterenol of T-lymphocyte nonimmune rosette formation with sheep erythrocytes

Absence of normal inhibition of epidermal mitosis by catecholamines in skin of patients with atopic dermatitis

Bronchospasm induced by beta-adrenergic blocking agents in asthmatics

CAUSE OF ATOPY

It is still not known exactly how an individual is predisposed to develop an atopic disease although some genetic basis is well established (see Chapter I). Among the possible causes is some abnormality of the mucosal barrier to antigens permitting them to enter the organism. There is evidence that atopic subjects differ from normal subjects by being more susceptible to sensitization by intranasal antigens, while there is no difference in susceptibility to sensitization by injection.[89] Atopic and nonatopic subjects have been reported not to differ in their capacity for demonstrating cutaneous P-K reactions after intranasal application of the allergens, however.[90]

Atopic subjects may differ from normal subjects in the ease with which information about antigen reaches plasma cells or in their production of specific IgE antibody. Differences in affinity of antibody for mast cells are possible, and these cells are known to differ in their numbers of IgE receptors.[29] Numerous possibilities of enzymatic differences and pharmacological differences which might affect the ease with which mediators are released from mast cells are already evident (see Fig. 2.2). It seems likely that various combinations of some of these possible abnormalities may help determine the presence of atopy, its specific manifestations, and its severity.

REFERENCES

1. Ramirez, M. A. : Horse asthma following blood transfusion. JAMA 73:984, 1919.
2. Prausnitz, C. , and Küstner, H. : Studien über die Überempfindlichkeit. Centralbl Bakteriol 1 Abt Orig 86:160, 1921.
3. Coca, A. F. , and Grove, E. F. : Studies in hypersensitiveness XIII. A study of the atopic reagins. J Imm 10:445, 1925.
4. Ishizaka, K. , Ishizaka, T. , and Hornbrook, M. M. : Physicochemical properties of human reaginic antibody IV. Presence of a unique immunoglobulin as a carrier of reaginic activity. J Imm 97:75, 1966.
5. Johansson, S. G. O. , Bennich, H. , and Wide, L. : A new class of immunoglobulin in human serum. Imm 14:265, 1968.
6. Devey, M. E. , and Panzani, R. : The IgG subclasses of antibodies to castor bean allergen in patients with allergic asthma: detection of a high incidence of antibodies of the IgG4 subclass. Clin All 5:353, 1975.
7. Devey, M. E. , Wilson, D. V. , and Wheeler, A. W. : The IgG subclasses of antibodies to grass pollen allergens produced in hay fever patients during hyposensitization. Clin All 6:227, 1976.
8. Shakib, F. , McLaughlan, P. , Stanworth, D. R. , Smith, E. , and Fairborn, E. : Elevated serum IgE and IgG4 in patients with atopic dermatitis. Brit J Derm 97:59, 1977.
9. Shakib, F. , Stanworth, D. R. , Smalley, C. A. , and Brown, G. A. : Elevated serum IgG4 levels in cystic fibrosis patients. Clin All 6:237, 1976.
10. Van der Giessen, M. , Homan, W. L. , van Kernebeek, G. , Aalberse, R. C. , and Dieges, P. H. : Subclass typing of IgG antibodies formed by grass pollen-allergic patients during immunotherapy. Int Arch All Appl Immunol 50:625, 1976.
11. Strober, W. , Krakauer, R. , Klaeveman, H. L. , Reynolds, H. Y. , and Nelson, D. L. : Secretory component deficiency. New Eng J Med 294:351, 1976.
12. Gleich, G. J. , Bieger, R. C. , and Stankievic, R. : Antigen combining activity associated with immunoglobulin D. Science 165:606, 1969.
13. Heiner, D. C. , and Rose, B. : A study of antibody responses by radioimmunodiffusion with demonstration of γ D antigen-binding activity in four sera. J Imm 104:691, 1970.
14. Vitetta, E. , and Uhr, J. W. : Immunoglobulin receptors revisited: a model for the differentiation of bone marrow derived lymphocytes is described. Science 189:964, 1975.

15. Bazaral, M., Orgel, H. A., and Hamburger, R. N.: IgE levels in normal infants and mothers and an inheritance hypothesis. J Imm 107:794, 1971.

16. Miller, D. L., Hirvonen, T., and Gitlin, D.: Synthesis of IgE by the human conceptus. J All Clin Imm 52:182, 1973.

17. Kjellman, N.-I. M., Johansson, S. G. O., and Roth, A.: Serum IgE levels in healthy children quantified by a sandwich technique (PRIST). Clin All 6:51, 1976.

18. Buckley, R. H., Wray, B. B., and Belmaker, E. Z.: Extreme hyperimmunoglobulinemia E and undue susceptibility to infection. Ped 49:59, 1972.

19. Patterson, R., Oh, S. H., Roberts, M., and Hsu, C. C. S.: Massive polyclonal hyperimmunoglobulinemia E., eosinophilia, and increased IgE-bearing lymphocytes. Am J Med 58:553, 1975.

20. Tada, T., and Ishizaka, K.: Distribution of γ E-forming cells in lymphoid tissues of the human and monkey. J Imm 104:377, 1970.

21. Bennich, H., and Johannson, S. G. O.: Structure and function of human immunoglobulin E. Adv Imm 13:1, 1971.

22. Ammann, A. J., Cain, W. A., Ishizaka, K., Hong, R., and Good, R. A.: Immunoglobulin E deficiency in ataxia-telangiectasia. NEJM 281:469, 1969.

23. Schwartz, D. P., and Buckley, R. H.: Serum IgE concentrations and skin reactivity to anti-IgE antibody in IgA deficient patients. NEJM 284:513, 1971.

24. Hobday, J. D., Cake, M., and Turner, K. J.: A comparison of the immunoglobulins IgA, IgG, and IgE in nasal secretions from normal and asthmatic children. Clin Exp Immunol 9:577, 1971.

25. Tse, K. S., Wicher, K., and Arbesman, C. E.: IgE antibodies in nasal secretions of ragweed-allergic subjects. J All 46:352, 1970.

26. Yunginger, J. W., and Gleich, G. J.: Seasonal changes in serum and nasal IgE concentrations. J All Clin Imm 51:174, 1973.

27. Donovan, R., Johansson, S. G. O., Bennich, H., and Soothill, J. F.: Immunoglobulins in nasal polyp fluid. Int Arch Allergy 37:154, 1970.

28. Katz, D. H.: Control of IgE antibody production by suppressor substances. J All Clin Immunol 62:44, 1978.

29. Ishizaka, T., Soto, C. S., and Ishizaka, K.: Mechanisms of passive sensitization. III. Number of IgE molecules and their receptor sites on human basophil granulocytes. J Imm 111:500, 1973.

30. Malveaux, F. J. , Conroy, M. C. , Adkinson, N. F. , Jr. ,
    and Lichtenstein, L. M. : IgE receptors on human basophils.
    J Clin Invest 62:176, 1978.
31. Zeiss, C. R. , Pruzansky, J. J. , Levitz, D. , and Wang, J. :
    The quantification of IgE antibody specific for ragweed anti-
    gen E on the basophil surface in patients with ragweed pol-
    lenosis. Immunol 35:237, 1978.
32. Cass, R. M. , and Andersen, B. R. : The disappearance
    rate of skin-sensitizing antibody activity after intradermal
    administration. J All 42:29, 1968.
33. Ishizaka, T. : "Functions and development of cell receptors
    for IgE" in Johansson, S. G. O. , and Strandberg, K. : Mo-
    lecular and Biological Aspects of the Acute Allergic Reaction,
    Plenum, New York, 1976.
34. Bach, M. K. , Block, K. J. , and Austen, K. F. : IgE and
    IgGA antibody-mediated release of histamine from rat peri-
    toneal cells. J Exp Med 133:752, 1971.
35. Reid, R. T. , Minden, P. , and Farr, R. S. : Reaginic acti-
    vity associated with IgG immunoglobulin. J Exp Med 123:
    845, 1966.
36. Levy, D. A. , and Carlton, J. A. : Influence of temperature
    on the inhibition by colchicine of allergic histamine release.
    Proc Soc Exp Biol Med 130:1333, 1969.
37. Gillespie, E. , and Lichtenstein, L. M. : Histamine release
    from human leukocytes: studies with deuterium oxide,
    colchicine, and cytochalasin B. J Clin Invest 51:2941,
    1972.
38. Kaliner, M. , and Austen, K. F. : Immunologic release of
    chemical mediators from human tissues. Ann Rev Pharm-
    acol 15:177, 1975.
39. Kaliner, M. , Orange, R. P. , and Austen, K. F. : Immuno-
    logical release of histamine and slow reacting substance of
    anaphylaxis from human lung. J Exp Med 136:556, 1972.
40. Tauber, A. I. , Kaliner, M. , Stechschulte, D. J. , and Aus-
    ten, K. F. : Immunologic release of histamine and slow re-
    acting substance of anaphylaxis from human lung. V.
    Effects of prostaglandins on release of histamine. J
    Immunol 111:27, 1973.
41. Coffey, R. G. , Hadden, J. W. , Hadden, E. M. , and Middleton,
    E. , Jr.: Increased adenosine triphosphatase in leukocytes
    of asthmatic children. J Clin Invest 54:138, 1974.
42. Bourne, H. R. , Melmon, K. L. , and Lichtenstein, L. M. :
    Histamine augments leukocyte adenosine 3', 5'-monophos-
    phate and blocks antigenic histamine release. Science 173:
    743, 1971.

43. Kaliner, M.: Human lung tissue and anaphylaxis: The effects of histamine on the immunologic release of mediators. Am Rev Resp Dis 118:1015, 1978.
44. Lichtenstein, L. M., and Gillespie, E.: The effects of the H1 and H2 antihistamines on "allergic" histamine release and its inhibition by histamine. J Pharmacol Exp Ther 192:441, 1975.
45. Lewis, R. A., Wasserman, S. I., Goetzl, E. J., and Austen, K. F.: Formation of slow-reacting substance of anaphylaxis in human lung tissue and cells before release. J Exp Med 140:1133, 1974.
46. Orange, R. P., Austen, W. G., and Austen, K. F.: Immunological release of histamine and slow-reacting substance of anaphylaxis from human lung. I. Modulation by agents influencing cellular levels of cyclic 3', 5'-adenosine monophosphate. J Exp Med 134:136S, 1971.
47. Lewis, R. A., Wasserman, S. I., Goetzl, E. J., and Austen, K. F.: Formation of SRS-A in human lung tissue and cells before release. J Exp Med 140:1133, 1974.
48. Mano, K., Akbarzadeh, A., Koesnadi, K., Sano, Y., Bewtra, A., and Townley, R.: The effect of hydrocortisone on beta adrenergic receptors in lung tissue. J All Clin Immunol 63:147, 1979.
49. Schayer, R. W.: Relationship of induced histidine decarboxylase activity and histamine synthesis to shock from stress and from endotoxin. Am J Physiol 198:1187, 1960.
50. Assem, E. S. K., Schild, H. O., and Vickers, M. R.: Stimulation of histamine-forming capacity in sensitized human leukocytes by antigen. J Physiol 216:67P, 1971.
51. Brocklehurst, W. E.: The release of histamine and formation of a slow reacting substance (SRS-A) during anaphylactic shock. J Physiol 151:416, 1960.
52. DeKock, M. A., Nadel, J. A., Zwi, S., Colebatch, H. J. H., and Olsen, C. R.: New method for perfusing bronchial arteries: histamine bronchoconstriction and apnea. J Appl Physiol 21:185, 1966.
53. Ash, A. S. F., and Schild, H. O.: Receptors mediating some actions of histamine. Brit J Pharmacol Chemother 27:427, 1966.
54. Black, J. W., Duncan, W. A. M., Durant, C. J., Ganellin, C. R., and Parsons, E. M.: Definition and antagonism of histamine H2-receptors. Nature 236:385, 1972.
55. Levi, R., and Capurro, N.: "Histamine H2-receptor antagonism and cardiac anaphylaxis," in Wood, C. J., and Simkins, M. A. (edd): International symposium on histamine H2-receptor antagonists, Smith, Kline & French Lab., Ltd., Welwyn Garden City, England, 1973.

56. Feldberg, W., and Kellaway, C. H.: Liberation of histamine and formation of lysocithin-like substances by cobra venon. J Physiol 94:187, 1938.
57. Brocklehurst, W. E.: "Pharmacological mediators of hypersensitivity reactions," in Gell, P. G. H., Coombs, R. R. A., and Lachmann, P. J. (edd): <u>Clinical aspects of immunology</u>, 3rd ed., Blackwell, Oxford, 1975, p 821
58. Wasserman, S. I., Goetzl, E. J., and Austen, K. F.: Inactivation of slow reacting substance of anaphylaxis by human eosinophil arylsulfatase. J Imm 114:645, 1975.
59. Kay, A. B., and Austen, K. F.: The IgE mediated release of an eosinophil leukocyte chemotactic factor from human lung. J Imm 107:899, 1971.
60. Wasserman, S. I., Goetzl, E. J., and Austen, K. F.: Preformed eosinophil chemotactic factor of anaphylaxis (ECF-A). J Imm 112:351, 1974.
61. Austen, K. F., and Orange, R. P.: Bronchial asthma: The possible role of the chemical mediators of immediate hypersensitivity in the pathogenesis of subacute chronic disease. Am Rev Resp Dis 112:423, 1975.
62. Newball, H. H., Lichtenstein, L. M., and Talamo, R. C.: Leukocyte arginine esterase-a potential new mediator of allergic reactions. J All Clin Imm 55:72, 1975.
63. Henderson, W. R., and Kaliner, M.: Immunologic and nonimmunologic generation of superoxide from mast cells and basophils. J Clin Invest 61:187, 1978.
64. Kellermeyer, R. W., and Graham, R. C., Jr.: Kinins-possible physiologic and pathologic roles in man. NEJM 279:754, 1968.
65. Weiss, A. S., Gallin, J. I., and Kaplan, A. P.: Fletcher factor deficiency. A diminished rate of Hageman factor activation caused by absence of prekallikrein with abnormalities of coagulation, fibrinolysis, chemotactic activity, and kinin generation. J Clin Invest 53:622, 1974.
66. Dolovich, J., Back, N., and Arbesman, C. E.: The presence of bradykinin-like activity in nasal secretions from allergic subjects. J All 41:103, 1968.
67. Mickel, B., Russell, T., Winkelmann, R. K., and Gleich, G. J.: Release of kinins during wheal and flare allergic skin reactions. J Clin Invest 47:68a, 1968.
68. Abe, K., Watanabe, N., Kumagai, N., Mouri, T., Seki, T., and Yoshinaga, K.: Circulating plasma kinin in patients with bronchial asthma. Exp 23:626, 1967.
69. Clark, R. A., and Kaplan, A. P.: Mediator release from human basophils. J All Clin Imm 55:85, 1975.

70. West, G. B.: Studies on the mechanism of anaphylaxis: a possible basis for a pharmacologic approach to allergy. Clin Pharmacol Ther 4:749, 1963.
71. Lichtenstein, L. M., Gillespie, E., Bourne, H. R., and Henney, C. S.: The effects of a series of prostaglandins on in vitro models of the allergic response and cellular immunity. Prostaglandins 2:519, 1972.
72. Piper, P. J., Walker, J. L.: The release of spasmogenic substances from human chopped lung tissue and its inhibition. Brit J Pharm 427:291, 1973.
73. Cox, J. S. G., Beach, J. E., Blair, A. M. J. N., Clarke, A. J., King, J., Lee, T. B., Loveday, D. E. E., Moss, G. F., Orr, T. S. C., Ritchie, J. T., and Sheard, P.: Disodium cromoglycate (Intal). Advan Drug Res 5:115, 1970.
74. Mathe, A. A., Hedqvist, P., Holmgren, A., and Svanborg, N.: Bronchial hyperreactivity to prostaglandin $F_2 \alpha$ and histamine in patients with asthma. Brit Med J 1:193, 1973.
75. Okagaki, T., Johnson, T. F., Reisman, R. E., Arbesman, C. E., and Middleton, E., Jr.: Plasma prostaglandin concentrations in allergic bronchial asthma. Int Arch All Appl Immunol 57:279, 1978.
76. Green, K., Hedquist, P., and Svanborg, N.: Increased plasma levels of 15-keto-13,14-dihydro-prostaglandin $F_2 \alpha$ after allergen-provoked asthma in man. Lancet 2:1419, 1974.
77. Strandberg, K., Mathe, A. A., and Yen, S. S.: Release of histamine and formation of prostaglandins in human lung tissue and rat mast cells. Int Arch All Appl Immunol 53:520, 1977.
78. Newball, H. H., Adkinson, N. F., Jr., Adams, G. K., Findlay, S. R., and Lichtenstein, L. M.: Mechanisms of anaphylactic release of prostaglandins from human lung. J All Clin Immunol 61:148, 1978.
79. Piper, P. J., Vane, J. R., and Wyllie, J. H.: Inactivation of prostaglandins by the lungs. Nature 225:600, 1970.
80. Szentivanyi, A.: The beta-adrenergic theory of the atopic abnormality in bronchial asthma. J All 42:203, 1968.
81. Zaid, G., and Beall, G. N.: Bronchial response to beta-adrenergic blockade. NEJM 275:580, 1966.
82. Zaid, G., Beall, G. N., and Heimlich, E. M.: Bronchial response to exercise following beta-adrenergic blockade. J All 42:177, 1968.
83. Nelson, H. S.: The effect of ephedrine on the response to epinephrine in normal men. J All Clin Imm 51:191, 1973.

84. Morris, H. G., Rusnak, S. A., Selner, J. C., Barzens, K., and Barnes, J.: Comparative effects of ephedrine on adrenergic responsiveness in normal and asthmatic subjects. J All Clin Immunol 61:294, 1978.
85. Kalisker, A., Nelson, H. S., and Middleton, E., Jr.: Drug-induced changes of adenylate cyclase activity in cells from asthmatic and nonasthmatic subjects. J All Clin Immunol 60:259, 1977.
86. Busse, W., Lee, T.-P., and Reed, C.: Decreased beta-adrenergic response in leukocytes in atopic eczema. J All Clin Immunol 57:234, 1976.
87. Kariman, K., and Lefkowitz, R. J.: Decreased beta-adrenergic receptor binding in lymphocytes from patients with bronchial asthma. Clin Res 25:503A, 1977.
88. Brooks, S. M., McGowan, K., Bernstein, I. L., Altenau, P., and Peagler, J.: Relationship between numbers of beta-adrenergic receptors in lymphocytes and disease severity in asthma. J All Clin Immunol 63:401, 1979.
89. Leskowitz, S., Salvaggio, J. E., and Schwartz, H. E.: An hypothesis for the development of atopic allergy in man. Clin Allergy 2:237, 1972.
90. Kontou-Karakitsos, K., Salvaggio, J. E., and Mathews, K. P.: Comparative nasal absorption of allergens in atopic and nonatopic subjects. J All Clin Immunol 55:241, 1975.
91. Sullivan, T. J., and Parker, C. W.: Possible role of arachidonic acid and its metabolites in mediator release from mast cells. J Immunol 122:431, 1979.
92. Henderson, W. R., Shelhamer, J. H., Reingold, D. B., Smith, L. J., Evans, R., III, and Kaliner, M.: Alpha-adrenergic hyperresponsiveness in asthma. New Eng J Med 300:642, 1979.
93. Szentivanyi, A., and Williams, J. F.: "The constitutional basis of atopic disease," in Bierman, C. W., and Pearlman, D. S. (edd): Allergic Diseases of Infancy, Childhood and Adolescence. Saunders, Philadelphia, 1980, p 173.

CHAPTER III | ASTHMA

DEFINITION AND CLASSIFICATION

No definition of asthma entirely acceptable to all interested physicians nor applicable to every patient seems possible. Nevertheless asthma is most widely understood to be a chronic pulmonary disease characterized by increased irritability of the tracheobronchial tree to a variety of stimuli manifested by recurrent episodes of more or less generalized airway obstruction usually reversible either spontaneously or following appropriate therapy.[1]

Atopic asthma, allergic asthma, or extrinsic asthma are terms applied to those subjects in whom exacerbations follow exposure to specific allergens. These usually have positive family histories for atopy (see Chapter I) and specific hypersensitivity is usually demonstrable by allergy skin testing, inhalation provocation testing, and/or radioallergosorbent testing.

Intrinsic asthma is largely a diagnosis of exclusion, including those asthmatics in whom specific allergens cannot be incriminated. Nonspecific factors such as infection, exercise, chemical or inert irritants in inhaled air, cold air itself, or psychic factors seem to provoke their asthmatic attacks. It is still unknown how the response to most of these agents is mediated. Reflex bronchoconstriction mediated by cholinergic pathways with interaction between acetylcholine and guanyl cyclase is probably the mechanism for some (see Fig. 2.2), because bronchoconstriction induced by inhalation of cold air, dust, histamine, or citric acid aerosols can be prevented by administration of atropine.[2]

Extrinsic asthma is mediated through the pathways described in Chapter II, but the site of the antigen-antibody reaction has been questioned because of the disparity between the size of many antigenic pollen grains (see Chapter XII) and the size of particles which reach the tracheobronchial tree. It is estimated that at least 95% of particles with a diameter larger than 15 μ are filtered out of inhaled air at the nose. Only particles small-

49

er than 3 μ penetrate as far as the respiratory bronchioles.[3] Since most allergenic whole pollen grains are larger than 15 μ in diameter few would be expected to reach the tracheobronchial tree in a subject breathing through his nose. Mouth-breathing may predominate in a patient with both allergic rhinitis and asthma, however. Photoscintigrams obtained following inhalation through the mouth of grass pollen grains (Kentucky bluegrass, average diameter 25 μ) bearing radioactive labels disclosed that none of the pollen reached the tracheobronchial trees of normal adults.[4] Pollen was deposited in the oropharynx and then swallowed. Inhalation of pollen extract, however, was followed by deposition of an estimated 10% in the lungs. Airway obstruction has been found to occur in asthmatics 6-10 hours after inhalation of whole grass pollen grains,[5] while it can begin within a few minutes after inhalation of pollen extract.[6] Application of ragweed pollen (average diameter 20 μ) to the nasal mucosa does not produce reflex bronchoconstriction in asthmatics. There is evidence, however, that during the ragweed season the atmosphere contains many particles smaller than 5 μ in diameter which are capable of reacting with ragweed reaginic antibody.[7] These particles, possibly plant fragments, would be well able to penetrate to much of the tracheobronchial tree. Thus, it seems most likely that the allergic reaction occurs at the mast cells in the lung of the asthmatic following inhalation of antigenic fragments, although gastrointestinal absorption of antigen is also possible.

Most asthmatic children seem to have a mixed form of asthma. Airway obstruction is triggered by the nonspecific factors responsible for intrinsic asthma, but specific allergens are also responsible for exacerbations.

PATHOPHYSIOLOGY

The actions of the chemical mediators released or formed following the reaction of antigen with reaginic antibody (see Chapter II) or as a result of nonspecific factors cause contraction of smooth muscle in the walls of the airways, tracheobronchial mucosal edema, and an increase in the rate of secretion of mucus by submucosal glands. (Goblet cells and Clara cells also secrete mucus). The result is both inspiratory and expiratory obstruction, but because the tracheobronchial tree normally becomes more narrow during expiration the obstruction is more extreme during expiration. The further consequences of this chain of events, illustrated in Fig. 3.1, include hyperinflation with a decrease in compliance. (Static compliance is the ratio of volume change to pressure change. At larger lung volumes greater changes in transpulmonary pressure are nec-

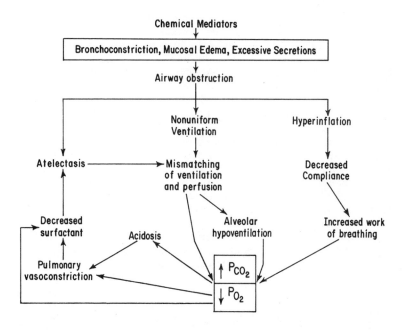

Fig. 3-1. Pathophysiology of asthma (modified from Siegel, Heimlich, and Richards). [1]

essary to cause the same change in volume.) The increased resistance to flow and decreased compliance increase the work of breathing, utilizing more of what may be a limited supply of oxygen. Accessory muscles of respiration may be called upon to help generate the further decrease in pressure necessary for inspiration. Contraction of expiratory muscles may be needed for the increased pressures necessary for expiration, and the increased transpulmonary pressures may cause narrowing or complete closure of some bronchioles due to the unevenness of the obstruction.

Anatomical dead space - that portion of each breath which remains in the upper airway and tracheobronchial tree, never reaching the gas exchanging units of the respiratory tract - is normally approximately equal in ml. to body weight in pounds. When ventilated parts of the lung are not perfused "physiological dead space" exceeds anatomical dead space. Nonuniform ventilation due to the airway obstruction and mismatching of ventilation and perfusion with increased physiological dead space contribute to alveolar hypoventilation. Abnormal ventilation-perfusion ($\dot{V}$/Q) relationships are often demonstrable in asthmatics even during remissions, but become more extreme early in asthmatic attacks.[6] Regions of the lung that are well ventilated may be poorly perfused, while other regions may be poorly ventilated but well perfused. Subsegmental, segmental, or even lobar atelectasis may occur with extreme airway obstruction, contributing further to the disturbed $\dot{V}$/Q relationship.

Initially the rising carbon dioxide tension in blood perfusing poorly ventilated parts of the lung can be compensated for by hyperventilation of other parts, but because the partial pressure of oxygen and oxyhemoglobin saturation cannot be improved much above the normal values while breathing room air, this mechanism cannot compensate for the hypoxemia which supervenes. If airway obstruction continues to progress, alveolar ventilation finally falls and hypercapnea may develop rapidly.

Hypoxia causes a metabolic acidosis by interference with conversion of lactic acid to carbon dioxide and water, while hypercapnia causes respiratory acidosis through the increase in carbonic acid and its dissociation into hydrogen ions and bicarbonate ions (Fig. 3.2).

$$CO_2 + H_2O \rightleftharpoons H_2CO_3 \rightleftharpoons H^+ + HCO_3^-$$

Fig. 3-2. Carbon dioxide-bicarbonate buffer system. An increase in the hydrogen ion concentration can occur: (1) by direct addition of hydrogen ions or by removal of bicarbonate ions, causing a shift of the reaction to the right by mass action (metabolic acidosis) or (2) by addition of carbon dioxide, causing a shift to the right by mass action (respiratory acidosis).

Hypoxia and acidosis can cause pulmonary vasoconstriction although sustained pulmonary hypertension with cor pulmonale is an uncommon complication of asthma.

Hypoxia and vasoconstriction may damage type II alveolar cells, diminishing production of surfactant, which normally stabilizes alveoli, tending to prevent atelectasis.[8]

Thus, if airway obstruction continues to progress, respiratory failure may supervene.

SYMPTOMATOLOGY AND MEDICAL HISTORY

The asthmatic child is subject to recurrent episodes of airway obstruction manifested by coughing, dyspnea, and wheezing, more pronounced on expiration than inspiration. The cough may be nonproductive but often sounds loose because of the increase in the amounts of tracheobronchial secretions present. Frequently the cough is productive of clear or white, mucoid sputum. When infection is present the sputum may be purulent. Coughing may be severe enough to provoke vomiting. Wheezing is often worse at night than during the daytime, possibly due to nocturnal exposure to environmental allergens (see Chapter XII), decreased ventilation during sleep, or circadian rhythms resulting in decreased plasma concentrations of adrenal corticosteroids at night, [9] or diurnal variations in catecholamine production, which may be decreased at night. [10]

The onset of wheezing may be gradual or sudden. It is often preceded by rhinorrhea with or without other symptoms of allergic rhinitis for a few hours or a few days. After wheezing has been present for some time, as respiratory and abdominal muscles tire, chest pain or abdominal pain may be noted.

The wheezing is usually reversible either spontaneously or following treatment with bronchodilators. In infants and less frequently in older children, some wheezing may persist between exacerbations of more severe airway obstruction, and pulmonary function testing often can disclose airway obstruction not extreme enough to cause wheezing during apparent remissions. Every effort should be made to establish the frequency, severity, and duration of previous asthmatic attacks, information vital to future assessment of response to treatment and also necessary to help determine the nature of the treatment program.

The medical history supplied by the parent is often one of recurrent or persistent "colds or bronchitis", and only after further questioning has elicited their association with the "continuity symptoms" of allergic rhinitis (excessive sneezing and nasal itching) and subclinical asthma (nocturnal coughing and coughing with exertion) is their allergic basis disclosed. [11]

Exacerbations of wheezing may be perennial, suggesting frequent or continual exposure to an allergen or multiple allergens, or seasonal, incriminating a specific pollen or group of pollens (see Chapter XII). A complete environmental history must be obtained to identify potential offending allergens (see Chapter XII). Frequently specific factors which have seemed to provoke asthmatic attacks can be identified by history, but these are more often "trigger" factors than allergens. (Fig. 3.3).

INFECTION

Although the nasal symptoms which frequently precede asthmatic attacks and are ascribed by parents to "colds" often are due to allergic rhinitis, true respiratory infections are among the commonest events which trigger asthmatic attacks.

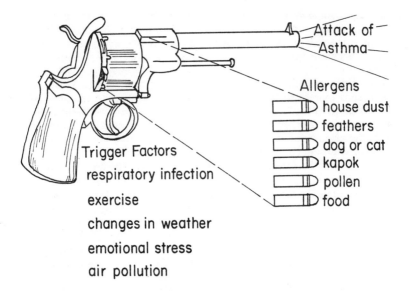

Fig. 3-3. Roles of trigger factors and allergens in eliciting asthmatic attacks (modified from Deamer). [11]

Current evidence indicates that respiratory viral infections often provoke exacerbations of asthma, but bacteria have only very rarely been implicated. [12-16] Respiratory viral infections (and infection with mycoplasma in one study[12]) may precipitate 1/3 of acute asthmatic attacks. The virus most commonly implicated in older children with asthmatic attacks has been rhinovirus. Influenza and parainfluenza have also been incriminated. Respiratory syncytial virus has been a frequent offender in children less than 5 years old, with coronavirus somewhat less frequently implicated. Coxsackie A9 has also been isolated occasionally.

The more severe and more extensive respiratory viral infections seemed most likely to be associated with wheezing in asthmatics in one study, while viral colonization without producing any symptoms of infection did not provoke wheezing. [15] Wheezing usually began the same day as the respiratory infection.

Virus infections have also been implicated as causes of airway obstruction in asthmatics by the demonstration of increased susceptibility to the induction of bronchospasm by methacholine inhalation in asthmatics following administration of influenza[17] or measles vaccine. [18]

There is evidence that the initial onset of allergic symptoms in children of allergic parents usually occurs within 6 weeks after an upper respiratory infection, associated with rising antibody titers to parainfluenza or respiratory syncytial virus.[19]

The mechanism through which infection provokes asthmatic attacks or the initial onset of allergic symptoms is unknown. Hypersensitivity to the infecting agent or its products is unlikely. Increased allergen penetration of the respiratory mucosa, and a nonspecific decrease in the threshold for stimulation of airway irritant receptors due to mucosal injury, or alteration of autonomic nervous system responses possibly by a metabolite of virus-infected cells may occur. Peripheral airway obstruction has been found in association with rhinovirus infections in normal adult smokers.[20] The possibility of a preferential depression of IgE-T suppressor lymphocytes due to viral infection has also been suggested.[19] Furthermore, viruses are known to enhance IgE-mediated histamine release from leukocytes of ragweed-allergic patients in association with interferon production, another possible mechanism through which viral infections may trigger asthmatic attacks.[21]

There is also evidence that asthmatic children have an increased susceptibility to viral respiratory infection.[22] Suppression of antibody-dependent cell mediated cytotoxicity has been found in asthmatics subject to triggering of exacerbations of asthma by respiratory infection, as compared with other asthmatics in whom infection was not usually known to provoke asthma, and with normal controls.[23] If this phenomenon is important in affording protection against viral infection, these observations might account for the increased susceptibility of some asthmatics to such infections.

Secondary bacterial respiratory infection may be superimposed upon asthma, probably because of impairment of mucociliary clearance by airway obstruction with accumulated secretions or as a further complication of atelectasis.

There is no conclusive evidence that distant foci of infection (such as otitis media) provoke asthmatic attacks with any substantial frequency, although paranasal sinusitis has occasionally been implicated.[24]

EXERCISE

Physical exertion is frequently reported by parents as a factor which precipitates wheezing in asthmatic children. Even when such a history is not obtained, airway obstruction is usually demonstrable by pulmonary function testing before and after suitable exercise.

Running for 1-2 minutes is often followed in asthmatics by a decrease in airway obstruction which returns to the preexercise baseline within a few minutes. This exercise induced bronchodilation is inversely related to pre-exercise peak expiratory flow rate (PFR) or forced expiratory volume in one second (FEV_1). If airway obstruction is already present before exercise, more bronchodilation usually follows brief exercise. Pretreatment with a bronchodilator followed by 1-2 minutes of exercise elicits more bronchodilation than either the bronchodilator or exercise alone.

If the asthmatic runs for at least 5 minutes, however, increased airway obstruction follows. This obstruction is usually most extreme 5-10 minutes after completion of exercise, and if severe enough may not return to the pre-exercise baseline until more than 1 hour later (Fig. 3.4).

The response is dependent upon the type of exercise as well as its duration. Exercise induced airway obstruction is more likely and more extreme following running than walking or cycling, and least likely to follow swimming.

Increased airway obstruction following exercise is most frequent and most extreme in asthmatics, but smaller changes in pulmonary function have been reported following exercise in children with cystic fibrosis and subjects with allergic rhinitis. Further study of such responses in children with allergic rhinitis is necessary to determine whether exercise testing may be a means of identifying those subject to subsequent development of asthma. These abnormal responses to exercise in asthmatics may persist for years after overt wheezing from other causes has subsided.

The mechanism through which exercise induces asthma remains unknown. A correlation with bronchoconstriction induced by inhalation of methacholine has been reported,[25] and exercise-induced airway obstruction has been inhibited by α-adrenergic blocking agents in some subjects.[26] Responses to exercise have been found usually to be unchanged by induction of adrenergic or cholinergic blockade, however, suggesting lack of mediation by the autonomic nervous system in most asthmatics.[27]

Data bearing upon other possible mechanisms have been equally contradictory. Different mechanisms may possibly act alone or in combination to cause exercise-induced asthma in different subjects.

Repetition of exercise at intervals of less than 2 hours is associated with a progressive diminution in the extent of post-exercise airway obstruction,[28] suggesting depletion of a store of a bronchoconstrictive substance, a precursor of such a substance, or an enzyme responsible for its release. The fact that

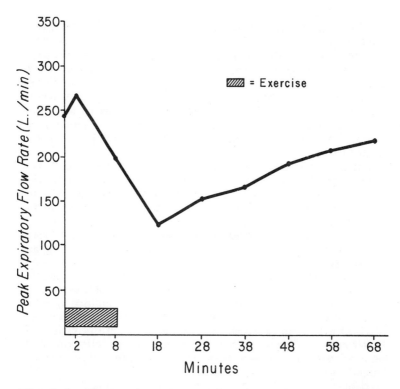

Fig. 3-4. Changes in peak expiratory flow rate in an asthmatic child during and after treadmill exercise (running, 3 miles per hour, 20% grade) showing the typical increase at 2 minutes of exercise, followed by exercise induced asthma becoming most severe 5-10 minutes after the completion of exercise.

exercise induced asthma is often inhibited by inhalation of cromolyn sodium 15-60 minutes before exercise also suggests that this abnormal response is caused by release of chemical mediators from mast cells.

Exercise-induced asthma is inhibited by inhalation of air at 90-100% relative humidity during exercise, and even the simple precaution of breathing through the nose to facilitate humidification and warming of the inspired air minimizes the abnormal response to exercise. [29,30] Obstructive changes in pulmonary function following exercise correlate well with respiratory heat exchange, which is dependent upon minute ventilation and the differences in water content and in temperature of inspired and expired air. [31] Apparently, cooling of mast cells due to increased ventilation with dry air during exercise can cause mediator release.

Exercise-induced asthma can be prevented, or its severity reduced by administration of a bronchodilator before exercise.[32] Oral theophylline, ephedrine, or metaproterenol is most effective if administered 30-60 minutes before exercise, but oral terbutaline is effective for 2-5 hours after administration, and the usual theophylline preparations afford some protection for as long as 6 hours. A sustained release theophylline preparation might be expected to be effective for 8-12 hours, as long as adequate serum concentrations are maintained, but an optimal effect cannot be expected after a single dose unless it is large enough to afford therapeutic serum concentrations. Aerosols of isoproterenol or metaproterenol are most effective in inhibiting exercise-induced asthma if inhaled within 15 minutes before exercise, but terbutaline aerosol is effective at 1 hour, and albuterol or fenoterol aerosols are effective for as long as 4-6 hours.

Inhalation of cromolyn inhibits exercise-induced asthma most effectively for 1 hour, but some effect is evident in patients for as long as 4 hours. Its relative freedom from side effects must be weighed against its relatively short duration of action.

Adrenal corticosteroids administered orally or by inhalation inhibit exercise induced asthma in rare patients, but are not indicated for its treatment because of the availability of safer drugs.

CHANGES IN WEATHER

Sudden changes in weather are often reported by parents to have been associated with asthmatic attacks, and several clinical studies have established correlations with some of these factors (Table 3.1). Inhalation of cold air is well established as a cause of bronchoconstriction in many asthmatics, and ex-

---

TABLE 3.1   WEATHER CHANGES REPORTED TO
PRECIPITATE ASTHMATIC ATTACKS

Decrease in temperature
Decrease in humidity
Increase in humidity
Decrease in barometric pressure
Increase in barometric pressure
Decrease in wind velocity

posure to cold air without its inhalation does not affect pulmonary function in susceptible subjects. Sudden changes in humidity, barometric pressure, and wind velocity have also been implicated.

It is evident that the effect of some of these factors upon asthmatics can be either direct or indirect through favoring increased atmospheric concentrations of allergens or industrial air pollutants. A decrease in wind velocity may favor increased atmospheric concentrations of both natural and industrial air pollutants, while rain is associated with decreased concentrations of pollens and most types of fungus spores. The greatest increase in frequency of asthmatic attacks have been associated with simultaneous changes in several of these factors.

AIR POLLUTION

Air pollution is known to aggravate many cardiac and respiratory conditions including asthma. The adverse effect of sudden exposure to very high concentrations of sulfur dioxide or other air pollutants upon asthmatics is well established. Almost all the asthmatics in Donora, Pennsylvania, suffered adverse effects during the episode of extreme pollution in 1948 (compared to 40% of the general population), [33] and significantly higher morbidity and mortality occurred among asthmatics as compared with the general population in the extreme air pollution episode of London in 1952. [34] Increases in the frequency or severity of asthmatic attacks associated with periods of increased air pollution have also been reported in other cities. The onset or aggravation of asthmatic symptoms has occurred in the Tokyo-Yokohama area in association with industrial air pollution. [35]

Inert dusts and irritant chemicals such as sulfur dioxide are known to cause reflex bronchoconstriction in asthmatics, a response mediated through vagal pathways and inhibited by atropine.

There is also evidence of some increase in the frequency of lower respiratory infections in children living in areas of Great Britain classified as being subject to higher levels of air pollution;[36] thus, air pollution might also elicit asthmatic attacks indirectly by causing respiratory infections.

The most ubiquitous source of local air pollution in the United States is cigarette smoking. An increased prevalence of cough has been reported in school children from homes where parents smoked, although the presence of respiratory symptoms in the children was better correlated with the presence of respiratory symptoms in the parents. [37] Thus, cross infection was thought to be a more important factor than inhalation of smoke by the children. Smoking parents were themselves more susceptible to respiratory disease, increasing the exposure of their children to infectious agents. On the other hand an increased frequency of illness in children in homes where someone smoked without an increased frequency of illness in the adults has also been reported.[38] Inhalation of sidestream cigarette smoke in concentrations comparable to those found in random samples from public facilities has been reported to cause significant airway obstruction in asthmatics within one hour.[39]

Strong fumes or odors as well as smoke are sometimes reported by parents to have provoked wheezing in asthmatic children. Such responses may be mediated either through a direct action upon irritant receptors or through triggering coughing which then causes reflex bronchoconstriction.

EMOTIONAL STRESS

Anger, excitement, anxiety, or depression are commonly reported by parents and asthmatic children to precipitate asthmatic attacks.[39] The fact that many asthmatic children improve quickly following admission to residential treatment centers where they are separated from the rest of their families, possible sources of conflicts resulting in some of these emotions, suggests that emotional factors can be very important in some children. Because other factors may also account for such responses - factors such as separation from environmental allergens - the effect of removal of the rest of the family from the asthmatic child's home has been studied.[40] In each case a substitute parent lived with the child for 2 weeks. Significant improvement occurred during the period of separation in 8 of 13 children whose parents had ranked emotional factors among the 3 factors most likely to trigger asthmatic episodes in their child, and improvement occurred in 3 of 12 children whose parents had not regarded emotional factors as so important. Anxiety and resentment aroused through discussion of stressful situations has been reported associated with an increased rate of secretion of bronchial mucus in an asthmatic.[41]

A history of sudden improvement when separated from the family during trips or hospitalizations should suggest the possible importance of emotional factors, among other things. Discussions evoking anxiety, anger, or depression have been found to elicit associated increases in rate or depth of respirations with or without asthma and can precipitate wheezing in some asthmatics.[42] Hyperventilation and stimulation of irritant receptors by a sudden, deep inspiration, coughing, or laughter, causing reflex bronchoconstriction, are some mechanisms through which emotions can provoke asthmatic attacks.

Although emotional stress is well established as an important trigger of asthmatic attacks, numerous clinical and experimental studies have failed to establish psychological factors as important to the pathogenesis of asthma. [43] Disturbed parent-child relationships may often complicate the management of the asthmatic child as they may the management of a child with any chronic disease, but the basic cause of the asthma must be sought elsewhere.

PHYSICAL FINDINGS

Physical findings depend upon the age of the child, the severity and chronicity of the asthma, and the timing of the examination with respect to remissions or exacerbations.

HEIGHT AND WEIGHT

Although most asthmatic children are within 2 standard deviations of the normal mean height and weight for children of their age according to growth data collected from comparable normal populations, severe asthma has been associated with inhibition of growth. [44] Both height and weight can be affected. Improvement in the control of the asthma is often followed by improvement in growth rate. [45]

Continuous treatment with adrenal corticosteroids is known to inhibit growth. [45] Growth suppression can also occur in severely ill asthmatic children not treated with corticosteroids probably as a result of poor nutrition (poor appetite) or chronic infection if there is associated bronchiectasis. In fact, improved growth has occasionally been observed when severe asthma has been brought under control with corticosteroid therapy.

RESPIRATORY RATE

Accurate determination of respiratory rate, pulse rate, and blood pressure is important even during symptomatic remissions, when they are usually normal, because of the possibility of unrecognized complications and to serve as a basis for comparison during exacerbations of asthma. The need for the child to be in a quiet, stable, resting state during the measurement of vital signs is obvious but often disregarded. Anxiety is one of the commonest causes of tachypnea as well as tachycardia and hypertension, but respiratory rate can usually be determined even without the child's knowledge by observation from across the room during the interview. If the child is young, this may be best accomplished while he is sitting quietly in the mother's lap. The respiratory rate should be compared with age-related normal values (Fig. 3.5).

Tachypnea is a useful sign of decreased lung compliance and restrictive pulmonary disease such as pneumonia, pleural effusion, or pneumothorax, when anxiety and other causes of increased respiratory rate can be excluded. These include exercise, fever, anemia, metabolic acidosis, and respiratory alkalosis.

GENERAL FEATURES

During an acute asthmatic attack the child is likely to prefer to stand or to sit, leaning forward somewhat. There may be evidence of recruitment of accessory muscles of respiration: flaring of the alae nasi. Intercostal and supraclavicular retractions are evident because of the abnormally great decrease in intrapleural pressure necessary for inspiration through the obstructed airways. In infants inspiratory retraction of the sternum may also be evident. Bulging of intercostal spaces may occur during expiration because of the abnormal increase

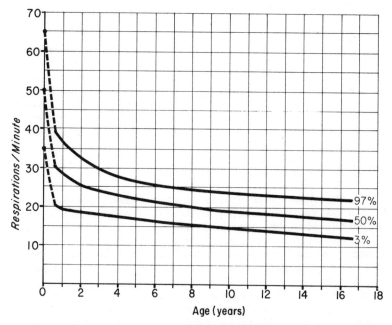

Fig. 3-5. Normal resting respiratory rates in infants and children. (Data of Iliff and Lee[46] and Miller[47]).

in intrapleural pressure necessary to force gas past the obstructions. Subcostal retractions, due to the action of a flattened diaphragm upon its sites of attachment to the walls of the thorax, are seen in extensive restrictive pulmonary disease as well as diffuse obstructive pulmonary disease. [48]

Head bobbing is described as a sign of dyspnea in infants. It can be observed with the infant lying in its mother's arms with the head unsupported except for the suboccipital area. Neck flexion with each inspiration occurs with contraction of scalene and sternocleidomastoid muscles, accessory muscles of respiration. [48]

Cyanosis may be evident if arterial oxygen saturation is less than 80-85%, but may not be present if the child is anemic.

Signs of allergic rhinitis (see Chapter IV) or atopic dermatitis (see Chapter V) often are also present.

CHEST CONFIGURATION

Chronic obstructive lung disease is known to be associated with the development of an increase in the antero-posterior diameter of the chest, the "barrel chest" deformity. This has been explained as an application of Pascal's principle, which states that pressure applied to an enclosed gas or liquid is transmitted, undiminished, in all directions. As pressure is increased within a malleable, non-spherical gas or fluid-filled object it will approach the shape of a sphere. [49] Thus, with the increased intrathoracic pressure caused by severe, persistent obstructive lung disease the thorax will tend to become spherical.

The chest of a newborn infant is almost circular in cross section, but as the child grows the depth (A-P diameter) increases less than the width (transverse diameter), so that by 2-3 years of age the depth-width ratio usually approximates 0.75. These parameters are more closely related to height than to age. Normal values have been published, 50-52 and graphs describing the normal relationships are readily available* (Fig. 3.6). Measurements can be made with obstetrical calipers or chest calipers (Fig. 3.7), during quiet tidal breathing. Children should be standing with their arms down. Maximum depth at the level of any horizontal plane between the xiphoid process and the sternal notch is measured from sternum to vertebral spinous process. Maximum width is measured from rib to rib at the midaxillary lines at the level of a horizontal plane between the xiphoid process and sternal notch. Plotting the point thus determined on the depth-width chart

* Medical Research Department, Mead Johnson Research Center, Evansville, Indiana 47721.

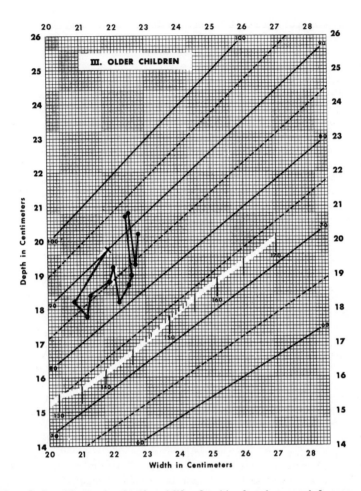

Fig. 3-6. Thoracic depth-width chart* showing serial measurements of the chest of an asthmatic boy obtained over a period of 15 months. Expected values for depth and width are found by locating the subject's height (cm.) on the curving, white regression line. Each large square on the checkerboard grid represents vertically 1 standard deviation of chest depth and horizontally 1 standard deviation of chest width for height. Diagonal lines indicate the thoracic index, each lying 1 standard deviation (5 units) from the next.

*Waring, W. W., Acker, S., Golladay, E. S., and Hilman, B. C. Reproduced with permission of Mead Johnson & Company.

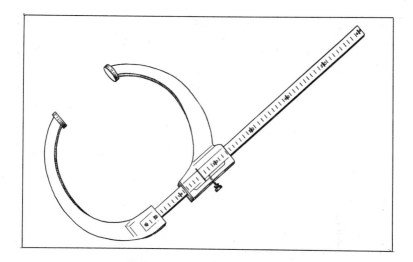

Fig. 3-7. Chest calipers, consisting of 2 plastic arms, one of which slides along the meter stick. Depth or width is read beneath line inscribed on the sliding segment.

permits immediate determination of the thoracic index ($\frac{depth}{width}$ x 100) and comparison with the values expected in normal children of the same sex and height.

Serial determination and plotting of chest measurements provides objective evidence of trends in chronic airway obstruction. Abnormal increases in thoracic index are rare in asthmatic children, occurring only in those with persistent, severe airway obstruction, and the abnormal chest configuration is reversible if the asthma can be brought under control. Children with severe pulmonary disease due to cystic fibrosis on the other hand may show a relentless increase in thoracic index, which often approximates 100 shortly before death. In asthmatics acute changes in chest configuration are evident during exacerbations.

DIGITAL CLUBBING

Digital clubbing was mentioned by Hippocrates as a sign of empyema,[53] and subsequently its association with a variety of other conditions has been recognized (Table 3.2). Hereditary clubbing often has its onset at or after puberty. The commonest pathological condition associated with digital clubbing in

TABLE 3.2   DISEASES ASSOCIATED WITH ACQUIRED
DIGITAL CLUBBING IN CHILDREN

PULMONARY	Bronchiectasis
	Pulmonary abscess
	Empyema
	Chronic pneumonia
	Neoplasms
CARDIAC	Cyanotic congenital heart disease
	Subacute bacterial endocarditis
HEPATIC	Biliary cirrhosis
GASTROINTESTINAL	Chronic ulcerative colitis
	Regional enteritis
	Chronic dysentery
	Multiple polyposis

children in the United States is probably cyanotic congenital heart disease; the commonest pulmonary condition is bronchiectasis, most often due to cystic fibrosis in white children. Minimal digital clubbing is only very rarely associated with uncomplicated asthma.[54] The presence of clubbing in an asthmatic should initiate a search for other conditions more frequently associated with it. Clubbing might be expected with bronchiectasis superimposed upon asthma.

The recognition of digital clubbing has usually depended upon largely subjective impressions gained from inspection of the finger, but accurate, objective assessment is possible utilizing measurements of finger casts.[55]

A cylinder formed from half of a 3 x 5 inch filing card sealed with masking tape and closed at one end with a gauze square can be filled with a smooth, thick paste prepared by addition of tap water to alginate dental impression powder.[*] The extended left index finger is inserted deeply into the freshly mixed material and kept immobile for 3 minutes until the mixture is firm. The finger is then removed, and the mold is filled with cement.[†] The mold is removed when the cast is dry (2 hours).

[*] Kalginate, Type 2 normal set, Teledyne Dental Products, 543 Warden Ave., Glendale, California 91202
[†] Duroc Miracle Stone, The Ransom and Randolph Co., P.O. Box 905, Toledo, Ohio 43691.

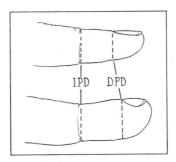

Fig. 3-8. Points of measurement of distal phalangeal depth (DPD) and interphalangeal depth (IPD) on casts of index fingers for assessment of digital clubbing. Normal ratio of DPD/IPD = 0.895 with a standard deviation of 0.041.

Measurements of the depth of the finger cast are made at the base of the nail (DPD) and at the distal interphalangeal joint (IPD) with a metric micrometer with a vernier scale (Fig. 3.8). A ratio of DPD/IPD greater than 1 is more than 2.5 standard deviations above normal and considered abnormal. This parameter has been found to be the most reliable from comparison of measurements in normal subjects and those with conditions commonly associated with digital clubbing.[55] It is independent of age, sex, and race.

At the bedside it is usually possible to determine by inspection whether DPD exceeds IPD. The cause of digital clubbing remains unknown.

CHEST PERCUSSION

A hyperresonant percussion note may be elicited during an acute asthmatic attack, but the percussion note is usually normal (resonant) during remissions. Percussion of the chest of a child normally elicits a note which is hyperresonant as compared with that elicited from an adult, however.

CHEST AUSCULTATION

Before the nineteenth century chest sounds were heard by immediate auscultation through placing the ear directly against the chest. This was rather unsatisfactory, and the significance of the little that could be heard was often misunderstood. In 1819 Laennec published his description of the first stethoscope, a wooden cylinder approximately 30 cm. long which transmitted sounds from the chest to one ear. [56] The binaural, flexible stethoscope was invented in the United States and first described in 1855. [57] The next important improvement, introduction of the differential stethoscope by S. Scott Alison in 1858, [58] has been slow to gain popularity.

The differential stethoscope (Fig. 3.9) consists of two identical chest pieces connected with the standard earpiece yoke by equal lengths of tubing. Alison ascribed its utility to the fact that when sound of the same character but different intensity is conveyed simultaneously to both ears, perception is limited to the ear receiving the louder sound. Thus, simultaneous auscultation of corresponding segments of the two lungs facilitates recognition of minimal suppression of breath sounds as well as differences in timing of inspiration or expiration. [48]

The lungs should be auscultated carefully over each of the 18 bronchopulmonary segments which can be examined (Fig. 3. 10). The position of the diaphragm is located by percussion,

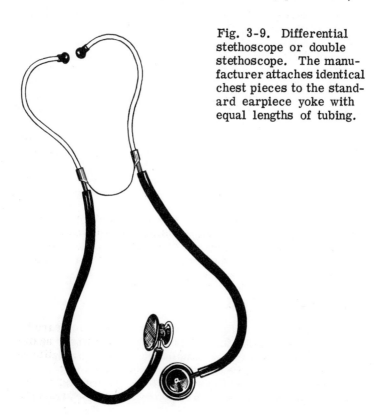

Fig. 3-9. Differential stethoscope or double stethoscope. The manufacturer attaches identical chest pieces to the standard earpiece yoke with equal lengths of tubing.

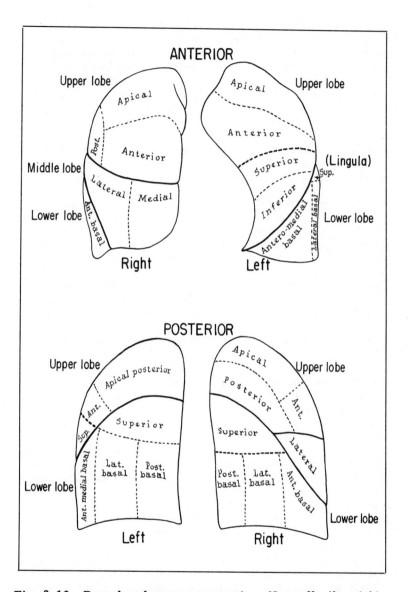

Fig. 3-10. Bronchopulmonary segments. Normally the right lung has 10 segments, one of which does not abut against the chest wall (medial basal segment of the lower lobe). The left lung has 8 or 9 segments, depending upon whether the apical and posterior segments of the upper lobe are considered separately.

and the normal locations of the segments can be learned quickly from reference to diagrams or models such as the Huber Lung Model*. Localization of abnormal findings is often helpful because certain conditions tend to involve certain segments, and it is essential for supplying appropriate instructions for postural drainage. It also permits closer correlation of physical findings with roentgenographic abnormalities.

Normally expiration takes slightly longer than inspiration, but the inspiratory phase heard by auscultation is normally longer than that of expiration by a ratio of 3:1. During an exacerbation of asthma both the time necessary for expiration and the duration of the expiratory phase of the breath sound are greatly prolonged. Even between overt exacerbations of asthma some prolongation of the expiratory phase may be present.

There is some disagreement and confusion over the classification of rales and rhonchi, a subject which can be clarified by reference to a program of recorded chest sounds correlated with a text. [59] Rales or crackles are usually classified as fine (crepitant), medium, or coarse. Fine rales are high pitched, crackling sounds resembling the crumpling of cellophane and ascribed to the popping apart of walls of alveoli held together by secretions. Medium and coarse rales are lower pitched sounds thought to originate in larger airways. Sibilant rales or rhonchi or wheezes are high pitched, continuous, musical sounds due to passage of air through narrowed airways, while sonorous rales or low pitched wheezes originate from larger airways. Even sibilant rales, however, must originate from airways large enough to be conducting air at sufficient velocity to produce a musical sound. [48]

During the acute asthmatic attack expiratory or inspiratory and expiratory sibilant rales are heard, but the expiratory wheezes are louder because of the increased obstruction during expiration. As the obstruction becomes more severe wheezing is audible even without the stethoscope. Wheezing may diminish with the most extreme airway obstruction due to lack of movement of sufficient air. During recovery from an asthmatic attack the sibilant rales may be replaced by sonorous rales or medium or coarse rales due to the presence of secretions in the large airways.

Between exacerbations of asthma it is often possible to elicit sibilant or sonorous rales as well as prolongation of the expiratory phases of the breath sounds with forced expirations or by assisting forced expirations by manual compression of the chest from front to back during auscultation.

* Clay-Adams Co., 299 Webrow Rd., Parsippany, New Jersey, 07054.

HYPOXIA AND HYPERCAPNIA

Mild hypoxia may be present without any associated clinical signs except those related to its cause. Signs of moderate and severe hypoxia include cyanosis, tachycardia, and either hypotension or hypertension (Table 3.3). One of the earliest neurological changes with hypoxia may be agitation. This must not be misinterpreted as an indication for sedation.

Hypercapnia and hypoxia are often present together. Signs of hypercapnia include tachycardia, hypertension, and miosis. If hypercapnia progresses confusion and a flapping tremor may supervene. With severe hypercapnia coma may occur and papilledema may be evident.

PULSUS PARADOXUS

Pulsus paradoxus, an exaggeration of the normal decrease in arterial blood pressure with inspiration, occurs in acute asthmatic attacks. The difference in systolic blood pressure during inspiration and expiration normally does not exceed 5 mm of mercury, but during asthmatic attacks the difference is often greater than 10 mm, and the extent of the pulsus paradoxus has seemed related to the severity of the airway obstruction.[60,61] The systolic pressure on expiration is determined by the highest level at which systolic pulse sounds are heard during expiration as the sphygmomanometer cuff is deflated; systolic pressure on inspiration, the highest level at which these sounds can be heard with every pulse beat throughout

TABLE 3.3   SIGNS AND SYMPTOMS
             OF HYPOXIA AND HYPERCAPNIA

HYPOXIA	HYPERCAPNIA
Cyanosis	Tachycardia
Tachycardia	Cardiac arrhythmias
Systemic hypotension or hypertension	Systemic hypertension
Pulmonary hypertension	Headache
Euphoria, agitation, or depression	Dizziness
Impairment of motor function and judgment	Confusion
Confusion, delirium	Drowsiness
Coma	Asterixis
	Coma
	Convulsions
	Miosis, papilledema

inspiration. The phenomenon has been ascribed to an increase in the volume of the pulmonary vascular bed during inspiration with diminished filling of the left heart and consequent reduction in left ventricular stroke volume. [60]

LABORATORY FINDINGS

EOSINOPHILIA

The differential white blood cell count may or may not reveal the presence of eosinophilia. The total leukocyte count must be considered in assessing the significance of the results of the differential count, and a total eosinophil count is more accurate than an estimate from the differential and total leukocyte counts. The normal mean eosinophil count in children is said to approximate 150 per cubic mm. with a range of 30-700, [62] but few data are available. A diurnal variation has been reported in children without adrenal insufficiency with a mid-morning nadir 20% below the 8:00 A.M. level and a maximal nocturnal increase 30% above the 8:00 A.M. level. [62]

Allergy is probably the commonest cause of eosinophilia in children in the United States. In one series reported from Great Britain as many as 85% of children with asthma had eosinophil counts of greater than 600 per cubic mm. [63] Eosinophilia has not usually seemed to correlate with the severity of asthma, but some data from adults show correlation with the severity of airway obstruction due to asthma. [64,65]

Asthmatic adults with eosinophilia have also been reported to respond better to treatment with bronchodilators than asthmatics with total eosinophil counts of less than 400 per cubic millimeter. [66]

Decreases in total eosinophil counts follow treatment with beta-adrenergic drugs (isoproterenol, epinephrine) and aminophylline. [67,68] Physical and mental stress have been associated with eosinopenia, and treatment with exogenous adrenal corticosteroids also suppresses total eosinophil counts. [65] Intercurrent infection in asthmatics is reputed to cause eosinopenia, a phenomenon said to be helpful in the diagnosis of infection superimposed upon asthma. [64] All of these factors must be considered in evaluating eosinophil counts in asthmatics.

Other causes of moderate eosinophilia (1,000-5,000 per cubic mm.) include parasitic infestations, exposure to drugs (usually without any other manifestation of hypersensitivity), and congenital immunodeficiency disorders (Table 3.4).

Extreme eosinophilia (30,000-100,000 per cubic mm.) in children is most commonly due to visceral larva migrans, but also occurs with the idiopathic hypereosinophilic syndrome and eosinophilic leukemia (Table 3.5).

TABLE 3.4   CAUSES OF MODERATE EOSINOPHILIA

Parasitic infestations (trichinosis, ascariasis, hookworm disease, strongyloidiasis, malaria, eosinophilic pneumonia, tropical eosinophilia)
Atopic allergy (asthma, allergic rhinitis, urticaria, atopic dermatitis)
Allergic bronchopulmonary aspergillosis
Drug exposure
Hodgkin's disease
Fanconi's anemia
Congenital sex-linked agammaglobulinemia
Thymic dysplasia (Nezelof's syndrome)
Hyperimmunoglobulinemia E with susceptibility to infection
(Buckley syndrome)
Chronic myelocytic leukemia
Polycythemia rubra vera
Postsplenectomy
Hypersensitivity angiitis
Periarteritis nodosa
Hepatic cirrhosis
Eosinophilic gastroenteritis
Metastatic neoplasms
Dermatitis herpetiformis
Radiation therapy
Peritoneal dialysis
Congenital heart disease (stenotic)
Hereditary eosinophilia

TABLE 3.5   CAUSES OF EXTREME EOSINOPHILIA[62]

Visceral larva migrans
Idiopathic hypereosinophilic syndrome
Eosinophilic leukemia
Conditions usually associated with only moderate eosinophilia:
    Trichinosis, hookworm disease, ascariasis, strongyloidiasis
    Hodgkin's disease
    Periarteritis nodosa
    Drug hypersensitivity

SPUTUM CYTOLOGY

Examination of sputum for eosinophiles may also be helpful when a suitable specimen can be obtained. Small children usually swallow any sputum produced. Material sufficient for examination can sometimes be collected on a cotton swab introduced into the pharynx above the larynx if a cough can be elicited.

The sputum may be clear, mucoid, or mucopurulent. Yellow sputum need not indicate the presence of infection, for an abundance of eosinophils can impart a macroscopic appearance similar to that associated with the presence of large numbers of neutrophils. Thus, microscopic examination is necessary.

Dried smears can be examined after staining with any one of a number of different stains such as Hansel's stain, designed to emphasize contrasts between eosinophils and other cells, or the same information can be obtained by examination of wet preparations. [69]

In addition to eosinophils, sputum obtained from an asthmatic may contain Charcot-Leyden crystals, needle-like crystals thought to be formed from degenerated eosinophils, and Curschmann spirals, bronchiolar casts composed of inspissated mucus and cellular debris. Creola bodies, clumps of bronchial epithelial cells, are found in subjects with viral respiratory infections as well as in asthmatics. [70] The exfoliation of ciliated epithelial cells with cytoplasmic degeneration, ciliocytophthoria, has been ascribed to the cytopathic effect of viruses, [71] while shedding of bronchial epithelial cells in asthmatics has been ascribed to mucosal edema. [70]

PULMONARY FUNCTION TESTING

Assessment of pulmonary function can supply additional objective data useful for diagnosis, indication of the severity of the airway obstruction at the time of the examination, evaluation of response to therapy, and prediction of responses to exercise.

Accurate measurement of most parameters of pulmonary function is not possible in children younger than 5 years of age because of the need for cooperation, and most reliable results are obtained in older children by a patient, understanding, enthusiastic technician, skilled at motivating children to compete with themselves in successive expiratory efforts.

Many instruments of varying sophistication and cost are available for measurement of lung volumes and flow rates. [72] One of the simplest is the Wright Peak Flow Meter (Fig. 3.11), which can be used to determine peak expiratory flow rate (PFR). This occurs early in the forced expiration and is effort

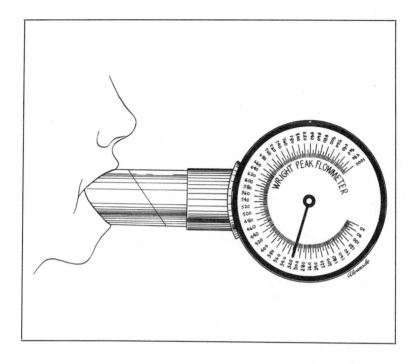

Fig. 3-11. Wright Peak Flow Meter (Armstrong Industries, Inc.,
Northbrook, Illinois 60062). The adult model (60-1000 liters/
minute) is suitable for most children at least 6 years of age; the
low range model (20-200 liters/minute) can be used for very
young children or those with low flow rates such as occur during
exacerbations of asthma. After a maximal inspiration the child
expires forcefully into the flow meter. Peak expiratory flow
rate can then be read directly from the meter.

dependent. Young children can more easily be taught how to
use the peak flow meter than a spirometer, because the flow
meter does not require a sustained effort. The best of 3-5 efforts which agree within 10% can be compared with normal value for the child's height (Fig. 3.12). Determination of PFR
is a satisfactory method of assessing airway obstruction although
less sensitive than determination of airway resistance. It is
especially useful when frequent determinations are necessary,
as in the evaluation of responses to exercise, where measurement of spirometric parameters every few minutes might cause
fatigue or provoke bronchospasm. Its simplicity also permits

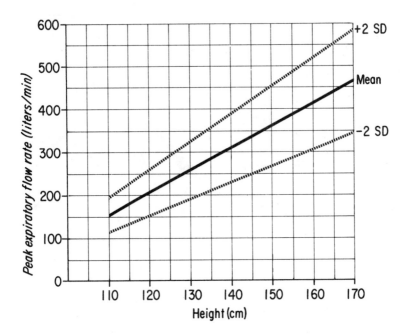

Fig. 3-12. Peak expiratory flow rate (Wright Peak Flow Meter, adult model) as a function of height in normal boys and girls. (Data collected by Polgar and Promadhat).[72]

$$PFR \text{ (L./min)} = 425.5714 + 5.2428 \times \text{Ht. (cm.)}$$

$$S. D. = 12.8\%$$

determination several times daily at home, and frequent measurement of PFR has been shown to supply more useful information about the variability and progression of airway obstruction due to asthma than less frequent use of more sophisticated techniques.[73]

Although decreases in PFR usually reflect airway obstruction, they also occur with reductions in vital capacity.

The lung volumes and their relationships to the spirogram obtained with a recording spirometer are indicated in Fig. 3.13. Instruments for recording single forced expirograms such as the portable Vitalor* or Pulmonor † produce somewhat different

* McKesson Appliance Co., Toledo, Ohio 43620
† Jones Medical Instrument Co., Oak Brook, Illinois 60521

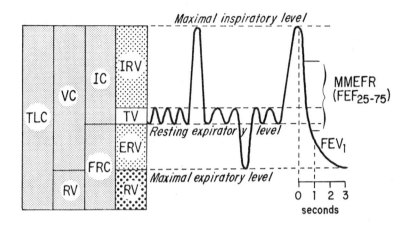

Fig. 3-13. Lung volumes and capacities and their determination from the tracing of a recording spirometer (modified from Comroe, et al).[74] TLC, total lung capacity; VC vital capacity, the maximal volume of gas that can be expelled from the lungs after a maximal inspiration; IC, inspiratory capacity, the maximal volume of gas that can be inspired from the resting expiratory level; FRC, functional residual capacity, the volume of gas remaining in the lungs at the resting expiratory level; TV, tidal volume, the volume of gas inspired or expired during each respiratory cycle; IRV, inspiratory reserve volume, the maximal additional gas that can be inspired after the tidal volume has been inspired; ERV, expiratory reserve volume, the maximal additional gas that can be expired after the tidal volume has been expired; RV, residual volume, the volume of gas remaining in the lungs after maximal expiration. FEV_1 is the volume expired during the first second of a forced expiration following maximal inspiration. MMEFR, maximal mid-expiratory flow rate, or FEF_{25-75}, forced expiratory flow rate from 25-75% of vital capacity, is the rate of flow during that portion of the expiration.

time-volume graphs (Fig. 3.14). A computer-printer available as an option with the Pulmonor as well as several other instruments provides automatic analysis of the forced expiration, printing the various parameters measured. An instrument which supplies a tracing is desirable to help assess the cooperation of the subject. A smooth, regular curve, resembling that of Fig. 3.14 should be obtained with the subject standing.

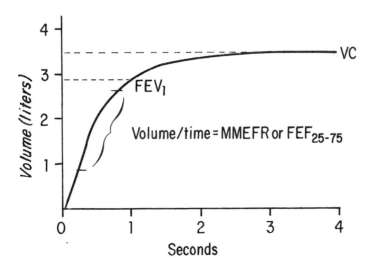

Fig. 3-14. Forced expirogram (Pulmonor) with determination of VC (vital capacity), FEV1 (forced expiratory volume in one second), and MMEFR or FEF25-75 (maximal mid-expiratory flow rate or forced expiratory flow rate from 25-75% of vital capacity). The best of three similar curves is usually analyzed.

Vital capacity should be compared with normal values for the child's height (Figs. 3.15, & 3.16). For a single determination only values more than 2 standard devaitions (26%) from the normal mean are considered abnormal. Vital capacity is reduced by restrictive pulmonary diseases such as pneumonia, tuberculosis, sarcoidosis, Hamman-Rich syndrome, atelectasis, lobectomy, pleural effusion, or pneumothorax. It is also reduced by non-pulmonary causes of limitation of respiratory movements or lung expansion such as neuromuscular disease (poliomyelitis, Guillain-Barre syndrome), recumbent position, painful respirations (fractured rib), kyphoscoliosis, diaphragmatic hernia or eventration, cardiac enlargement, or intrathoracic tumors. With obstructive pulmonary disease such as asthma, vital capacity is often normal but may be reduced if airway obstruction is extreme enough to occlude completely some bronchioles. The commonest cause of reduced vital capacity in children is insufficient cooperation.

Forced expiratory volume in one second (FEV1), a measurement of obstructive pulmonary disease, can also be compared with normal values for the child's height (Fig. 3.17). If VC is reduced, however, FEV1 will also be reduced. Because of

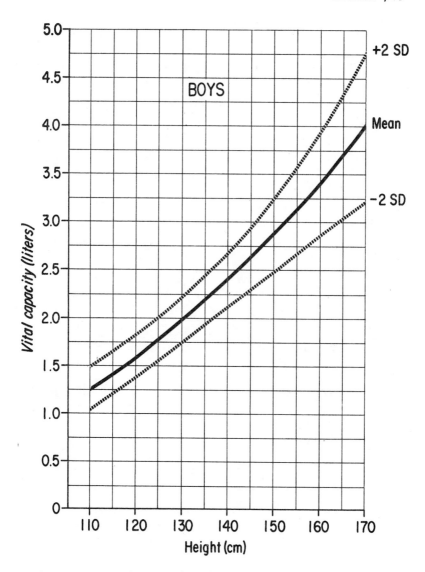

Fig. 3-15. Vital capacity as a function of height in normal boys (data collected by Polgar and Promadhat).[72]

$$VC_{boys} \; (ml.) = 4.4 \times 10^{-3} \times Ht. \; (cm.)$$

$$S.D. \; = approx. \; 13\%$$

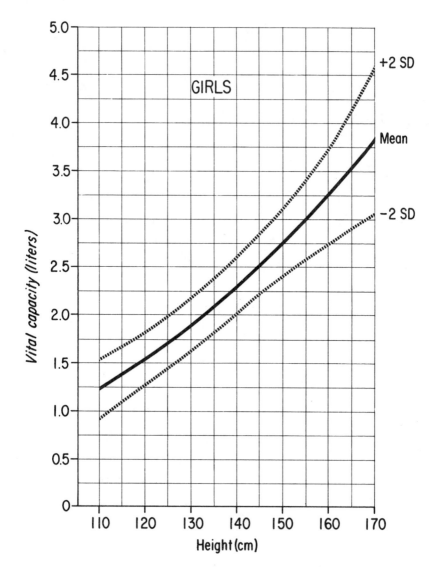

Fig. 3-16. Vital capacity as a function of height in normal girls. (Data collected by Polgar and Promadhat).[72]

$$VC_{girls} \text{ (ml.)} = 3.3 \times 10^{-3} \times Ht. \text{ (cm.)}$$

$$S.D. = \text{approx. } 13\%$$

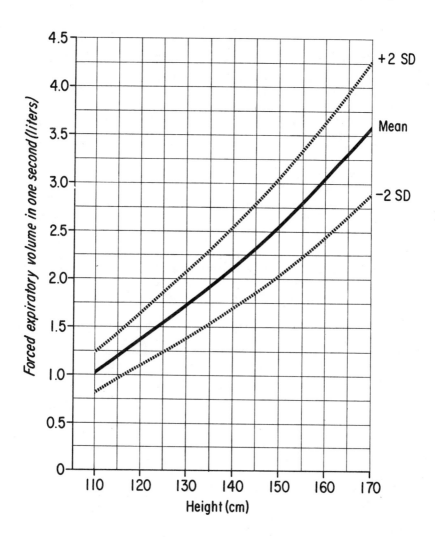

Fig. 3-17. Forced expiratory volume in one second as function of height in normal boys and girls. (Data collected by Polgar and Promadhat).[72]

$$FEV_1 \text{ (ml.)} = 2.1 \times 10^{-3} \times Ht.\ 2.80 \text{ (cm.)}$$

$$S. D. = 10\%$$

this the ratio of FEV_1/VC is more useful as an indicator of air-way obstruction. This ratio is usually expressed as per cent. The normal mean ratio of $\frac{FEV_1 \times 100}{VC}$ in children is 86% (S. D.

= 7%),[72] while that for adults is 83%. Thus, the lower limit of normal in children is 72%. A reduction in the ratio of FEV_1/VC occurs with airway obstruction as seen with asthma, cystic fibrosis, bronchial foreign body, or airway compression by an aberrant blood vessel or enlarged lymph node.

Maximal mid-expiratory flow rate (MMEFR, MMF, FEF_{25-75}), mean flow rate calculated over the middle 50% of the forced expiratory volume (see Figs. 3.13 & 3.14), has been considered the most sensitive parameter derived from the forced expirograms for detection of airway obstruction. It is less effort dependent than FEV_1 or PFR. Induced bronchospasm producing a decrease in vital capacity has been shown sometimes to be associated with an increase in MMEFR, however, calling into question its reliability as an index of acute airway changes when not adjusted for change in lung volume.[75] Normal values are available for children (Fig. 3.18), but the normal range as a function of height is more variable than for other parameters based upon presently available data.

Functional residual capacity (FRC) and residual volume (RV) can be determined by gas dilution or plethysmographic techniques and airway resistance can be measured using a body plethysmograph.[74] All of these are increased during acute asthmatic attacks.

Flow volume loops can be obtained using a pneumotachograph, a transducer, and a recorder or oscilloscope. Most useful information is derived from the maximum expiratory flow volume (MEFV) curve, and the inspiratory curve can be omitted to simplify the maneuver for the child (Fig. 3.19). Determination of flow rates at various points of the curve or loop is possible, and these are indicated as flow at a certain percent of total lung capacity (if this has also been determined) or vital capacity. The lung volumes usually measured by spirometry can also be determined from the MEFV curve. Flow rates below 2/3 maximal expiration are relatively less dependent upon effort, a consideration especially important in the evaluation of children. Decreased flow rates at low lung volumes have been found useful in the detection of obstruction of peripheral small airways (2 mm or less in internal diameter), which contribute so little to total airway resistance that significant obstruction may be present despite normal spirometric parameters. Small airway obstruction is often present in asthmatics, and maximum expiratory flow rate ($\dot{V}max$) at 25-50% VC or 50% TLC have been reported to be the most sensitive indices of airway obstruction.[76] Others have reported MMEFR equally sensitive when expressed

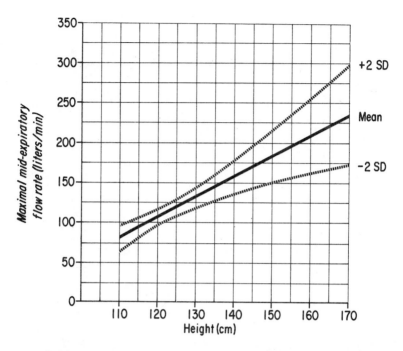

Fig. 3-18. Maximal mid-expiratory flow rate as a function of height in normal boys and girls. (Data collected by Polgar and Promadhat).[72]

MMEFR (L./min.) = 207.70 + 2.621 x Ht. (cm.)
S.D. = 8-16% up to 150 cm. in height, more above that height.

as VC per second to relate it to lung volume.[77] Normal values for $\dot{V}$max are not yet available for children, but it has been estimated that $\dot{V}$max at 50% VC should approximate 1 TLC/sec at 6-18 years of age.[78] Convexity toward the volume axis of the descending MEFV curve indicates airway obstruction. This can be quantitated by measuring the distances to the flow volume curve and to the abscissa from a straight line drawn between peak flow and RV (see Fig. 3.19).[79] This curvilinearity score $\left(\dfrac{\text{Distance to FV curve}}{\text{Distance to abscissa}}\right)$ could underestimate convexity toward the abscissa if effort-dependent peak flow were low, however.

Acute asthmatic attacks are associated with decreases in $\dot{V}$max, MMEFR, FEV_1, FEV_1/VC, and PFR. The VC may also be reduced with occlusion of airways. There are increases in airway resistance, FRC, RV, and TLC. These parameters

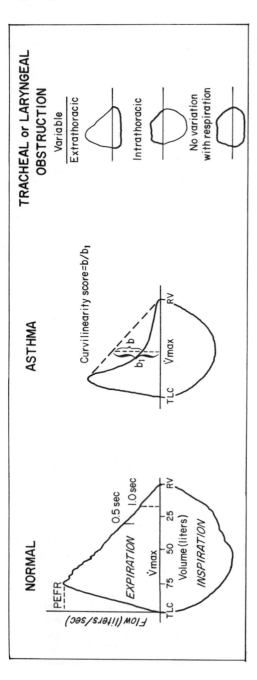

Fig. 3-19. Flow volume loop with determination of peak expiratory flow rate (PFR), forced expiratory volume in one second (FEV$_1$), and flow rates ($\dot{V}$max) at 75, 50, and 25% of vital capacity. Flow rates may also be expressed as % total lung capacity when known. Forced expiration begins at total lung capacity (TLC) and ends at residual volume (RV). Vital capacity is TLC - RV. Inspiration begins at RV and ends at TLC. Airway obstruction causes convexity of the expiratory flow volume curve toward the volume axis. This is measured by the curvilinearity score. A fixed extrathoracic obstruction to the airway causes a plateau in the inspiratory portion of the loop; intrathoracic obstruction, a plateau in the expiratory curve. Circumferential obstructive lesions which do not vary with respiration cause plateaus in both inspiratory and expiratory curves.

all tend to return toward normal with improvement after treatment, but usually are still distinctly abnormal when symptoms
of wheezing and dyspnea have subsided. When expiratory wheezing during quiet breathing is no longer detectable by auscultation,
airway resistance usually is nearly normal, but substantial abnormalities of the other parameters may still be present. [80]
Indeed, abnormalities of $\dot{V}$max, FRC, RV, and spirometric
parameters have often been demonstrated during remissions of
asthma.[76,77] Mild hypoxemia has also been found in asymptomatic asthmatics. [81]

Demonstration of airway obstruction is of less diagnostic
value than demonstration of its reversibility following administration of a bronchodilator. Administration of isoproterenol by
inhalation is well tolerated by most children. Safe, effective
doses are 0.01 ml/Kg of 1:200 isoproterenol by nebulization or
150 mcg delivered from a freon-propelled metered-dose inhaler.[81] The transient increase of 10% in pulse rate immediately
after treatment confirms that the drug has reached the heart
and a satisfactory dose has probably reached the lungs. An
improvement of at least 15% in PFR or FEV_1 should usually be
demonstrated 5-15 minutes after treatment if reversible airway
obstruction was present. In normal adult subjects inhalation of
isoproterenol or isoetharine has been found to elicit no significant change in forced VC or FEV_1, or improvement of less than
5% in FEV_1, [82] although it has been followed by significant increases in MMEFR (mean 15%) and significant decreases in airway resistance.

When no significant airway obstruction is demonstrated at
the time of initial testing, airway obstruction can be induced in
asthmatics by exercise. Treadmill running (3-4 miles per hour,
15-20% grade) for 6-8 minutes is a reliable method of eliciting
the response and permits constant observation of the subject.
Pulmonary function is measured before exercise, immediately
after exercise, and 5 and 10 minutes later (see Fig. 3.4). A
decrease in PFR or FEV_1 of 15% following treadmill running
indicates an abnormal response, and a decrease of 10% after 8
minutes of treadmill walking is significant. Decreases of as
much as 50% are not uncommon in asthmatics. Bronchodilators
or cromolyn administered before testing may inhibit exercise-
induced asthma, so they should be withheld for at least 8 hours
if possible. Sustained release theophylline preparations must
be withheld for 12 hours or more. Exercise testing should be
deferred when significant airway obstruction is already present.

Measurement of pulmonary function before and after inhalation of a cholinergic agent has also been proposed as a procedure useful in the diagnosis of asthma. Successive inhalation
of aerosols of methacholine solutions varying in concentration

from 0. 15 mg/ml - 25 mg/ml if necessary has been followed
by decreases in FEV1 of at least 15-20% in almost all asthmatics within 5 minutes. After the positive response has been
elicited, further administration of the higher concentrations of
methacholine is discontinued. Decreases in FEV1 of less than
15% may follow inhalation of methacholine in normal subjects,
but larger decreases occur in only 15% of normal subjects[83].
Abnormal responses have also followed methacholine inhalation
in nonasthmatic subjects with hay fever and normal subjects
with respiratory infection, but the responses in these have been
less extreme than those seen in most asthmatics.

Measurement of pulmonary function before and after inhalation of aerosols of antigen solutions has proved helpful in the
identification of specific allergens (see Chapter XIII).

BLOOD GASES

Blood gases and acid-base balance are usually normal during remissions of asthma, but mild hypoxemia has sometimes
been found in asymptomatic asthmatics. Their determination
is essential to appropriate evaluation of status asthmaticus.[1,
84-86]

Arterial blood can be obtained from radial, brachial, fe-
moral, or temporal arteries after infiltration of the skin and
subcutaneous tissue with a local anesthetic. Use of a local anesthetic is often unnecessary when the radial artery is used.
Blood is collected in a 2 ml syringe in which the dead space has
been filled with a heparin solution (1, 000 U/ml) to prevent clot-
ting and contact of the specimen with air. Subsequent mixing
of blood and heparin is facilitated by introduction of mercury
into the syringe, and the specimen is immediately placed in ice
and analyzed within a few minutes. Pressure is applied to the
puncture site for at least 5 minutes after withdrawing the needle
to minimize hematoma formation.

The commonest complications of arterial puncture are
thrombosis with distal ischemia, hemorrhage, or formation of
a false aneurysm. These occur most frequently following puncture of a relatively large artery, and radial artery puncture
has been found to be a safe procedure.[87]

Analysis of "arterialized" capillary specimens obtained by
finger, heel, or ear-lobe puncture after warming the extremity
or ear for 10 minutes has shown that pH, P_{CO2}, and P_{O2} usually agree closely with those of arterial blood even in infants
older than 3 hours of age unless peripheral circulation is poor.
Reliance upon capillary specimens for determination of P_{O2} is
especially likely to be misleading in an ill child with poor capillary perfusion or when arterial P_{O2} is > 90 mm Hg due to ad-

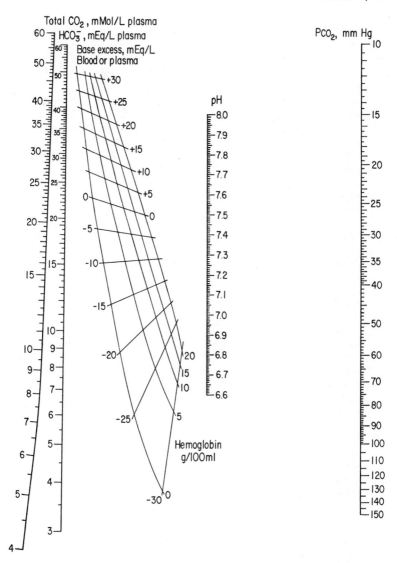

Fig. 3-20. Blood acid-base alignment nomogram (modified from Siggaard-Andersen[89]). Related values are indicated by a straight line passing through any two known values, such as pH and P_{CO2}.

ministration of oxygen. Good correlation between arterial and earlobe capillary P_{O2}, P_{CO2} and pH has been reported in "normotensive" children with status asthmaticus when hyperemia of the earlobe had been induced by application of thurfyl nicotinate (Trafuril). [88]

When arterial pH and P_{CO2} have been determined, these can be plotted on the Siggaard-Andersen alignment nomogram (Fig. 3.20) to find base excess, the deviation of buffer base from normal. Base excess is thus an index of the metabolic component of the acidosis or alkalosis. Its relationship to bicarbonate and the hazards of overemphasizing the significance of the base excess are discussed in detail elsewhere. [90]

Normal values for blood gases and acid base balance in children are indicated in Table 3.6. Early in the asthmatic attack hypocapnea may occur with respiratory alkalosis due to hyperventilation. Hypoxemia results in a superimposed metabolic acidosis due to accumulation of lactic acid and other organic acids. As airway obstruction continues or progresses, arterial P_{CO2} returns to normal and then increases further, resulting in respiratory acidosis.

TABLE 3.6   BLOOD GASES AND ACID-BASE BALANCE

NORMAL VALUES IN CHILDREN (ARTERIAL BLOOD)	
pH	7.35 to 7.45
P_{CO2}	35 to 45 mm Hg
P_{O2}	>85 mm Hg (sea level, room air)
Standard Bicarbonate	22 to 28 mEq/L
Base excess	-3 to +4

CHEST ROENTGENOLOGY

Chest roentgenograms obtained during acute exacerbations of asthma show evidence of generalized hyperinflation which may include hyperlucency, depression of the diaphragm, increase in the anteroposterior diameter of the chest with anterior bowing of the sternum and kyphosis, and an increase in the size of the retrosternal radiolucency of the lateral view. The heart may appear small.

With extreme airway obstruction bulging of intercostal spaces may be evident and sites of costal insertions of the diaphragm may be seen as "scalloping" of the diaphragm.

A mild or moderate increase in the peribronchial markings is often seen in children with chronic asthma, and an increase in the size of hilar vessels relative to the size of the peripheral pulmonary vasculature has been reported.[91] Roentgenographic pulmonary infiltrates have been reported in 20-30% of children hospitalized for asthma or status asthmaticus.[84, 92] Atelectasis or pneumonia can occur as a complication of an acute asthmatic attack, and their differentiation is often difficult. Lobar and segmental consolidation appears as a dense, more or less homogeneous opacification usually occupying the normal position of a lobe or segment without significant displacement of contiguous fissures, mediastinum, or hilum. The presence of an air bronchogram rules out obstructive atelectasis, but its absence does not rule out consolidation.

Accurate localization of the involved lobe or segment is necessary to permit appropriate postural drainage. Roentgenographic localization is often facilitated by the relationship of a radiodensity to interlobar septa or fissures (Fig. 3. 21). Fissures may be incomplete anatomically, obscured by other structures, or distorted by normal or pathologic variations in the size, shape, or position of a lobe. Nevertheless their locations are dependable enough to be useful frequently in localization of disease.

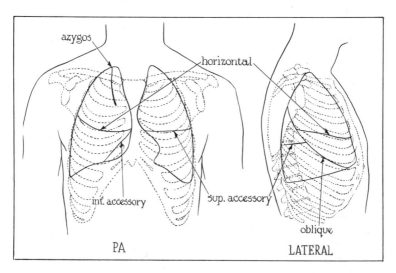

Fig. 3-21. Interlobar septa or fissures.

The oblique fissure or major fissure is not usually seen in the PA view. In the lateral view at least part of it is generally seen. It usually parallels the sixth rib from the level of the vertebral end of the fifth rib or fifth interspace posteriorly to the diaphragm up to several centimeters behind the anterior costophrenic angle.

The horizontal fissure or minor fissure is found between the right middle lobe and right upper lobe. It is seen in the lateral view in more than half of normal subjects and in the PA view in approximately half of normal adults but somewhat less frequently in children. [93] It usually meets the oblique fissure in the midaxillary line at the level of the fifth rib or interspace and extends to the level of the anterior end of the fourth rib. Rarely a left middle lobe and left horizontal fissure are present.

A superior accessory fissure, separating the superior segment of the lower lobe from the basal segments, has been recognized in approximately 5% of normal subjects, usually on the right. [93] An inferior accessory fissure, separating the medial basal segment of the lower lobe from the other basal segments, has been recognized in PA views of 5-10% of patients in the right lung and less than 1% in the left lung. [93]

The azygous fissure is a comma-shaped density in the upper lobe, almost always in the right lung. It is due to an abnormal relationship between the lung and azygous vein during development.

The roentgenographic appearance of consolidation of the various bronchopulmonary segments is indicated in Fig. 3.22 and 3.23. Atelectasis can be differentiated from consolidation by displacement of adjacent fissures, mediastinum, or hilum, elevation of the diaphragm, and narrowing of intercostal spaces. Compensatory hyperinflation of other lobes may be evident. Crowding of vascular markings may be seen in a partially collapsed lobe. Lobar atelectasis is illustrated by Fig. 3.24.

Atelectasis of the right upper lobe is evident from elevation of the horizontal fissure and right hilum with shift of the trachea toward the collapsed lobe. Anterior displacement of the superior half of the oblique fissure is evident on the lateral view. The dense, collapsed lobe itself may blend with the superior mediastinum. The apical segment of the right upper lobe also collapses against the mediastinum and may be indistinguishable from it.

The lower border of the anterior segment of the right upper lobe is the horizontal fissure, which forms a well defined boundary to consolidation of this segment. Boundaries are not so distinct with consolidation of the posterior segment except for the lower border formed by the oblique fissure in the lateral view (see Fig. 3.22).

CONSOLIDATION

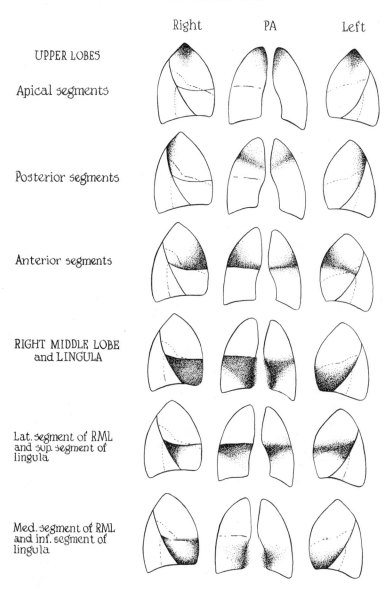

Fig. 3-22. Roentgenographic appearance of consolidation of segments of the upper lobes and right middle lobes.

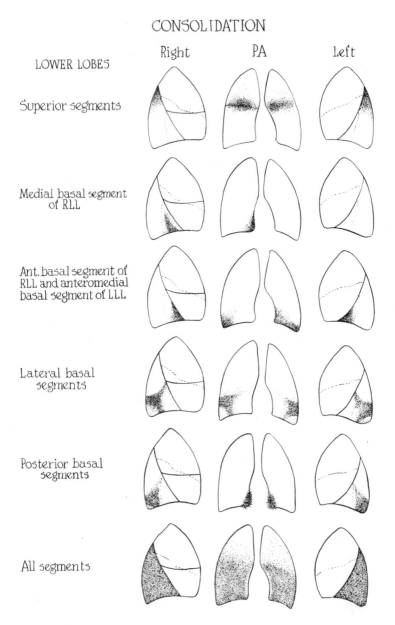

Fig. 3-23. Roentgenographic appearance of consolidation of segments of the lower lobes.

ATELECTASIS

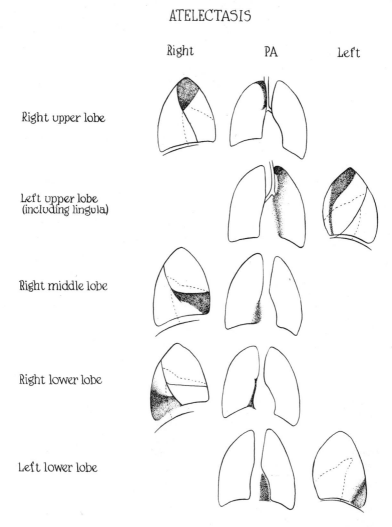

Right   PA   Left

Right upper lobe

Left upper lobe
(including lingula)

Right middle lobe

Right lower lobe

Left lower lobe

Fig. 3-24. Roentgenographic appearance of lobar atelectasis.

Since there is only rarely a horizontal fissure in the left lung, consolidation of the anterior segment of the left upper lobe presents no sharply defined lower border, and consolidation of the superior segment of the lingula is associated with no well defined upper border (see Fig. 3.22).

Collapse of the left upper lobe usually includes the lingula and presents as an anterior radiodensity in the lateral roentgenogram. The radiopaque wedge extending to the hilum may also be evident on the lateral view. Herniation of the overexpanded right lung across the midline may be evident as a radiolucency anterior to the collapsed lobe on the lateral and adjacent to the trachea on the PA view (see Fig. 3.22).

Consolidation or atelectasis of the lingula and consolidation of the medial segment of the right middle lobe or atelectasis of the right middle lobe obliterates the adjacent cardiac border on the PA view. With atelectasis the PA view may appear normal except for this obliteration of the cardiac border, or there may be slight hilar displacement. The lateral view discloses anterior displacement of the lower half of the oblique fissure with atelectasis. Collapse of the right middle lobe also causes downward displacement of the horizontal fissure (see Fig. 3.24).

Consolidation of the superior or posterior basal segments of the lower lobes or medial basal segment of the right lower lobe does not obliterate the adjacent cardiac borders (see Fig. 3.23). Consolidation of a basal segment obliterates the adjacent portion of the diaphragm on the lateral view, and this silhouette sign may indicate which lung is involved. The left hemidiaphragm is usually distinguishable from the right on the lateral view because of its relationship to the gastric air bubble and its obliteration anteriorly by contact with the heart when the heart is in its normal position.

The lower lobe collapses downward, posteriorly, and medially, obliterating adjacent portions of heart and diaphragm on the lateral view (see Fig. 3.24). Cardiac borders remain distinct on the PA view. Left lower lobe atelectasis presents as a wedge of increased density on the PA view.

Accurate identification and localization of segmental disease usually requires both PA and lateral roentgenograms.

Other complications of asthma which may be identified in chest roentgenograms include pneumomediastinum and pneumothorax. Pneumomediastinum is manifested as radiolucent streaks outlining mediastinal structures and often dissecting into the neck and over the chest wall where it may be evident as subcutaneous emphysema in the axillae in the PA chest roentgenogram. Pneumothorax presents as a uniform radiolucency of variable size lateral to or surrounding the lung which collapses medially and posteriorly with a large pneumothorax.

Chest roentgenograms are also helpful in ruling out the presence of other conditions which must be considered in the differential diagnosis of asthma, including bronchial foreign bodies and airway obstruction due to vascular anomalies or enlarged lymph nodes.

Bronchography can demonstrate bronchospasm, irregular bronchial dilatation, retained secretions and mucous plugging of small airways, and bronchial mucosal irregularities in chronic asthmatics, but these changes are usually generalized and some may be evident on the conventional chest roentgenograms. Bronchography in such children rarely supplies new information necessary to direct treatment, so it is rarely necessary.

IMMUNOGLOBULIN E

Serum IgE concentrations are frequently but not always elevated in children with asthma. Their significance and the identification of specific allergens by the radioallergosorbent test are discussed in Chapter XIII.

ALLERGY SKIN TESTING

Allergy skin testing is frequently useful for the identification of specific allergens. Techniques, interpretation, and limitations are discussed in Chapter XIII.

DIFFERENTIAL DIAGNOSIS

The clinical features of asthma are usually so typical that its diagnosis is not difficult in the older child. Diagnosis is more difficult in the infant and young child, whose small airways more easily become sufficiently obstructed to produce wheezing and in whom wheezing is often less responsive to treatment than in older children.

Many conditions can cause or simulate wheezing and merit consideration in the differential diagnosis of asthma. (Table 3.7)

FOREIGN BODY

Airway obstruction can be due to the presence of a foreign body in the hypopharynx, larynx, trachea, bronchus, or esophagus. Death can occur quickly due to asphyxia, but unrecognized bronchial foreign bodies may be present for years, causing chronic bronchitis and bronchiectasis. Unsuspected esophageal foreign bodies resulting in tracheal compression apparently have caused recurrent wheezing associated with respiratory infections without evident dysphagia for as long as one year. [95]

TABLE 3.7 DIFFERENTIAL DIAGNOSIS OF ASTHMA
IN INFANTS AND CHILDREN

I. Foreign Bodies (hypopharyngeal, esophageal, laryngeal, tracheal, bronchial).

II. Supraglottic Conditions

Retropharyngeal abscess or tumor, peritonsillar abscess, flaccid epiglottis, epiglottitis.

III. Laryngeal Conditions

Croup, angioedema of larynx, laryngeal stenosis, laryngomalacia, vocal cord paralysis, neoplasm, tetany.

IV. Tracheal Conditions

Tracheomalacia, tracheitis, external compression by vascular ring, enlarged lymph nodes, or neoplasm.

V. Bronchial Conditions

Bronchiolitis, bronchitis, bronchiectasis, bronchial stenosis, external compression by enlarged lymph nodes.

VI. Pulmonary Conditions

Pneumonia, cystic fibrosis, tuberculosis, histoplasmosis, pertussis, atelectasis, congenital lobar emphysema, pneumothorax, allergic bronchopulmonary aspergillosis, hypersensitivity pneumonitis, Loeffler's syndrome, hemosiderosis.

VII. Primary Abnormality Outside Respiratory Tract

Congestive heart failure, vascular ring, alpha-1-antitrypsin deficiency, gastroesophageal reflux, tetany, hyperventilation.

Prompt diagnosis and removal of a foreign body from the respiratory tract is important to minimize the likelihood of complicating infection with resultant tissue damage and to forestall the possibility of movement to a site where it may cause more complete obstruction or from which it may be more difficult to remove.

If aspiration has occurred during observation of the child there is usually a history of choking or coughing. Chronic coughing, wheezing, or dyspnea may date from that episode or may begin a few days later after edema or suppuration has occurred. Peanuts and some other foreign bodies of vegetable origin produce oils which are especially irritating to the tracheobronchial mucosa, causing extensive inflammation and edema. Furthermore, beans, peas, corn, or seeds can absorb water, increasing to many times their initial size.

The cough is often flat or brassy and usually nonproductive. Stridor may be present. A slap or thud may be heard as a tracheal foreign body strikes the narrow subglottic area on expiration. Wheezing is heard best at the open mouth. Localized wheezing is helpful in the diagnosis of a bronchial foreign body, but reflex bronchospasm may cause generalized wheezing, and wheezing is often readily transmitted throughout the small chest of a child. Use of a differential stethoscope is especially helpful in detecting localized airway obstruction.

Chest roentgenograms will disclose the signs of atelectasis if complete obstruction of a bronchus has occurred (see Fig. 3.24). If the foreign body has formed a check valve, permitting inspiration but preventing expiration from a lung or lobe, comparison of inspiratory and expiratory films is helpful. The obstructed lung or lobe can be identified as the one which remains hyperinflated following expiration, causing mediastinal shift toward the opposite side, while the intercostal spaces remain widened and the hemidiaphragm depressed as compared with the hemithorax containing the unaffected lung. Right and left decubitus films are also helpful. The dependent lung shows less evidence of inflation unless obstructive hyperinflation is present.

LARYNGEAL OBSTRUCTION

The inspiratory stridor due to airway obstruction at the larynx or supraglottic obstruction is usually easily differentiated from the wheezing of asthma, which is usually more severe on expiration than inspiration. Poorly supported supraglottic or glottic structures tend to collapse with inspiration, causing airway obstruction. Expiratory narrowing of intrathoracic airways on the other hand causes more extreme obstruction when the lesion is intrathoracic, resulting in wheezing which is more extreme during expiration.

Laryngotracheitis or laryngotracheobronchitis may be confused with asthma, but the harsh, barking cough typical of croup is usually heard and inspiratory stridor usually predominates although expiratory sonorous or sibilant rales may also be present.

TRACHEOMALACIA

Tracheomalacia is a congenital absence of the cartilaginous tracheal rings or an abnormal increase in their pliability resulting in collapse during expiration. It may be associated with laryngomalacia. The symptoms, cough, wheezing, stridor, and sometimes cyanosis, usually begin within the first 4-6 weeks of life and are often aggravated by an increase in tracheobronchial secretions associated with respiratory infections. Expiratory prolongation is evident. Suprasternal and intercostal retractions may be present. The diagnosis is made by demonstration of abnormal mobility of the tracheal wall by careful bronchoscopy or cinefluorography and exclusion of other causes of tracheal obstruction. Variable degrees of narrowing of the trachea with expiration occur normally in infants, and roentgenograms commonly disclose buckling of the pliable infantile trachea at the cervico-thoracic junction. Thus, demonstration of tracheal narrowing on a single lateral chest roentgenogram is insufficient to establish the diagnosis of tracheomalacia.

Symptoms of tracheomalacia usually improve by 6 months of age and subside by 12-18 months of age.

VASCULAR RING

Partial tracheal obstruction from a vascular abnormality is usually due to a right aortic arch with left ligamentum arteriosum or persistent ductus arteriosus, double aortic arch, anomalous innominate or left carotid artery, or aberrant right subclavian artery (Fig. 3.25). The last of these is least likely to cause respiratory symptoms, although it may cause dysphagia.

Typical symptoms include an inspiratory "crow", expiratory wheezing, and a brassy cough. Respiratory distress may be more extreme during feedings or with respiratory infections, and there may be dysphagia. There may be recurrent pneumonia and atelectasis. An opisthotonic position is often maintained, probably to facilitate displacement of the obstructing vessels by the rigid, anterior portion of the trachea. Forcible flexion of the neck may cause apnea. In rare patients symptoms may not be recognized until well beyond infancy.

Roentgenographic examination of the barium-filled esophagus discloses a horizontal indentation at the level of the third or

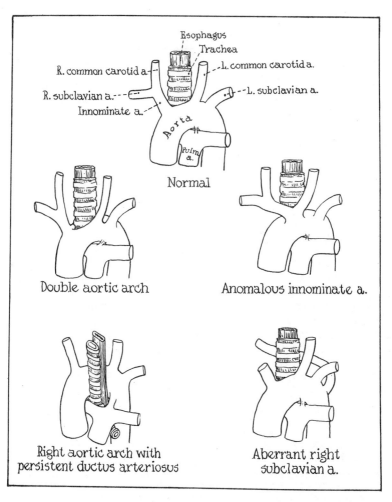

Fig. 3-25. Vascular causes of tracheal obstruction and normal relationships of trachea and esophagus to the great vessels.

fourth vertebra if there is a double aortic arch or right aortic arch with persistent ductus arteriosus. A posterior, oblique indentation of the barium-filled esophagus is seen with an aberrant right subclavian artery. Tracheal compression by an anomalous innominate artery causes a curvilinear indentation of the anterior trachea which may be evident on lateral chest roentgenograms with or without radiopaque contrast material in the trachea, but the esophagram is normal.

BRONCHIOLITIS

Acute bronchiolitis is one of the commonest conditions in infants which may be very difficult or initially impossible to differentiate from asthma. It occurs usually in infants less than six months of age and almost always less than two years of age. It is commonest in the winter or early spring, often occurring in epidemics. Respiratory syncytial virus is the commonest cause; adenoviruses and parainfluenza have sometimes been implicated. Bronchiolar obstruction is due to edema of the walls and mucous plugs and cellular debris within the bronchioles. Alveolar hyperinflation results and there may be focal atelectasis. Hypoxemia is usual and hypercapnea can occur.

Coryza may be present for several days or only a few hours before the sudden development of coughing, which may be paroxysmal, and wheezing. Irritability and inability to sleep are common, and coughing and respiratory difficulty interfere with feeding. Tachypnea and tachycardia are present, but the temperature is usually only slightly elevated or even normal. Cyanosis may be present. Intercostal and sternal retractions may be evident. Auscultation discloses fine, crepitant and sibilant rales during inspiration and expiration, diminishing if obstruction progresses and ventilation becomes very poor. Physical and roentgenographic signs of hyperinflation are present. Chest films may also disclose pulmonary infiltrates, subsegmental or segmental atelectasis, and bronchiolar thickening, or they may appear normal except for evidence of hyperinflation. There is usually no leukocytosis.

Most of these clinical features can also occur in the asthmatic infant, but the infant with bronchiolitis may appear more dyspneic and toxic. A positive immediate family history for atopic diseases and absence of concurrent illness in the rest of the family favor a diagnosis of asthma. A history of recurrent similar episodes is more consistent with asthma, but at least two episodes of bronchiolitis may occur in the same child.[96] A history of the onset of symptoms shortly after exposure to a potential allergen may be important. Symptoms or signs of allergic rhinitis (see Chapter IV) or atopic dermatitis (see Chapter V) would also suggest asthma. Eosinophilia is not associated with bronchiolitis, but it is not always present in asthmatics.

Substantial improvement within 20 minutes after administration of a bronchodilator such as Bronkephrine would strongly suggest asthma; only slight improvement or no change in airway obstruction follows administration of sympathomimetics to infants with bronchiolitis.[97] On the other hand infants with asthma may not improve dramatically following administration of a sympathomimetic, so a failure to respond is not very helpful in the differential diagnosis. Administration of many repeated or excessive doses of sympathomimetics to infants with bronchiolitis is unwise because of resultant cardiac stimulation.

Identification of respiratory syncytial virus in nasopharyngeal secretions by the immunofluorescent antibody technique would strongly suggest bronchiolitis.[98] Reports that 25-32% of infants with bronchiolitis later develop asthma and as many as 49% develop asthma or nasal allergy have only rarely been based upon data including viral isolation.[96,99] Some data suggest that exacerbations of wheezing associated with isolation of respiratory syncytial virus from infants are most likely to occur only once and do not indicate a predisposition to the development of asthma,[100] but respiratory syncytial virus has also been associated with exacerbations of asthma,[13,14] and others have reported recurrent wheezing in infants with bronchiolitis associated with isolation of respiratory syncytial virus.[101]

It is not known whether later development of asthma in children who have had bronchiolitis is a consequence of the bronchiolitis or due to misdiagnosis of the initial exacerbation of asthma.

ASTHMATIC BRONCHITIS

Asthmatic bronchitis, allergic bronchitis, or infectious asthma are terms usually used to describe episodes of wheezing which seem to occur only in association with respiratory infections, usually in children less than 5 years of age. Symptoms include rhinorrhea, nasal congestion, and fever followed by coughing and wheezing, often responsive to bronchodilators. Subsequent diagnosis of asthma has been reported in 5-50%.[102,103]

The clinical distinction between mild bronchiolitis and "asthmatic bronchitis" is arbitrary, and some of the same features are helpful in predicting which of the children bearing these diagnoses will later be found to have asthma: recurrent episodes of wheezing, onset beyond 18 months of age, family history of atopic diseases, eosinophilia. Elevated serum concentrations of IgE probably also indicate children likely to have asthma.[104]

Specific allergens often can be identified in children with asthmatic bronchitis, and it seems likely that many if not most of the children bearing this diagnosis are mild asthmatics in whom respiratory infections have provoked wheezing. Appropriate treatment is especially important in these infants and young children, whose small airways increase the risk of complications.

CYSTIC FIBROSIS

A history of chronic cough or wheezing, recurrent bronchitis or pneumonia, or atelectasis should suggest the possibility of cystic fibrosis. Although symptoms of malabsorption are usually also present (frequent, bulky, foul-smelling stools, protuberant abdomen, poor weight gain despite a large appetite), they may be absent in as many as 20% of children with cystic fibrosis. [105] There is often a history of noisy breathing, and the cough may produce thick, tenacious mucus which the infant is unable to expel from his pharynx. There is often no family history of cystic fibrosis because it is transmitted as an autosomal recessive disorder. An increase in the anteroposterior diameter of the chest and digital clubbing are common. Chest roentgenograms may disclose hyperinflation; sub-segmental, segmental, or lobar atelectasis; and peribronchial infiltrate, often in the upper lobes of infants.

The diagnosis is established by analysis of sweat collected following pilocarpine iontophoresis with quantitative determination of chloride by titration and sodium with a flame photometer. [106] Screening methods are not definitive and should not be used in an attempt to rule out the possibility of cystic fibrosis. A sweat chloride concentration greater than 60 mEq/L in a child and based upon analysis of at least 50 mg. or preferably 100 mg. sweat is diagnostic of cystic fibrosis when reported from a reliable laboratory whose technicians are familiar with the technique.

ALLERGIC BRONCHOPULMONARY ASPERGILLOSIS

Although allergic bronchopulmonary aspergillosis has been reported only rarely in children, its features so closely resemble those of asthma that it merits consideration in the differential diagnosis. Typical histories include recurrent wheezing with low grade fevers, expectoration of brown plugs in which the organisms can usually be found, eosinophilia in the peripheral blood or sputum, and transient or migratory pulmonary infiltrates. Very high serum concentrations of IgE are usually present. [107] Serum precipitins have usually but not always been reported. Allergy skin testing with aspergillus elicits the usual immediate reaction typical of Type I hypersensitivity followed by a "late" reaction evident at 3-8 hours. It is not known whether asthmatics exhibiting such "dual" skin tests and weak serum precipitin concentrations but lacking clinical features of the syndrome should be considered to have mild or early allergic aspergillosis.

HYPERSENSITIVITY PNEUMONITIS

Hypersensitivity pneumonitis or extrinsic allergic alveolitis includes a group of disorders which result from sensitization against inhaled organic dusts, including moldy hay (farmer's lung) moldy sugar cane (bagassosis), bird droppings (pigeon breeder's disease), and dust from heating and air conditioning systems contaminated with thermophilic actinomycetes such as Micropolyspora faeni or Thermoactinomycetes vulgaris. Humidifiers and vaporizers have also been implicated. 108, 109

In atopic subjects bronchospasm or rhinorrhea may occur initially following brief exposure. In both atopic and nonatopic subjects, cough, dyspnea, chills, fever, myalgia, and malaise occur 4-6 hours after exposure in association with fine crepitant rales heard by auscultation and subside after another 8-12 hours until reexposure. 110 Wheezing has sometimes been heard. Rales may persist for several days. Exacerbations are associated with leukocytosis, but little or no eosinophilia. Chest roentgenograms may disclose fine, nodular densities and peripheral infiltrates.

Prolonged rather than intermittent exposure is associated with continual, progressive symptoms of dyspnea, cough, anorexia, fatigue, and weight loss. Chest roentgenograms may be normal or show evidence of fibrosis.

Precipitating IgG antibodies specific for the offending antigen are found in the serum, but precipitins at lesser titers are also found in asymptomatic subjects exposed to the same antigen. Skin testing may elicit both immediate and late (4-6 hour) reactions when inhaled serum proteins are responsible for the reaction, but testing with thermophilic actinomycetes is unreliable because of nonspecific reactions due to irritation. Pulmonary function testing may disclose restrictive and less frequently obstructive changes.

Hypersensitivity pneumonitis has usually been ascribed to a Type III reaction, but the mechanism is not completely understood, and a Type IV reaction has also been implicated.

Hypersensitivity pneumonitis has been reported more frequently in adults but also occurs in children.

HYPOGAMMAGLOBULINEMIA

Hypogammaglobulinemia or dysgammaglobulinemia can be ruled out as possible causes of recurrent pneumonia or bronchiectasis by quantitative determination of serum immunoglobulin concentrations and comparison of the results with normal values for the child's age. 111

CARDIAC ASTHMA

Pulmonary edema in infants can result from either left ventricular failure or obstruction of pulmonary venous return due to a congenital cardiac abnormality. Tachypnea is one of the earliest signs. Both fine, crepitant rales and sibilant inspiratory and expiratory rales may be present, and there may be a history of previous, similar episodes lasting several hours and treated as asthma. A cardiac murmur may be absent or obscured by the noisy respirations. Hepatomegaly may not be present, or when present, may be erroneously ascribed to the downward displacement of the liver common in infants with depressed diaphragms due to obstructive pulmonary disease. Tachycardia occurs with hypoxemia and hypercapnea as well as congestive heart failure.

Roentgenographic evidence of cardiac enlargement suggests primary cardiac disease, but alveolar hypoventilation due to upper airway obstruction can also present with cardiomegaly.[112] Furthermore, the heart may be of normal size despite the presence of pulmonary edema due to total anomalous pulmonary venous return, cor triatriatum, or mitral atresia. In such cases chest roentgenograms disclose a diffuse, hazy, groundglass appearance over the lung fields with perihilar accentuation.

An increase in arterial oxygen tension of more than 25 mm Hg following administration of oxygen is generally thought to indicate pulmonary rather than cardiac disease, but the color of occasional infants with severe pulmonary disease may not improve with oxygen administration, and increases in P_{O2} can also follow oxygen administration to infants with large left to right shunts and associated pulmonary insufficiency.[112]

Cardiac catheterization and angiocardiography may be necessary to establish the diagnosis.

ALPHA-1-ANTITRYPSIN DEFICIENCY

Alpha-1-antitrypsin, the major component of α_1 globulin, is normally present in serum at a concentration of 180-280 mg%.[113] Severe deficiency of alpha-1-antitrypsin (10-15% normal concentrations) is usually inherited as an autosomal recessive disorder, while some heterozygotes may have 30-60% normal concentrations. Most subjects with severe deficiency and some heterozygotes have developed progressive emphysema before 40 years of age, occasionally beginning in childhood as early as 18 months of age.

Symptoms in children have included chronic cough, wheezing, increasing dyspnea, and poor growth. There may be recurrent pneumonia and atelectasis. Digital clubbing may be present.

Examination of the chest may disclose an increase in the anteroposterior diameter and hyperresonance to percussion. Chest roentgenograms disclose emphysematous changes, which may predominate in the lower lobes, and evidence of the recurrent pneumonia.

Alpha-1-antitrypsin deficiency has also been associated with neonatal hepatitis followed by cirrhosis. [113] In one family both hepatic and pulmonary disease have occurred in two of three siblings. [114]

Alpha-1-antitrypsin concentrations normally increase during bacterial infections, but temporary decreases have been measured during respiratory distress syndrome in infants with normal phenotypes, apparently due to adsorption to hyaline membranes. [115]

Several methods are available for the diagnosis of alpha-1-antitrypsin deficiency. It was first detected by serum protein electrophoresis from an absence of the α_1 globulin band. Alpha-1-antitrypsin can be measured by radial immunodiffusion using commercially available kits. These are satisfactory for identification of very low concentrations, but may be unsatisfactory for detection of heterozygotes. Genetic typing has been found to be more reliable for diagnosis, but it is not yet widely available.

GASTROESOPHAGEAL REFLUX

Gastroesophageal reflux can at least trigger acute asthmatic attacks. It has been found in children with severe asthma, especially when associated with nocturnal coughing or recurrent pneumonia or atelectasis. [116] Most infants with gastroesophageal reflux have histories of vomiting. Measurement of esophageal intraluminal pH with a probe (Tuttle test) is the most reliable method available for detection of gastric acid reflux. Esophageal manometry is useful for the evaluation of lower esophageal sphincter function. Esophagrams and technetium scans have often been normal in children with gastroesophageal reflux. Theophylline has been reported to decrease lower esophageal sphincter pressure in humans, so it should be discontinued if possible before studies of gastroesophageal reflux are undertaken, unless the effect of the drug itself is to be evaluated. [117] Reflex bronchoconstriction may occur in asthmatics with gastroesophageal reflux even without aspiration. [118] Response to limitation of evening feedings, elevation of the head of the bed, and antacids has not been encouraging.

COMPLICATIONS

PNEUMOMEDIASTINUM AND PNEUMOTHORAX

Increased intraalveolar pressure during acute asthmatic attacks may cause tissue damage which permits air to dissect along vascular sheaths to the hilum and mediastinum.[94] Further dissection may occur along fascial planes permitting air to reach the neck and subcutaneous tissues over the chest.

Extreme air hunger, tachypnea, anxiety, and restlessness are the commonest symptoms of pneumomediastinum. There may be substernal pain. A sudden disappearance of cardiac dullness to percussion may be noticed, and subcutaneous crepitus is often present. Hamman's sign, a crunching sound caused by cardiac movements, is heard only rarely by auscultation.[94] The diagnosis is usually made from the appearance of the chest roentgenogram.

Pneumomediastinum is usually a benign complication except in infants or very young children in whom the pressure is less readily relieved by dissection of air into the neck and subcutaneous tissues. Compression of the trachea and great vessels may occur, resulting in reduced venous return to the heart, decreased cardiac output, hypotension, and tachycardia. Cyanosis may be especially evident over the upper part of the body. Occasionally aspiration by needle or even cervical mediastinotomy may become necessary. Administration of increased concentrations of oxygen facilitates resorption of pneumomediastinum.

Pneumomediastinum is reported to occur more frequently as a complication of asthma in children older than 9 years of age, and only very rarely in those less than 2 years old.[92] Its occurrence is not restricted to children with severe or chronic asthma.[94] Paroxysmal coughing and use of intermittent positive pressure breathing have been implicated as causes.

Pneumothorax is a very rare complication of asthma, sometimes associated with pneumomediastinum but usually ascribed to rupture of a pleural bleb.[94] Symptoms include chest pain of sudden onset, dyspnea, tachypnea, and cyanosis. A large pneumothorax causes hyperresonance to percussion and diminished breath sounds. The heart and mediastinum may be shifted toward the opposite side of the chest. A small pneumothorax may resolve without intervention, but a tension pneumothorax may necessitate immediate decompression. Evacuation by closed thoracotomy followed by continuous drainage through a water sealed chest tube is indicated.

ATELECTASIS

Subsegmental, segmental, or lobar atelectasis can occur in an asthmatic after complete obstruction of a bronchus or bronchiole with secretions, edema, and bronchospasm. Continued perfusion of the obstructed portion of lung with absorption of the trapped gas is followed by collapse. Atelectasis is also favored by alterations in surfactant induced by hypoxia and vasoconstriction.[8,119]

Lobar atelectasis in asthmatic children most commonly involves the right middle lobe, and atelectasis of this lobe may be associated with recurrent wheezing whether the child is atopic or not. Anatomic features which predispose the right middle lobe to obstruction are well recognized: a relatively small lobe supplied with a long, narrow bronchus emerging at an acute angle from the bronchus intermedius. Lymph nodes surrounding the bronchus are potential sources of obstruction.

Atelectasis has been reported in as many as 7% of children requiring hospitalization for asthma[119] and 5.6% of asthmatic children who were not acutely ill.[120] It has even been recognized in asymptomatic asthmatic children. Atelectasis is probably most common in young asthmatic children, whose airways are still relatively small.

Cough, wheezing, and dyspnea are the commonest symptoms of atelectasis. Massive atelectasis may cause cyanosis. Localized diminished breath sounds, sibilant rales, or dullness to percussion suggest atelectasis, but complete atelectasis of a segment or the right middle lobe may be present with entirely normal physical findings because hyperinflated adjacent segments occupy space previously filled by the obstructed lobe or segment.

The diagnosis is usually made by chest roentgenograms (see Fig. 3-24) but roentgenographic evidence of atelectasis is often overlooked or mistakenly ascribed to pneumonitis. Prompt treatment with bronchodilators, antibiotics, and postural drainage is indicated to facilitate reexpansion and to forestall the development of bronchiectasis. Recurrent atelectasis of the same lobe or segment is especially common in young children.

INFECTION

Viral respiratory infections are known to provoke many asthmatic attacks,[12-16] but there is also evidence of an increased susceptibility to viral respiratory infection in asthmatic children.[20]

Bacterial pneumonia has also occurred as a complication

of asthma, probably due to multiplication of pathogenic organisms in secretions distal to obstructing bronchiolar mucous plugs. Bronchopulmonary infection has been evident at the time of postmortem examination in one half of victims reported in surveys of death from asthma in children in the United States.[121-123]

Bronchiectasis is a rare complication of asthma, usually following recurrent or persistent atelectasis with chronic infection. The commonest symptom is coughing, sometimes productive of purulent sputum. Hemoptysis may occur. Physical examination may reveal digital clubbing. There may be dullness to percussion over the involved lobe or segment, and auscultation may disclose diminished breath sounds or rales. Chest roentgenograms may disclose circular radiolucencies, but selective bronchography following a period of intensive treatment with bronchodilators and postural drainage may be necessary to establish the diagnosis. Surgery is rarely necessary, so the importance of the information to be gained from bronchography must be weighed against the risks of the procedure.

STATUS ASTHMATICUS

Status asthmaticus is persistent, severe wheezing, unresponsive to 1:1000 aqueous epinephrine, Bronkephrine, or terbutaline administered at doses usually considered adequate. A few authors include lack of response to intravenous aminophylline as a criterion for the diagnosis of status asthmaticus.

Factors implicated as causes of status asthmaticus include the presence of mucosal edema and inspissated tracheobronchial secretions which do not respond promptly to bronchodilators as bronchospasm does. Such changes have very commonly been found at the time of postmortem examination in children who have died during status asthmaticus.[121-123]

Evidence of bronchopulmonary infection has also been common in such children, and it is possible that infection may contribute to status asthmaticus through its effect upon the nature of tracheobronchial secretions or the mucociliary escalator. Viral infection may favor the development of status asthmaticus by the same mechanism through which it provokes asthmatic attacks.[12-16]

The acidosis so frequently found in status asthmaticus has been implicated as a possible cause of the poor response to epinephrine by both experimental and clinical evidence. Guinea pig tracheal smooth muscle has been found to respond to epinephrine or aminophylline with more relaxation in alkaline solutions than in acid solutions.[124] Correction of acidosis alone has sometimes relieved airway obstruction in subjects with status asthmaticus, an effect ascribed to restoration of normal responsiveness to endogenous epinephrine.

Overuse of nebulized isoproterenol or epinephrine has sometimes been associated with the development of status asthmaticus.[125] A cause and effect relationship has not been well established, but repeated administration of β-adrenergic stimulents or their use in large doses has been followed by decreased responsiveness.[126] A metabolite of isoproterenol is 3-methoxyisoproterenol, a weak β-adrenergic blocking agent, but this cannot account for the appearance of resistance to the effects of other β-adrenergic stimulants, and the mechanisms are unknown.

Obstruction due to mucosal edema or inspissated tracheobronchial secretions, infection, acidosis, and overuse of sympathomimetics probably vary in importance in the development of status asthmaticus in different children or even in the same child at different times.

All of these diverse factors must be considered in evaluating the child with status asthmaticus. In addition to the clinical features of asthma discussed earlier in this chapter, the state of hydration should be assessed from the history of oral intake, vomiting, frequency and volume of urination, and recent changes in weight as well as the usual clinical signs of dehydration: dry skin and mucous membranes, poor skin turgor, sunken eyeballs or fontanel. Respiratory difficulty interferes with oral intake and coughing or medications may provoke vomiting. Because theophylline is a diuretic as well as a bronchodilator, its use may contribute to dehydration.

Fever or purulent nasopharyngeal or tracheobronchial secretions may suggest the presence of infection, but fever can also occur during asthmatic attacks without evident infection,[84] possibly due to dehydration, and secretions may appear purulent because of an abundance of eosinophils.

Details concerning medications previously administered (sympathomimetics, theophylline, adrenal corticosteroids) are essential for safe, effective therapy.

Assessment of the adequacy of ventilation has been discussed earlier in this chapter, but a more formal approach utilizing clinical scoring systems has been found useful in grading the severity and following the progression of the airway obstruction (Table 3.8).[86,127]

Status asthmaticus is a medical emergency necessitating immediate hospitalization to facilitate further evaluation, therapy, and observation. Initial laboratory procedures should include determinations of hemoglobin or hematocrit, leukocyte count and differential, serum electrolytes, and arterial pH, P_{CO_2} and P_{O_2}. Moderate leukocytosis may be due to dehydration or recent administration of epinephrine. [84]

Lateral and PA chest roentgenograms should be obtained as soon as possible without delaying therapy. These should be promptly examined for evidence of complications such as atelectasis, pneumonia, pneumomediastinum, or pneumothorax.

Frequent additional determinations of arterial blood gases and pH may be necessary to evaluate responses to treatment and to indicate any need for modification of therapy depending upon the child's clinical response. Hypoxemia is usually present in status asthmaticus, but respiratory alkalosis is also often present initially. With progression of the airway obstruction pH and P_{CO_2} gradually return to normal, and hypercapnia and respiratory acidosis may then supervene. It has been suggested that respiratory failure is established by the presence of an arterial P_{CO_2} of 65 mm Hg or more with two or three of five clinical signs: cyanosis in 40% oxygen, decreased or absent inspiratory breath sounds, severe inspiratory retractions and use of accessory muscles of respiration, depressed level of consciousness and diminished response to pain, or poor skeletal muscle tone. [127, 128] Respiratory failure is often also associated with arterial P_{O_2} of less than 50 mm Hg and pH less than 7.25. Its diagnosis has been facilitated by the development of clinical scoring systems (see Table 3.8).

TREATMENT

The most effective form of treatment is elimination of exposure to the offending allergen (see Chapters IX and XII). When allergens which cannot be avoided are identified - allergens such as pollens and atmospheric molds - immunotherapy is often beneficial (see Chapter XIV). Appropriate use of pharmacologic agents is essential in management of the acute asthmatic attack and often is necessary for control of symptoms while awaiting response to other forms of therapy.

SYMPATHOMIMETICS

The sympathomimetic amines have chemical structures resembling that of epinephrine, but individual differences alter their activity (Fig. 3.26). Some of these differences are due to interaction with different receptors. This concept was suggested by differences in the relative potency of various sympathomimetics in producing certain actions (Table 3.9). Isoproterenol acted predominantly on β-adrenergic receptors

TABLE 3.8   CLINICAL SCORING SYSTEM FOR
             CHILDREN WITH STATUS ASTHMATICUS[127]

	0	1	2
P_{O_2} or	70-110 in air	≤ 70 in air	≤ 70 in 40% O_2
Cyanosis	None	In air	In 40% O_2
Inspiratory Breath Sounds	Normal	Unequal	Decreased or absent
Use of Accessory Muscles of Respiration	None	Moderate	Maximal
Expiratory Wheezing	None	Moderate	Extreme or none because of poor air exchange
Cerebral Function	Normal	Depressed or agitated	Coma

Total score of 5 suggests impending respiratory failure.
Score of 7 with arterial $P_{CO_2} \geq 65$ mm Hg indicates respiratory
failure.

and had almost no action on α receptors, while norepinephrine
was a potent α receptor agonist but had very little β receptor
activity.[129] Epinephrine was active on both α and β receptors,
but less active than isoproterenol in producing bronchodilation.
Further study indicated the presence of two different types of
β adrenergic receptors.[130] The β_1 adrenergic receptors
mediate cardiac contraction, while β_2 receptors mediate bronchodilation. The theory was further supported by the discovery
and development of blocking agents with specificity for α, β_1,
or β_2 adrenergic receptors.

Interaction of a β-adrenergic agonist such as isoproterenol
with adenyl cyclase catalyzes the formation of cyclic adenosine
monophosphate from adenosine triphosphate. Increases in the
intracellular concentration of cyclic AMP cause bronchodilation
and inhibition of release of chemical mediators from the mast
cell. Stimulation of α-adrenergic receptors, on the other hand,
is followed by a decrease in intracellular cyclic AMP concentration (see Chapter II).

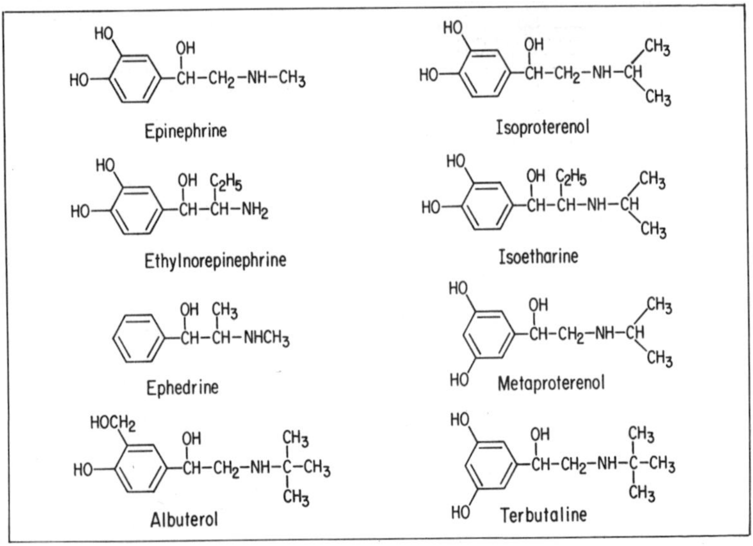

Fig. 3-26. Chemical structures of sympathomimetic bronchodilators.

EPINEPHRINE

Epinephrine, long regarded as the drug of choice for treatment of the acute asthmatic attack, is active upon both α and β-adrenergic receptors. It can be administered by subcutaneous injection or inhalation and usually produces bronchodilation within a few minutes. Vasoconstriction resulting from α adrenergic stimulation may relieve bronchial mucosal congestion.

If necessary the initial dose of 1:1000 aqueous epinephrine administered by subcutaneous injection (Table 3.10) can be repeated twice at 20 minute intervals. Relief of wheezing usually follows the initial injection and almost always follows the second. Rarely improvement occurs only after the third injection. Failure to respond to three adequate doses of 1:1000 aqueous epinephrine administered at 20 minute intervals would establish the diagnosis of status asthmaticus and the need for hospitalization and treatment with other agents.

If satisfactory relief has followed an injection of 1:000 aqueous epinephrine, 1:200 epinephrine suspension (Sus-Phrine) can be administered 30 minutes later. In this preparation 20% of the epinephrine is present in solution for an immediate effect, while the rest, initially present in crystalline form, provides more sustained relief.

TABLE 3.9   CLASSIFICATION OF ADRENERGIC
RECEPTORS

α	β_1	β_2
Vasoconstriction	Cardiac contraction	Bronchial smooth muscle relaxation
Ureteral contraction	Coronary arterial smooth muscle relaxation	Arterial smooth muscle relaxation (skeletal muscle)
Uterine contraction		Uterine relaxation
Intestinal relaxation (smooth muscle)	Intestinal relaxation (smooth muscle)	Skeletal muscle tremor
Pupillary dilatation	Lipolysis	Glycogenolysis
Gastrointestinal sphincter contraction		Glycolysis
Splenic capsule contraction		

The maximal adult dose of 1:1000 aqueous epinephrine is 0.5 ml, but more than 0.3 ml is rarely necessary in adolescents, and larger doses are associated with an increase in the frequency and severity of side effects.

The diversity of side effects is due to the activity of epinephrine on α, β_1, and β_2 adrenergic receptors. Subarachnoid hemorrhage and hemiplegia have followed subcutaneous injection of 0.5 ml of 1:1000 aqueous epinephrine in young adults. [131]

ETHYLNOREPINEPHRINE

Ethylnorepinephrine hydrochloride (Bronkephrine) is an effective bronchodilator with less α adrenergic activity than epinephrine. Consequently fewer side effects have usually been reported with use of ethylnorepinephrine, and it may be safer than epinephrine for use in infants or subjects with hypertension.

TABLE 3.10   BRONCHODILATOR DOSAGE AND SIDE EFFECTS

Epinephrine, 1:1, 000, aqueous	0. 01 ml/Kg (SC) (Max. 0. 3 ml) q 20 min. x 3 if necessary May repeat in 4 h	Tachycardia, hypertension, precordial discomfort, headache, nausea, vomiting, vertigo, muscle tremor, nervousness, excitement, pallor, drowsiness.
Epinephrine, 1:200, aqueous suspension (Sus-Phrine)	0. 005 ml/Kg (SC) (Max. 0. 3 ml) May repeat in 8 h	
Ethylnorepinephrine (Bronkephrine)	0. 01-0. 02 ml/Kg (SC) (Max. 0. 5 ml) May repeat in 20 min.	Same as those for epinephrine but less frequent and less severe.
Ephedrine	0. 5-1 mg/Kg (o) q4-6h	Insomnia, nervousness, irritability, tachycardia, palpitations, tremor, headache, vertigo, anorexia, nausea, vomiting, epigastric pain.
Isoetharine, 1%, or Isoproterenol, 1:200	0. 01 ml/Kg (Inh) (Max. 0. 5 ml) q4-8h, diluted in saline and nebulized	Tachycardia, palpitations, excitation, flushing, weakness, headache, tremor, insomnia.
Metaproterenol,	0. 5 mg/Kg (o) q6-8h (Max. 20 mg. qid) >12 y.o.: 1.3- 1. 95 mg (Inh) q4-8h	Same as those for isoproterenol but less frequent, and drowsiness.
Terbutaline*	12-15 yrs: 0. 075 mg/ Kg (o) or 2. 5 mg q6h t. i. d. Adult dose: 5 mg. q6h t. i. d. (o) 0. 01 mg/Kg (SC) (Max. 0. 25 mg) May repeat in 20 min (Max. 0. 5 mg in 4 h)	Tachycardia, nervousness, headache, nausea, tremor.

o - orally
Inh - by inhalation
SC - by subcutaneous injection
*Not approved by Food and Drug Administration for use in children

EPHEDRINE

The absence of the hydroxyl substituents on the benzene ring of ephedrine (see Fig. 3.26) decreases its bronchodilator activity as compared with that of epinephrine, but it also permits activity following oral administration because it is not subject to inactivation by catechol-0-methyltransferase. The methyl substitution on the α-carbon atom blocks oxidation by monoamine oxidase, resulting in a longer duration of action (4 hours), ephedrine's other advantage over epinephrine.

Ephedrine's usefulness is often limited by insomnia, nervousness, and irritability resulting from central nervous system stimulation, as well as other side effects (see Table 3.10).

Treatment of normal subjects with ephedrine has sometimes been found to suppress metabolic and cardiovascular responses to epinephrine.[132] Implications regarding possible effects upon response to bronchodilators in asthmatics have not been fully explored, but administration to children at usual doses for 8 weeks has been reported not to induce tolerance.[133]

ISOPROTERENOL

Isoproterenol is very active on both $\beta 1$ and $\beta 2$ adrenergic receptors. Doses effective in producing bronchodilation also cause appreciable cardiac stimulation and may cause other side effects (see Table 3.10).

Following inhalation or oral administration it is rapidly metabolized by catechol-o-methyltransferase to 3-methoxyisoproterenol, a weak beta-adrenergic blocking agent.[134] Oral administration is also followed by inactivation by intestinal and hepatic sulfatase. Consequently it usually is administered by inhalation, although it can also be given by intravenous injection and may be effective following sublingual absorption.

The prompt but relatively brief bronchodilation which follows inhalation of isoproterenol may tend to encourage its overuse, especially when administered from a convenient, self-propelled nebulizer.

Airway obstruction has been found to be aggravated in some asthmatics by inhalation of isoproterenol.[135,136] In these a temporary improvement in pulmonary function has been followed by increasing airway obstruction within one hour. Symptomatic improvement has followed discontinuation of aerosol treatment in such patients.

Inhalation of therapeutic doses of isoproterenol has frequently been followed by a decrease in arterial P_{O2} despite a lessening of airway obstruction.[137,138] This has been associated with an increase in the alveolar-arterial oxygen tension gradient, and the phenomenon is probably due to a reversal of compensatory pulmonary vasoconstriction aggravating further the ventilation perfusion imbalance so often present during acute asthmatic attacks. Decreases in arterial P_{O2} have also followed subcutaneous injection of epinephrine, and intravenous administration of aminophylline, as well as inhalation of albuterol aerosol. Some authors have reported a lack of decrease in arterial P_{O2} following albuterol inhalation, however.[138] Inhalation of an aerosol containing both isoproterenol and phenylephrine is not followed by decreases in arterial P_{O2}, probably because of the vasoconstrictor activity of phenylephrine. Significant decreases in arterial P_{O2} do not usually follow bronchodilator administration, and most decreases in P_{O2} do not exceed 5-10 mm Hg., but rare patients have been reported in whom inhalation of isoproterenol has been followed by a decrease in arterial P_{O_2} of as much as 25 mm Hg.[137] This response can be prevented or minimized by administration of supplemental oxygen.

There is evidence that isoproterenol and other sympathomimetics with beta-adrenergic activity can induce tachyphylaxis and tolerance or subsensitivity to some extent in some patients. Incubation with isoproterenol has been reported to have induced definite tachyphylaxis in bronchial strips from 7 of 12 patients.[139] Responsiveness to the drug was found to have been suppressed. in these. Possible mechanisms include reduced affinity of receptors for the drug or a reduction in the number of receptors. An 85% decrease in the number of beta-adrenergic receptors on polymorphonuclear leukocytes has been demonstrated after administration of terbutaline, 2.5 mg q.i.d. for as few as 6 days, with restoration of the number of receptors present before treatment, within 7 days after discontinuation of treatment, but not within 1 day.[140] The clinical significance remains uncertain because despite similar findings in asthmatics treated for months with oral terbutaline, discontinuation of the drug was followed by an increase in the need for other drugs for control of symptoms. Tolerance to oral terbutaline or albuterol has been reported, but the clinical significance of the small differences in pulmonary response has been questioned, and others have found no tolerance after months of treatment with oral terbutaline or metaproterenol.[141-144]

Overuse of isoproterenol has been implicated as a possible factor contributing to deaths from asthma.[125, 145] It is unknown whether this is related to production of the metabolite with weak beta-adrenergic blocking properties, the unexplained aggravation of airway obstruction which occurs in rare patients, hypoxemia which occasionally follows isoproterenol inhalation, induction of tolerance to the drug, or deferral of other forms of treatment until they are unable to overcome severe airway obstruction. It is possible that the deaths have not been due to use of isoproterenol, but that the severe airway obstruction responsible for the death has also led to overuse of the bronchodilator in a futile attempt to reverse it.

Use of epinephrine in conjunction with isoproterenol shortly before death during an asthmatic attack has occasionally been reported. [146] Administration of excessive doses of isoproterenol can apparently elicit tachycardia and extrasystoles, ventricular fibrillation, or bradycardia followed by asystole. [147] It is not well established that the risk of arrhythmias is substantially increased by concomitant use of epinephrine and isoproterenol, but it may be prudent to avoid administration of these drugs within 2 hours of each other.

The usual dose of 1:200 isoproterenol recommended for delivery by nebulization is 0.01 ml/Kg, but there is evidence that comparable bronchodilation can be elicited with less tachycardia with a dose of 0.005 ml/Kg. [81] Peak bronchodilation occurs at 5-15 minutes, and duration of action is 60-90 minutes.

ISOETHARINE

The first clinically important sympathomimetic selective for β-2 adrenergic receptors was isoetharine. [130] It differs from isoproterenol by the presence of an α-alkyl ethyl substituent (see Fig. 3.26). It has a short duration of action (1 1/2 - 2 hours) and can cause the same side effects which can follow use of isoproterenol, including only slightly less tachycardia than follows isoproterenol when administered by inhalation. [81] It offers no other substantial advantage over isoproterenol.

METAPROTERENOL

Metaproterenol is an effective bronchodilator which differs from isoproterenol only in the position of one of the phenolic hydroxyl groups (see Fig. 3.26), but this change prevents inactivation by catechol-O-methyl transferase, permitting a much longer duration of action (at least 4 hours after inhalation). It is also less susceptible than isoproterenol to inactivation by sulfatases and therefore active following oral administration. There is evidence that treatment with oral metaproterenol and theophylline affords more bronchodilation than treatment with theophylline alone, at least at modest serum theophylline concentrations. [148] Side effects are less frequent following inhalation of metaproterenol than isoproterenol. The commonest side effect, tachycardia, has been reported in approximately 7% of patients treated with oral metaproterenol.

TERBUTALINE

Terbutaline differs from metaproterenol by the addition of a methyl group to the N-alkyl substituent (see Fig. 3.26), a change which confers upon terbutaline greater selectivity for $\beta 2$ adrenergic receptors[149] and an even longer duration of action reported following inhalation, [150] subcutaneous injection, [149] or oral administration. [151] The longer duration of action has been ascribed to decreased susceptibility to the action of monoamine oxidase.

Inhalation of terbutaline at doses which usually cause no tachycardia or other side effects is followed within 5 minutes by bronchodilation which may be maintained for 5 hours. [150] A dose of 4-5 mg by nebulization or 0.5-0.75 mg by metered-dose aerosol has been recommended for adults. [152] Administration by intermittent positive pressure breathing has been found to offer no advantage over simple nebulization.

Prompt bronchodilation, lasting as long as 4-5 hours, has also been reported following administration of terbutaline by subcutaneous injection. Terbutaline has not always been found to have a longer duration of action than aqueous epinephrine by this route, but more bronchodilation may follow terbutaline than epinephrine at recommended doses. [153]

Oral terbutaline has elicited significant bronchodilation within 15-30 minutes, persisting for at least 7 hours. [154] Use of both terbutaline and theophylline in usual doses has been reported to elicit more bronchodilation than either alone. [155]

Side effects have included slight increases in heart rate and systolic blood pressure, headache, nervousness, nausea, dizziness, and tremor. These have been more common after oral or subcutaneous administration of the drug, but small increases in heart rate, headache, tremor, and nervousness have been reported in occasional patients after inhalation of terbutaline. [152]

ALBUTEROL (SALBUTAMOL)

The N-tertiary butyl substituent in the side chain of albuterol results in selectivity for $\beta 2$ adrenergic receptors as in terbulatine (see Fig. 3.26). Substitution of $CH_2 OH$ at the 3 position of the phenolic ring prevents inactivation by catechol-O-methyl transferase, resulting in a long duration of action of at least 5 hours. Albuterol also elicits bronchodilation within 30 minutes following oral administration and persisting for 6-8 hours, but muscle tremors occur more frequently following oral administration than inhalation. [156]

Decreases in arterial PO_2 have occasionally followed inhalation of albuterol[157] and terbulatine, [158] but may occur less frequently than following inhalation of isoproterenol. [138, 159]

METHYLXANTHINES

Methylxanthines such as theophylline (1-3 dimethylxanthine) and aminophylline (theophylline ethylenediamine) are effective bronchodilators which act through inhibition of the phosphodiesterase responsible for conversion of cyclic adenosine monophosphate to adenosine monophosphate (see Fig. 2.2). Because the action of theophylline is not mediated by β adrenergic receptors, an additive effect can be expected when it is used in conjunction with sympathomimetics, and aminophylline often relieves bronchospasm in subjects who have failed to respond to adrenergic drugs.

Theophylline can be administered orally, intravenously, or rectally. Because of its poor solubility in water, alleged erratic absorption from the gastrointestinal tract, and associated side effects, including nausea and vomiting, theophylline has been marketed in a number of different preparations (Table 3.11). Ethylenediamine increases the solubility of theophylline in water, and oxtriphylline is said to be more soluble, more stable, better absorbed from the gastrointestinal tract and less irritating to the gastric mucosa than aminophylline.[160] Dihydroxypropyltheophylline, which is not converted to theophylline in the body, is said to cause less gastric irritation than most theophylline compounds. There is evidence that bioavailability of the various preparations other than dihydroxypropyltheophylline is actually determined only by the anhydrous theophylline content or equivalence (see Table 3.11).[161]

Measurement of blood or plasma theophylline concentrations following administration of various oral preparations has indicated more rapid absorption of liquid preparations than tablets.[162] Therapeutic blood levels have often been reached within 10-15 minutes after oral administration of liquid preparations, and absorption from aqueous solutions seems as rapid and as complete as absorption from hydroalcoholic solutions.[163] Nausea and abdominal pain due to gastric irritations may be less frequent with hydroalcoholic solutions of theophylline.[163] Absorption of tablets of micronized theophylline is usually as rapid as absorption of liquid preparations.[164]

Rectal administration of theophylline in suppositories has been followed by slow, erratic absorption, but somewhat faster absorption has followed use of rectal solutions.[165]

One consequence of the availability of three routes for administration of theophylline has been numerous toxic reactions, some ending in death. Theophylline dosages followed by death have usually been very excessive. The drug has often been administered rectally and sometimes simultaneously by two or three different routes. In one review the drug was reported to

TABLE 3.11   XANTHINE CONTENT OF ORAL BRONCHODILATORS

Preparation	Generic Name	Content (mg)	Anhydrous Theophylline Equivalent (mg)
Aerolate III capsule *	Theophylline (anhydrous)	65	65
Aerolate Jr. capsule *	Theophylline (anhydrous)	130	130
Aerolate Sr. capsule *	Theophylline (anhydrous)	260	260
Aerolate Liquid	Theophylline (anhydrous)	160/15cc	160
Aminodur Dura-Tabs*	Aminophylline	300	236
Aminophylline Tablets	Aminophylline	100, 200	85, 170
Asbron Elixir or Tablet	Theophylline sodium glycinate	300/15cc or tab	150
	Guaifenesin	100	
Brondecon Elixir	Oxtriphylline	100/5cc	64
	Guaifenesin	50/5cc	
Brondecon Tablet	Oxtriphylline	200	128
	Guaifenesin	100	
Bronkodyl capsule†	Theophylline (anhydrous)	100, 200	100, 200
Bronkodyl Elixir	Theophylline (anhydrous)	80/15cc	80

Table 3.11 (cont'd.)

Bronkolixir	Theophylline (anhydrous)	15/5cc	15
	Ephedrine	12	
	Guaifenesin	50	
	Phenobarbital	4	
Bronkotabs	Theophylline (anhydrous)	100	100
	Ephedrine	24	
	Guaifenesin	100	
	Phenobarbital	8	
Choledyl Elixir	Oxtriphylline	100/5cc	64
Choledyl Tablet	Oxtriphylline	100, 200	64, 128
Elixicon Suspension	Theophylline (anhydrous)	100/5cc	100
Elixophyllin Caps or Elixir	Theophylline (anhydrous)	100, 200 80/15cc	100, 200 80
Elixophyllin SR Caps*	Theophylline (anhydrous)	125, 250	125, 250
Lufyllin Tablet	Dihydroxypropyl-theophylline	200, 400	
Lufyllin GG Tab or Elixir	Dihydroxypropyl-theophylline Guaifenesin	200/tab or 30cc 200	
Marax Syrup	Theophylline (anhydrous)	32.5/5cc	32.5
	Ephedrine	6.25	
	Hydroxyzine	2.5	
Marax Tablet	Theophylline (anhydrous)	130	130
	Ephedrine	25	
	Hydroxyzine	10	
Mudrane Tablets	Aminophylline	130	110.5
	Potassium iodide	195	
	Phenobarbital	8	

Table 3.11 (cont'd.)

Quadrinal Suspension	Theophylline calcium salicylate	65/5cc	32.5
	Ephedrine	12	
	Phenobarbital	12	
	Potassium iodide	160	
Quadrinal Tablet	Theophylline calcium salicylate	130	65
	Ephedrine	24	
	Phenobarbital	24	
	Potassium iodide	320	
Quibron Capsule or Liquid	Theophylline (anhydrous)	150/cap or 15cc	150
	Guaifenesin	90	
Quibron-300 Capsule	Theophylline (anhydrous)	300	300
	Guaifenesin	180	
Slo-Phyllin Gyrocaps*	Theophylline (anhydrous)	60, 125, 250	60, 125, 250
Slo-Phyllin Tabs or Syrup	Theophylline (anhydrous)	100, 200/tab	100, 200,
		80/15cc	80
Slo-Phyllin GG Caps or Syrup	Theophylline (anhydrous)	150/cap or 15cc	150
	Guaifenesin	90	
Sustaire Tablets*	Theophylline (anhydrous)	100, 300	100, 300
Tedral Elixir	Theophylline (anhydrous)	32.5/5cc	32.5
	Ephedrine	6	
	Phenobarbital	2	
Tedral Suspension	Theophylline (monohydrate)	65/5cc	58.5
	Ephedrine	12	
	Phenobarbital	4	

Table 3.11 (cont'd.)

Tedral Tablet	Theophylline (anhydrous)	130	130
	Ephedrine	24	
	Phenobarbital	8	
Tedral SA Tablet*	Theophylline (anhydrous)	180	180
	Ephedrine	48	
	Phenobarbital	25	
Theo-Dur Tablets*	Theophylline (anhydrous)	100, 200, 300	100, 300, 300
Theolair Tablets †	Theophylline (anhydrous)	125, 250	125, 250
Theolair SR Tablets*	Theophylline (anhydrous)	250, 500	250, 500
Theophyl Chewable	Theophylline (anhydrous)	100	100
Theophyl-225 Tab or Elixir	Theophylline (anhydrous)	225/tab or 30cc	225
Theophyl SR Capsules*	Theophylline (anhydrous)	125, 250	125, 250
Verequad Suspension	Theophylline calcium salicylate	65/5cc	32.5
	Ephedrine	12	
	Guaifenesin	50	
	Phenobarbital	4	
Verequad Tablet	Theophylline calcium salicylate	130	65
	Ephedrine	24	
	Guaifenesin	100	
	Phenobarbital	8	

* Sustained release preparations

† Micro-pulverized or micronized preparations absorbed as rapidly as liquid preparations

have been administered rectally to 91 of 104 children with theophylline toxicity, including 84 who had received it by this route alone.[166] The earliest symptoms of theophylline toxicity are usually restlessness, nausea, and vomiting. Other symptoms include irritability, headache, epigastric pain, hematemesis, twitching, convulsions, pallor, fever, and coma. It is possible for convulsions to occur without milder antecedent symptoms, however. The diuretic action of theophylline and vomiting may cause dehydration. Albuminuria may be present. Occasionally cardiac arrest has followed injection of aminophylline through central venous catheters.

Both toxic symptoms and therapeutic response have been found to be closely related to plasma concentrations of theophylline. The therapeutic range has been found to be 5-20 μ g/ml plasma or serum, with most patients requiring concentrations of at least 10 μ g/ml for most effective bronchodilation. Toxic symptoms may occur with serum levels of 13 μ g/ml, but increase sharply in frequency at concentrations exceeding 20 μ g/ml.

Pharmacokinetic studies have disclosed important differences in the rates of metabolism of theophylline in different patients,[167] with plasma half-life following intravenous injection varying from 70-600 minutes in asthmatic children. Thus, it is possible for a dose of theophylline which may be ineffective in one patient to cause toxicity in another.

Ninety percent of the drug is usually eliminated from the body by biotransformation by hepatic microsomal enzymes, so plasma half-life is prolonged in the presence of heart failure, possibly due to decreased perfusion of the liver, or hepatic dysfunction, such as cirrhosis.[168,169] Approximately 65% of plasma theophylline is usually bound to protein, but a decrease in binding to a s little as 32% has been found in some patients with cirrhosis.[169] This doubling of the free fraction of theophylline might alter the quantitative response to a given serum concentration of theophylline. A direct relationship between serum protein binding and pH has also been reported with 30% theophylline bound at pH 7.0 and 65% bound at 7.8.[170]

A mean increase of 68% in plasma theophylline half-life has been reported in 6 asthmatic children during the acute stages of upper respiratory tract illnesses due to influenza or adenovirus, as compared with plasma half-life one month later.[171] No changes were found during febrile illnesses in children without serological evidence of virus infections.

Increases of 50% in plasma theophylline half-life have been reported to follow administration of the macrolide antibiotic, troleandomycin, probably due to an effect upon liver function, and a similar effect of erythromycin salts has been reported in a few patients.[172,173]

Cigarette smoking, on the other hand, causes a decrease in the plasma half-life of theophylline, and ingestion of charcoal-broiled beef has a similar effect, probably due to stimulation of hepatic microsomal enzymes by polycyclic hydrocarbons. [174, 175]

Other facets of the diet can also affect theophylline metabolism. Diets high in protein have been associated with a decrease in plasma theophylline half-life, while diets high in carbohydrate and low in protein can cause prolongation of the half-life. [176]

Daily administration of phenobarbital for 4 weeks has been found to increase clearance of theophylline from the serum, an effect also ascribed to induction of hepatic microsomal enzymes, but administration of phenobarbital for only 2 weeks has not elicited significant changes in clearance. [177, 178]

Optimal therapy with safe, efficacious doses of theophylline is assured only if the rate of elimination from the plasma is estimated by determination of plasma concentrations. A spectrophotometric method has been used most commonly, but gas chromatographic methods permit use of a smaller sample size (1 ml serum) and caffeine, theobromine and barbiturates, which cause overestimation of theophylline concentrations determined by the spectrophotometric method, do not interfere with the gas chromatographic determination. Methods utilizing high pressure cation exchange chromatography are specific for theophylline, permit a further reduction in sample size to 0.1 ml serum, and are more rapid (30 minutes). The enzyme multiplied immunoassay technique (EMIT) is also rapid and specific, and requires only small volumes of serum. [179] Results from whatever method is used must be correlated with clinical findings, and occasional validation of results at another laboratory is desirable.

Aminophylline can be safely administered intravenously to most children at a dose of 5 mg/Kg body weight if the recommended dosage interval has elapsed since the last dose of theophylline, and if previous dosage has not been excessive. An interval greater than the usual dosage interval may be necessary in patients receiving continual treatment with sustained release preparations, but determination of the serum theophylline concentration before administration of the intravenous aminophylline assures use of appropriate doses. The dose should be diluted and administered by slow injection or infusion over 10-20 minutes. For optimal therapy a constant infusion can be administered at a rate determined for each patient to maintain his plasma concentration at $10-20 \mu g/ml$. If administration by constant infusion is impossible, the initial dose can be repeated safely at 8 hour intervals for most children. Larger doses of intravenous aminophylline have sometimes been recommended, but it is prudent to avoid use of larger doses unless plasma theophylline concentrations are monitored. The optimal infusion rate can be inferred often from serum theophylline concentrations obtained previously during status asthmaticus or during treatment with oral theophylline. Allowance must be made for the fact that aminophylline dihydrate is only 78.9% anhydrous theophylline, however. Rates of clearance of theophylline are usually reported to remain stable in children for at least as long as 6-8 months.[180]

Theophylline dosage requirements to maintain serum concentrations of 10-20 μ g/ml at steady state vary with age. Average doses recommended for children more than 3 months old are:

<9 years old	24 mg/Kg/24 hours
9-12 years old	20 mg/Kg/24 hours
12-16 years old	16-18 mg/Kg/24 hours
>16 years old	12-13 mg/Kg/24 hours

Maintenance dosage calculations for obese patients should be based upon ideal body weight.[181] Modification of the dosage is also necessary in the presence of cardiac failure, hepatic dysfunction, or other factors known to alter theophylline metabolism. A need for modification is also evident when clinical response seems inadequate or when signs or symptoms of possible toxicity occur. The necessary change in dosage is indicated by peak serum theophylline concentrations found $1\frac{1}{2}$-$2\frac{1}{2}$ hours after administration of the usual oral theophylline preparation, 4-8 hours after administration of most sustained release preparations, or 6-10 hours after TheoDur, and "trough" concentrations obtained immediately before the next scheduled dose. Peak concentrations may occur as early as $\frac{1}{2}$-$1\frac{1}{2}$ hours after a liquid preparation or a capsule or tablet containing micronized theophylline (Bronkodyl, Theolair). Peak serum theophylline concentrations are useful in determining a need for increase in dosage only if obtained at steady state, after 5 half-lives (usually within 20-36 hours after regular administration has begun). Recommended alterations in dosage are indicated in Table 3.12. Determination of serum theophylline concentration, again after steady state has been reached following the change in dosage or earlier if signs or symptoms of toxicity are present, is recommended.

The usual theophylline preparations must be administered to most children at 6 hour-intervals if they are to maintain adequate serum concentrations. Use of sustained release preparations at 8 hour (Slo-Phyllin Gyrocaps, Theolair SR, Theophyl SR) or 12 hour (Theo-Dur tablets) intervals is preferable

TABLE 3.12   THEOPHYLLINE DOSING ADJUSTMENTS
INDICATED BY PEAK SERUM THEOPHYLLINE
CONCENTRATIONS
(modified from Hendeles, et al.[182])

Peak Theophylline Concentration (μ gm/ml)	Dosing Adjustment In Total Daily Dose
<5	100% increase in 2-4 equal increments at 2 day intervals
5-7.5	50% increase in 2 equal increments at 2 day intervals
8-10	20% increase
11-13	10% increase if necessary for control of symptoms
14-20	10% decrease if side effects present
21-25	10% decrease
26-30	25% decrease after omitting next dose
31-35	33% decrease after omitting next dose
>35	50% decrease after omitting next 2 doses

because of smaller fluctuations in serum theophylline concentrations and improved compliance due to the longer dosing intervals.[183] Children too young to swallow capsules or tablets often will accept the granules from sustained release capsules as a sprinkle on strained or chopped food; this does not alter absorption characteristics of these preparations. The granules should not be dissolved before administration, however, and no attempt should be made to administer any fraction of the contents of a capsule, because many of the granules may contain no drug. One can compensate for the initial delay in increase in serum concentrations by administration of a rapidly absorbed preparation, such as Theolair tablets at a dose of 2-4 mg/Kg, with the first dose of the sustained release preparation.[184]

Numerous oral preparations containing both theophylline and ephedrine are available, and there is evidence of a partially additive effect of the combination. [133,185,186] The drawback of such convenient preparations is the fixed ratio of the two drugs. Often this ratio is not optimal for the patient. For one drug to be given at an effective dose, a toxic dose of the other might be necessary. The ratio of the ingredients in such preparations should be compared and allowance must be made for each patient's tolerance for the ingredients. Often it may be desirable to start treatment with oral theophylline alone until its optimal dose is determined. Later terbutaline, metaproterenol, or ephedrine can be added if necessary, with continued observation for possible side effects.

Oral administration of theophylline or theophylline and ephedrine is very helpful in the management of mild asthmatic attacks. Continued treatment for 5-7 days after symptoms have subsided may help prevent what might otherwise have been an earlier recurrence, because pulmonary function may remain abnormal for several days after symptoms have subsided. Children with symptoms as often as every 2-3 days often respond to continual treatment with oral bronchodilators.

Theophylline can be administered rectally at a dose of 7 mg/Kg every 12 hours, but there is considerable uncertainty concerning the optimal dose and interval between doses by this route. Peak concentrations are found at 1-2 hours. Because toxicity has so often followed rectal administration, parents must be carefully instructed to avoid simultaneous administration of oral theophylline, and it may be safest to use the rectal route only when monitoring of serum theophylline levels is possible.

Careful observation for signs and symptoms of toxicity is necessary whenever theophylline is used, whatever the route of administration.

EXPECTORANTS

The tiniest, inhaled, airborne particles are exhaled without having been deposited. Larger particles are removed from the inhaled air and then cleared from the airways. The site of removal is largely dependent upon the size of the particle (Fig. 3.27). At least 95% of particles larger than 15 μ in diameter and some as small as 4.5 μ are removed at the nose by filtration and impaction upon the mucous blanket covering the ciliated epithelium. Most other particles more than 2-3 μ in diameter are removed by impaction on the mucous blanket of the pharynx, larynx, trachea, bronchi, and bronchioles. Particles between

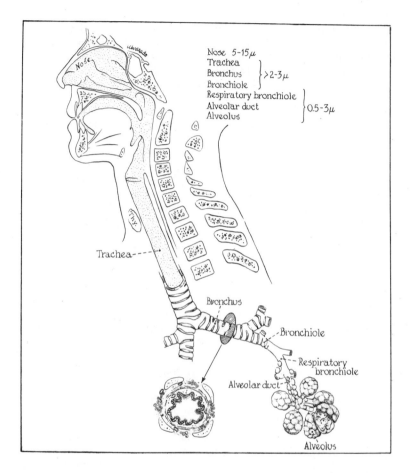

Fig. 3-27. The effect of size upon site of deposition of inhaled particles in the normal respiratory tract.

0.5 and 3 μ in diameter are collected in the respiratory bronchioles, alveolar ducts, and alveoli by gravitational settling and brownian movement. Particles less than 0.5 μ in diameter may be exhaled.[187] Particles deposited on the alveolar fluid are carried toward the respiratory bronchioles or engulfed by macrophages. Particles carried to the larger airways or deposited in them are cleared by the mucociliary escalator.

The mucus, consisting of 95% water and 2% glycoproteins as well as other proteins, lipids, and inorganic materials, is produced mostly by submucosal glands, goblet cells, and Clara

cells with the addition of some alveolar fluid.[187] The glycoproteins, averaging 1,000,000 in molecular weight, consist of
coiled polypeptide chains which determine the sputum viscosity.
The mucous blanket is approximately 5μ thick. Its thin,
outer, gel-like layer entraps particles and rests upon the tips
of the cilia. The lower, aqueous layer of mucus bathes the
cilia, permitting them to move freely. The coordinated, continuous beat of the cilia propels the mucus of the lower respiratory tract toward the glottis.[187]

An expectorant is an agent which promotes the clearance
of mucus or exudate from the tracheobronchial tree by lique-
faction or stimulation of the secretion of mucus. It is unlikely
that a great alteration in the normal characteristics of this
mucus would be desirable because this might interfere with these
clearance mechanisms. Pathologic alterations in the characteristics of tracheobronchial secretions are undesirable, however, and agents which would minimize or prevent such changes
would be helpful.

WATER

Children often limit their fluid intake during acute asthmatic attacks because of dyspnea. There may be loss of fluid
through vomiting caused by medications or paroxysms of coughing. Diuresis induced by theophylline may cause further fluid
loss. Air reaching the terminal airways is normally fully saturated with water through humidification by the upper respira-
piratory tract, trachea, and bronchi. Dehydration as well as
nasal obstruction due to allergic rhinitis, may interfere with
humidification of inspired air, causing inspissation of tracheobronchial secretions which then cause further airway obstruction.
Evidence of this has usually been found at the time of postmortem
examination of children who have died during status asthmaticus.[121-123] Sputum viscosity is increased by a humidity of
50% or less, and low humidity inhibits ciliary movement.

An increase in the oral intake of fluids has been reported
to reduce the viscosity of sputum.[188] Early in an asthmatic
attack it may be possible to maintain hydration by encouraging
oral intake of fluids, but this may aggravate vomiting, and over-
ly enthusiastic efforts to maintain hydration by this route may
cause gastric dilatation and further impairment of ventilation.
Intravenous administration of hypotonic fluids containing glucose and electrolytes is safer if the usual precautions regarding the volume and constitution of such fluids are observed.
The need for some caution in the administration of intravenous
fluids to prevent water intoxication is emphasized by evidence
of an increased rate of secretion of antidiuretic hormone during
status asthmaticus.[189]

Inhalation is apparently not an effective route of administration for water. Only very small volumes of aerosol are deposited in the lower respiratory tract. Mist tent therapy can have a deleterious effect upon pulmonary function even in children with cystic fibrosis, and inhalation of nebulized saline can provoke bronchospasm in asthmatic children.

GLYCERYL GUAIACOLATE

There is little objective evidence of efficacy of the few pharmacologic agents marketed as expectorants, possibly partly due to the lack of homogeneity of sputum, difficulty in obtaining specimens suitable for analysis, and lack of agreement upon techniques suitable for measuring changes in sputum consistency.

Study of glyceryl guaiacolate has disclosed inconsistent effects on respiratory tract secretions. Evidence of enhancement of mucous secretion has been equivocal. There is some evidence that glyceryl guaiacolate may prevent decreased surface tension of tracheobronchial secretions, an effect which may be important in enhancing expectoration.[190]

Very little evidence of toxicity has been reported. A slight inhibitory effect upon platelet aggregation has not been found to have clinical significance. The toxic dose must greatly exceed the dose of 100 mg three times daily usually recommended for children.

IODIDES

Although iodides are generally regarded as more effective expectorants than glyceryl guaiacolate there is also a dearth of objective evidence of their efficacy. One study comparing oral doses of 100 mg. three times daily with 300 mg three times daily in 8-16 year old asthmatic children disclosed improvement at the higher dose (mean dose 24 mg/Kg/day) in some children.[191] Dramatic improvement reported in a very few asthmatics has been ascribed to some unknown mechanism other than expectorant activity.[192]

Sodium iodide can be added to intravenous fluids but there is no evidence of its efficacy.

The chief limitation to use of potassium iodide has been numerous associated side effects, including acneiform skin eruptions (occurring mostly in adolescents), urticaria, erythema nodosum, and other cutaneous eruptions which sometimes respond to reductions in dosage. Painful swelling of the parotid and submandibular salivary glands, which may be associated with swelling of the upper half of the face (possibly due to lacrimal gland involvement), has also sometimes responded to reductions in dosage.[193] Gastrointestinal side effects have included anorexia, nausea, vomiting, epigastric pain, and diarrhea. Rhinorrhea is common and headache has occurred.

Thyroid enlargement is one of the commonest side effects of iodide therapy, and hypothyroidism has been reported with and without evident increases in the size of the gland.[194] Small but significant decreases in serum concentrations of thyroxine and triiodothyronine and increases in thyrotropin have followed administration to normal men of as little as 1 drop of saturated solution of potassium iodide twice daily for 11 days.[195] Thyrotropin concentrations sometimes increased after only 4 days of treatment. Although it has been claimed that iodinated glycerol causes fewer side effects than potassium iodide, hypothyroidism and goiters have also been associated with its use.[196]

Because of the great frequency of associated side effects and the lack of objective evidence of substantial benefit to most patients it is most prudent to avoid use of iodides in asthmatic children. If used at all it may be wise to prescribe intermittent treatment, discontinuing use of the drug for 3 days each week or 1 week each month.

N-ACETYLCYSTEINE

N-acetylcysteine has been shown to be highly effective in decreasing the consistency of sputum in vitro, an effect ascribed to the action of its free sulfhydryl group in opening disulfide bonds present in mucus and disruption of polymerization bonds of desoxyribonucleic acid.[197, 198] Its effectiveness is related to concentration: the 20% solution is more effective than 10% or 5%.[197] Selective delivery of a small volume to a bronchus or bronchiole obstructed with mucus followed immediately by suction or postural drainage of the involved bronchopulmonary segment to remove the liquefied secretions could be expected to be beneficial. The efficacy of N-acetylcysteine aerosol delivered by inhalation has not been established, however. The site of deposition of the aerosol is determined largely by particle size.[199] The drug should be inhaled through the mouth to prevent deposition in the nose, but even with this precaution it may be difficult to deliver sufficient drug to the peripheral airways where it is most likely to be needed. Treatments should be followed immediately with postural drainage to remove secretions.

Its use in asthmatics is considered contraindicated by some because of the bronchospasm which it often provokes in such subjects. In asthmatics administration of a nebulized mixture of 0. 25 ml of 1:200 isoproterenol and 3 ml of 10% N-acetylcy-stein may be better tolerated than N-acetylcysteine alone. Stomatitis also occurs as a side effect.

ADRENAL CORTICOSTEROIDS

Adrenal corticosteroids are very effective for the treatment of asthma, but their use is limited by numerous undesirable side effects.

The mechanism through which glucocorticoids benefit asthmatics is not fully known. The steroid apparently pene-trates the cell membrane and binds to receptor proteins. The steroid-receptor complex binds to the cell nucleus and can in-fluence ribonucleic acid and protein synthesis.[200] Proteins which are than synthesized mediate the biologic effects of the steroid. The 6-12 hours required before clinical effects of ad-ministered corticosteroids become evident is probably related to the time necessary for these intracellular events to occur. There is evidence suggesting that hydrocortisone may cause a delay in the resynthesis of histamine following its secretion by mast cells.[201]

There is also evidence that corticosteroids may potentiate the activity of catecholamines upon adenyl cyclase; restoration of responsiveness of leukocyte adenyl cyclase to isoproterenol stimulation has been demonstrated in asthmatics,[202] rever-sal of the increased leukocyte and platelet adenosine triphos-phatase activity typical of asthmatics has occurred,[203] and an increase in the number of beta-adrenergic receptors in rat lung has been reported.[204] Furthermore, corticosteroids may in-hibit formation of cyclic guanosine monophosphate.[205]

Cortisol (hydrocortisone) is the glucocorticoid naturally produced by the adrenal cortex at a rate of 12 mg/M^2/day after the neonatal period, or about 4 mg/day for a 7 Kg infant and 20 mg/day for a 70 Kg adult. Other steroids must be converted by the liver to cortisol before they become biologically active (Fig. 3. 28). Certain modifications of the chemical structure of cor-tisol cause variations in the biologic properties of the various synthetic analogues, most resulting in increased anti-inflam-matory activity and less sodium and water retention than occurs with cortisol or cortisone. Doses of cortisol and its analogues equal in potency of anti-inflammatory action, however, are also equally potent in eliciting side effects due to catabolic activity (Table 3. 13).

Most circulating cortisol is inactive due to binding to transcortin, an alpha-1-globulin.[206] Some is loosely bound to albumin - small amounts at physiological concentrations, but larger amounts when total cortisol concentration is elevated as

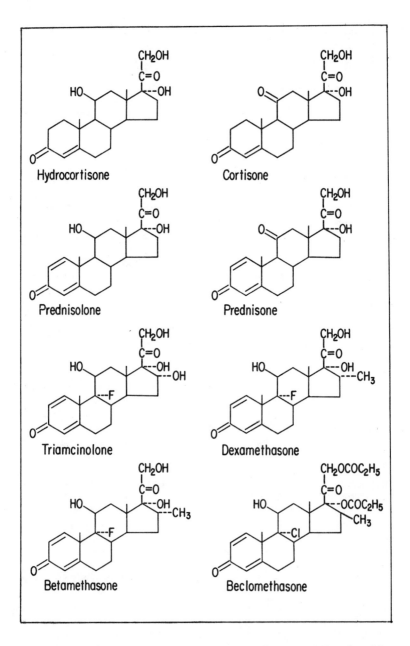

Fig. 3-28. Chemical structures of some adrenal corticosteroids.

TABLE 3.13 ADRENAL CORTICOSTEROIDS AND SOME SYNTHETIC ANALOGUES					
COMPOUND	EQUIVALENT DOSES (Mg)	PLASMA HALF-LIFE (MINUTES)	ORAL FORMS TABLETS (Mg)	LIQUIDS (mg/5ml)	INJECTABLE FORMS (Mg/ml)
Cortisone	25.0	30	5, 10, 25		25, 50 (susp)
Hydrocortisone	20.0	90	5, 10, 20	10 (susp)	5, 10, 25, 50, 100, 250, 500, 1000 mg/vial (powder)
Prednisone	5.0	60	1, 2, 5, 5, 10, 20, 25, 50		
Prednisolone	5.0	200	1, 2, 5, 5		20, 25, 50, 100 50 mg/vial (powder)
Methylprednisolone	4.0	200	2, 4, 16		20, 40, 80 40, 125, 500, 1000 mg/vial (powder)
Triamcinolone	4.0	200	1, 2, 4, 8, 16	2, 4, (syrup)	5, 10, 25, 40 (susp)
Dexamethasone	0.75	300	0.25, 0.5, 0.75, 1.5	0.5 (elixir)	4, 8
Betamethasone	0.6	300	0.6	0.6 (syrup)	6 (susp)

it is following exogenous administration. It has been estimated that 25% of the albumin-bound cortisol is freely diffusable and metabolically active. Normally only 5-10% of circulating cortisol is unbound and thus free to enter cells and to express its metabolic activity, but more is free when total cortisol concentration is increased. [206]

The synthetic corticosteroids are less effectively bound to transcortin than cortisol is, and the synthetic analogues are metabolized more slowly, resulting in a longer plasma half-life and increased effective tissue concentrations. Plasma half-life of cortisol administered by intravenous infusion to normal subjects has been reported to be 1.3-1.9 hours[207] while the plasma half-life of prednisone is 60 minutes and that of dexamethasone is 300 minutes. Oral administration of prednisone, however, is also reported to have been followed by peak plasma steroid concentrations within 1 hour and continued elevations of plasma levels for 4-8 hours. [208] Steroids may be metabolized more rapidly in patients who have been treated daily with prednisone for at least 1 year, [209] and less rapidly in patients with liver disease. [207]

Metabolic activity of steroids persists much longer than their elevated plasma concentrations. Dexamethasone is active for as long as 72 hours after administration; prednisone, prednisolone, or methylprednisolone, for 36 hours or less.

The major effects which corticosteroids can have on most tissues of the body result in numerous possible side effects (Table 3.14). [210,211] Adrenal suppression is the most common side effect. Its extent is related to dosage and duration of treatment. Adrenal suppression can occur within 24 hours of administration of a glucocorticoid[206,212] and has been reported within 2 hours following single doses of prednisolone. [213] As little as 2.5 mg. prednisone daily can at least maintain adrenal suppression in children. [214] It is uncertain how long adrenal suppression persists after discontinuation of treatment with steroids, and there is variability among patients, but postoperative adrenal insufficiency has occurred as long as 24 months after steroid therapy had been stopped. [215] Recovery occurs more frequently within 9 months, [216] and plasma cortisol concentrations have been found to return to normal within 2 weeks after discontinuation of daily prednisone in asthmatic children treated for more than 6 months. [214]

Some of the uncertainty regarding the duration of suppression is due to the use of different methods for assessing adrenal function. Determination of morning plasma cortisol concentration has been found to provide a reliable index of adrenal function, but one which may not correlate with ability to respond to stress. [214] The cortisol response to hypoglycemia induced by

---

TABLE 3.14   POSSIBLE COMPLICATIONS OF THERAPY
WITH ADRENAL CORTICOSTEROIDS

ACCEPTABLE COMPLICATIONS

Excessive weight gain	Insomnia
Edema	Headache
Polyphagia	Euphoria
Facial mooning	Fatigue
Development of "buffalo hump"	Increased urinary fre-
Acne	quency and nocturia
Ecchymoses	Leg cramps
Striae	Abdominal pain
Hypertrichosis	Leukocytosis

SERIOUS COMPLICATIONS

Endocrine
  Hypothalamic-pituitary-adrenal
    suppression
  Diabetes

Central nervous system
  Psychosis
  Pseudotumor cerebri
  Convulsions
  Neuritis

Cardiovascular
  Hypertension
  Thromboembolism
  Arteritis
  Congestive heart failure

Gastrointestinal
  Peptic ulcer
  Pancreatitis

Adverse effects on infection
  Enhancement of virulence
  Masking of signs and symptoms
  Activation of latent infections

Allergic

Hematopoietic
  Agranulocytosis

Musculoskeletal
  Growth suppression
  Myopathy
  Tendon rupture
  Osteoporosis
  Aseptic necrosis

Ocular
  Subcapsular cataracts
  Glaucoma
  Exophthalmos

Serum electrolytes
  Hypokalemia

Cutaneous
  Erythema nodosum
  Dermatitis

Subcutaneous
  Panniculitis

Fetal
  Adrenal insufficiency

administration of insulin may be the most reliable indicator of ability to respond to stress.[217] The metyrapone test, measurement of the increased urinary excretion of 11-hydroxycorticosteroids resulting from increased ACTH secretion following administration of an inhibitor (metyrapone) of the 11-β-hydroxylase necessary for synthesis of cortisol, is a more sensitive test of response of the hypothalamic-pituitary-adrenal axis. It is often abnormal even in subjects who can respond normally to stress.[218] Measurement of plasma cortisol before and after administration of ACTH is relatively insensitive on the other hand, assessing only the response of the adrenal gland itself.

Children who have received long term treatment with adrenal corticosteroids must be considered subject to adrenal insufficiency when faced with stress, and it may be prudent to supply additional corticosteroids even if steroid therapy has been discontinued as long as 9 months before the stress. Sudden discontinuation of steroid therapy can also cause potentially fatal adrenal insufficiency with symptoms including abdominal pain, vomiting, shock and coma.

Impairment of linear growth may also be a serious consequence of long term corticosteroid therapy in children. Growth suppression may occur when the steroid dosage is more than twice the normal daily secretion rate of cortisol (12 mg/M^2).[219] Severe asthma can also suppress growth, however, and initiation of therapy with corticosteroids has occasionally been followed by a growth spurt as the asthma was brought under control.[220]

Substitution of therapy with adrenocorticotropic hormone for corticosteroids has been reported to induce less inhibition of growth,[221] but others have been unable to confirm this.[222] Treatment with ACTH has also been reported to cause less hypothalamic-pituitary-adrenal suppression than treatment with corticosteroids, but adrenal suppression can follow treatment with ACTH.[223] Another possible advantage of ACTH for the treatment of asthma is a direct relaxing effect upon bronchial smooth muscle which has been demonstrated in vitro.[224]

An important disadvantage of treatment with ACTH is limitation by the secretory capacity of the adrenals to lower concentrations of circulating corticosteroids than may be desired. It may be especially hazardous to rely upon ACTH in a patient who may have adrenal suppression from previous treatment with steroids.

Because ACTH stimulates androgen production its use may cause acne and hirsutism more frequently than therapy with corticosteroids, and it may cause earlier epiphyseal maturation. Hyperpigmentation may occur from treatment with ACTH due to melanophore stimulation.

Allergic reactions, including systemic anaphylaxis, have occurred much more frequently following administration of ACTH than with steroids, [225] although anaphylactic reactions to steroids have also been reported very rarely. [226] This disadvantage of ACTH therapy can be largely obviated by the use of synthetic corticotropin. [227] Because of these disadvantages, ACTH therapy generally seems less desirable than treatment with corticosteroids.

Administration of a steroid in a single morning dose on alternate days has been found effective in minimizing undesirable side effects, including growth inhibition and adrenal suppression. [205, 220, 228] Administration of the steroid soon after arising in the morning mimics the natural diurnal variation in plasma cortisol concentrations, which are maximal then. [9, 229]

Long acting steroids such as dexamethasone or betamethasone can cause adrenal suppression even when administered on alternate days, but satisfactory control of asthma with little or no adrenal suppression is usually possible with use on alternate days of a steroid with intermediate duration of action such as prednisone, prednisolone, or methylprednisolone. [228] Alternate day therapy with prednisone can maintain significant adrenal suppression which has followed previous daily treatment with steroids, however. [230]

Duration of action is affected by the nature of the conjugate as well as the chemical structure of the steroid itself when it is administered by intramuscular injection. Acetates, diacetates, acetonides, and tertiary butylacetates are very slowly absorbed from the injection site, resulting in low plasma concentrations and persistence of effects, including adrenal suppression, for weeks. Hemisuccinates and phosphates, on the other hand, have a rapid onset of action and a duration of action similar to the usual plasma half-life of the steroid.

Efforts to minimize side effects associated with the use of corticosteroids have included administration by inhalation of steroids with greater topical anti-inflammatory activity than cortisol. Inhalation of dexamethasone four times daily is known to be highly effective in controlling asthma but also causes adrenal suppression. [231] Inhalation of betamethasone 17-valerate (200 μ g q. i. d.), beclomethasone dipropionate (100 μ g b. i. d. - q. i. d.) and triamcinolone acetonide (100-400 μ g q. i. d.) has been found to be very effective in controlling asthma at doses which usually cause no significant adrenal suppression. [232, 233] Larger doses have been associated with adrenal suppression, and this may account for data suggesting similar adrenal suppression from inhalation of beclomethasone dipropionate and oral administration of prednisone on alternate days. [234, 235] The deaths of 3 children, apparently due to adrenal insufficiency during acute asthmatic attacks, 5-6 months after substitution of inhalation of beclomethasone for daily oral administration of corticosteroids, emphasizes the risk for such children if adequate systemic steroids are not supplied at times of stress. [236]

Oral or laryngeal candidiasis has occurred occasionally as a complication of inhalation of corticosteroids. Such monilial infections have responded to treatment with antifungal agents or discontinuation of steroid inhalation. Bronchial biopsies obtained during bronchoscopy from asthmatics treated with beclomethasone by inhalation for 6 months have disclosed only changes which could be ascribed to the asthma. [237]

Long term therapy with adrenal corticosteroids should not be started without careful consideration of the attendant hazards. In a very few asthmatic children, incapacitated despite all other effective forms of therapy, steroids may be necessary to permit some semblance of normal function. The initial dose should be large enough to be effective. Prednisone or prednisolone at a dose of 2 mg/Kg/day (minimum dose 20 mg, maximum dose 80 mg) in four divided doses has been recommended as a suppressive dose. [210] The dose should then be reduced as symptoms improve. Some asthmatic children respond to smaller doses than this. Treatment for as few as 3 days is often sufficient to cause a relief of acute symptoms which may not recur before other forms of management may become effective.

If prolonged therapy is necessary, inhalation of beclomethasone dipropionate aerosol (Beclovent or Vanceril), 50-100 μ g b. i. d. -q. i. d. , may be preferable to administration of oral corticosteroids. If inhaled beclomethasone at the maximum total daily dose of 500 μg (1, 000 μ g for an adult) does not afford adequate control prednisone, prednisolone, or methylprednisolone should be administered as a single morning dose on alternate days. When alternate day therapy is being substituted in a patient who has previously been receiving daily oral therapy, twice the dose he has been receiving daily is initially administered on alternate days. Since even alternate day therapy can maintain adrenal suppression previously induced by daily therapy, [230] it is preferable to start with alternate day therapy if possible. In rare patients asthmatic symptoms may not be satisfactorily controlled by administration of a steroid on alternate days.

Whatever regimen is used, the dose should be the smallest which affords satisfactory symptomatic control, and duration of treatment should be as short as possible. Dosage reductions must be gradual when steroids have been used for more than a few days. This can usually be accomplished by changing the dose of prednisone by decrements of 2. 5-5 mg on alternate days at 1-2 week intervals until it can be discontinued. A severe exacerbation of asthma within a few months after discontinuation of long term steroid therapy is a definite indication for prompt treatment with corticosteroids because of the likelihood of adrenal suppression.

In children old enough (5-6 years) to be taught how to inhale medication effectively, inhalation of beclomethasone, betamethasone, or triamcinolone may permit effective symptomatic control with fewer side effects than occur with oral administration of steroids. Beclomethasone (50-100 μ g. t. i. d. -q. i. d.) is approved for use in children at least 6 years old, but these other preparations are still available only for experimental use in children in the United States. Occasional supplemental therapy with oral corti costeroids for a few days has been necessary in many patients treated with steroids by inhalation and is essential if adrenal suppression is present.

CROMOLYN SODIUM (DISODIUM CROMOGLYCATE)

Cromolyn sodium (Fig. 3. 29) affords protection against airway obstruction induced by experimental inhalation of allergen in many asthmatics. [238] It is neither a bronchodilator nor an antihistamine and has no anti-inflammatory activity. [239] It has no effect upon mucociliary clearance. [240] It does not prevent the reaction between antigen and specific IgE antibody, [239] but prevents release of chemical mediators from sensitized mast cells following this antigen-antibody reaction. Pretreatment with cromolyn has been found to inhibit airway obstruction induced by voluntary hyperventilation, [241] exercise, [242] exposure to cold air [243] and Type III reactions. [244] In some children it inhibits the induction of bronchoconstriction by inhalation of methacholine or histamine. [245] It has usually been found to be more efficacious in the treatment of extrinsic asthma than intrinsic asthma, however.

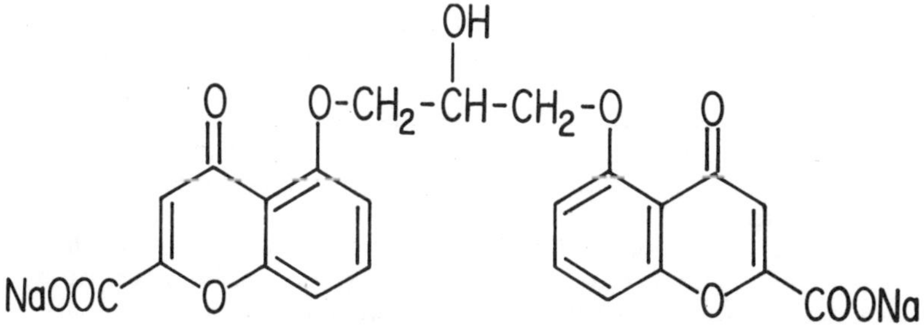

Fig. 3-29. Chemical structure of cromolyn sodium.

Only 1% of orally administered cromolyn is absorbed from the gastrointestinal tract so it must be administered by inhalation. It is supplied as a crystalline powder with 50% of the particles by weight ranging in size from 2-6 μ (mass median diameter 2.6 μ) in gelatin capsules containing 20 mg cromolyn and 20 mg lactose.[246] It has been estimated that following inhalation from the special inhaler 1-2 mg of this dose reaches the alveoli[247] and 9% of the 20 mg of inhaled drug is systemically absorbed [246] and excreted in urine and bile.[239]

Treatment with 20 mg q.i.d. has been followed by improvement in most asthmatic children, but 20-25% have not seemed to benefit from its use. Children who will not respond to cromolyn therapy cannot be identified without a therapeutic trial, but factors implicated in treatment failures include emotional instability, infection, and failure to use the drug or to inhale it properly. An increased frequency of treatment failures has also been reported among black children. Improvement usually occurs within the first two weeks of treatment - a decrease in the frequency or severity of symptoms or a decrease in the need for corticosteroids or bronchodilators to maintain satisfactory symptomatic control. If no improvement can be recognized after 4 weeks of inhalation of cromolyn at a dose of 20 mg q.i.d., the drug should be discontinued as a failure.

Children younger than 5 years of age usually cannot be taught how to inhale cromolyn properly, and it is not recommended by the U.S. Food and Drug Administration for that age group. Administration of nebulized cromolyn (20 mg in 2-2.5 ml) has been reported effective in children of this age, however, and nebulized cromolyn has been found to inhibit exercise-induced asthma.[248-250] Cromolyn is not helpful in the treatment of acute asthmatic attacks since it is effective only when administered before antigenic challenge and cannot be inhaled effectively during episodes of dyspnea and severe wheezing.

The most common side effect has been throat irritation due to deposition of powder. This can be obviated by following treatments with a few swallows of liquid. Coughing or wheezing sometimes provoked by inhalation of the powder can be prevented or minimized by pretreatment with a bronchodilator. Cromolyn therapy has occasionally caused maculopapular and urticarial eruptions or angioedema. Nasal congestion and pulmonary infiltrates with eosinophilia have rarely been reported as possible side effects.[251]

Use of cromolyn is indicated for prevention of asthma when unavoidable exposure to an offending allergen can be anticipated in a patient who responds to its use, and a 4-week trail is indicated in patients with perennial asthma necessitating frequent or continual use of bronchodilators or corticosteroids. A trial of cromolyn is recommended by some in preference to continual treatment with bronchodilators because of the paucity of side effects. Its use should be continued beyond 4 weeks if a beneficial effect has been evident. Subsequent maintenance with 20 mg t. i. d. or even less is sometimes possible. Cromolyn is also helpful for inhibition of exercise induced asthma and can be administered 15-30 minutes before anticipated exercise.

Its use should be temporarily discontinued during acute asthmatic attacks or status asthmaticus and resumed when dyspnea and wheezing have subsided. Discontinuation during bronchial infections has also been recommended.

Patients must be carefully instructed in how to inhale the drug. The technique should be demonstrated, and the first dose should be administered in the presence of the physician or a trained assistant.

ANTIHISTAMINES

Antihistamines have not generally been found useful for the treatment of asthma despite occasional reports of subjective improvement in a few asthmatics.[252] Airway obstruction has seemed aggravated by administration of antihistamines to occasional patients,[252] and there is experimental evidence that some antihistamines can cause bronchoconstriction.[253] Antihistamines have generally been considered contraindicated in status asthmaticus because of their potential for causing inspissation of tracheobronchial secretions, although diphenhydramine has been reported to have no effect upon volume or viscosity of tracheobronchial secretions in experimental animals.[254]

One antihistamine, thiazinamium, has been found to cause bronchodilation and to afford protection against the induction of bronchospasm by allergen inhalation.[255]

Objective assessment of the effects of continuous treatment with therapeutic doses of diphenhydramine, chlorpheniramine, and tripelennamine in children with severe, perennial asthma who were also receiving bronchodilators has failed to reveal any evident adverse responses although administration of promethazine was associated with a significant increase in the use of bronchodilators.[256] At double the usually prescribed dose of diphenhydramine and chlorpheniramine for 2 weeks each, significant decreases in peak expiratory flow rate, measured three times daily, occurred in some children, while significant increases occurred in others. Treatment with chlorpheniramine of patients with mild asthma has also been associated with significant clinical improvement.[257]

Variability in response to antihistamines is further evidence of the heterogeneity of asthma. Chemical mediators other than histamine are probably of greater importance in most asthmatics. It seems safe to prescribe antihistamines for the treatment of allergic rhinitis even in patients with asthma, but it may be prudent to recommend discontinuation of their use whenever severe wheezing supervenes until it has responded to therapy.

PHYSICAL THERAPY

It seems reasonable that gravity-assisted postural drainage with cupping or percussion over the chest should be of assistance in the removal of excessive tracheobronchial secretions. Such measures have been shown to increase the volume of sputum produced by coughing in subjects with cystic fibrosis over short periods of time.[258] Improvement in pulmonary function has been demonstrated for 30-45 minutes after postural drainage in patients with cystic fibrosis, asthma, or chronic bronchitis. [259-261] Improvement in flow rates at low lung volumes has sometimes been more substantial than improvement in FVC or FEV_1. The procedure is usually well tolerated by asthmatic children when only mild or moderate airway obstruction is present, but it may aggravate wheezing if attempted when severe airway obstruction is present. It is likely to be poorly tolerated by those asthmatic children in whom coughing often provokes airway obstruction.

Indications for segmental postural drainage include any condition with excessive tracheobronchial secretions: pneumonia, bronchitis, bronchiectasis, or an ineffective cough as well as asthma when airway obstruction is not severe. It may be especially helpful in the treatment of lobar or segmental atelectasis due to retained secretions. Contraindications include pulmonary hemorrhage with hemoptysis and multiple rib fractures.

For most effective drainage the child should be placed successively in the several different positions in which gravity can be expected to facilitate drainage of the various bronchopulmonary segments (Fig. 3.30 to Fig. 3.38). Infants can be supported with pillows on the lap of the therapist or parent; older children should lie on a flat, firm surface such as that of an ironing board resting upon a couch with one end supported by books or the arm of the couch to the desired elevation. Vigorous clapping with the cupped hand over the segment to be drained for 1-3 minutes should be painless yet effective. Slow, deep breaths followed by coughing and expectoration are encouraged during and following therapy in each position to be used. Chest physiotherapy for 1 minute to each segment 2-3 times daily may be helpful during convalescence from acute asthmatic attacks.

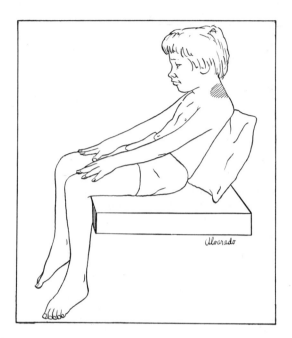

Fig. 3-30. Position for segmental bronchial
drainage of apical segments of upper lobes:
bed flat and child leaning back at 30° angle
against pillow and therapist. Therapist claps
with cupped hand over area between clavicle
and top of scapula on each side (modified from
Waring). [87]

Treatment for 2-3 minutes of one or two involved segments three
times daily may be more beneficial when atelectasis or localized rales are evident.

TREATMENT OF ACUTE ASTHMATIC ATTACKS

Most asthmatic attacks of mild or moderate severity can be
effectively controlled by the administration of an oral bronchodilator such as theophylline, ephedrine, metaproterenol, albuterol,
or terbutaline.   The child should be observed for possible
side effects (see above).   If neither theophylline alone nor
a sympathomimetic alone affords satisfactory relief, combination of theophylline with a sympathomimetic is likely to be
more efficacious.

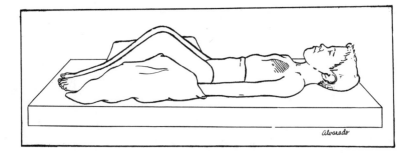

Fig. 3-31. Position for segmental bronchial drainage of anterior segments of upper lobes: bed flat and child supine with pillow supporting knees. Therapist claps between clavicle and nipple on each side (modified from Waring). [87]

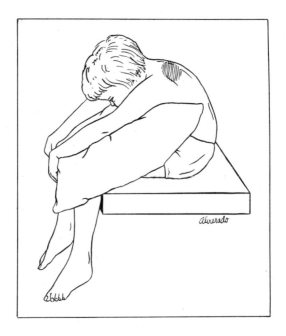

Fig. 3-32. Position for segmental bronchial drainage of posterior segments of upper lobes: bed flat and child leaning forward at 30^0 angle over folded pillow. Therapist claps over upper back on both sides (modified from Waring). [87]

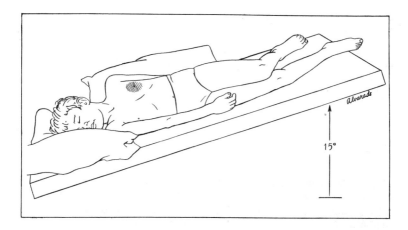

Fig. 3-33. Position for segmental bronchial drainage of lingular segments of left upper lobe: feet elevated 15⁰, child lying on right side and rotated 1/4 turn backward, knees flexed. Therapist claps over left nipple (or lateral and inferior to breast when there is breast development) (modified from Waring). [87]

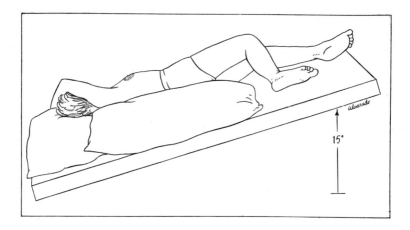

Fig. 3-34. Position for segmental bronchial drainage of right middle lobe: feet elevated 15⁰, child lying on left side and rotated 1/4 turn backward, knees flexed. Therapist claps over right nipple (or lateral and inferior to breast when there is breast development) (modified from Waring). [87]

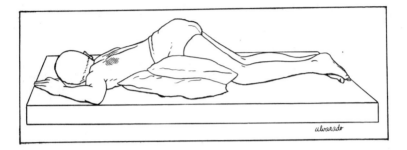

Fig. 3-35. Position for segmental bronchial drainage of superior segments of lower lobes: bed flat, child prone with hips supported by 2 pillows. Therapist claps over middle of back at tip of scapula on each side of spine (modified from Waring).[87]

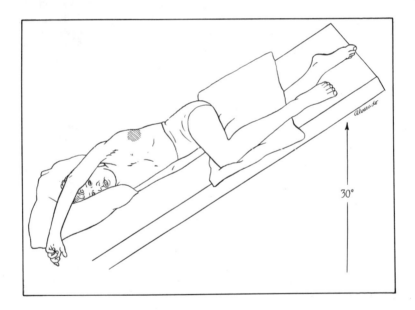

Fig. 3-36. Position for segmental bronchial drainage of anterior basal segments of lower lobes: feet elevated 30°, child lying on side with pillow supporting upper knee. Therapist claps over lower ribs. (Reverse position for opposite lung) (modified from Waring). [87]

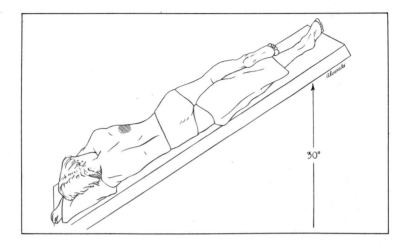

Fig. 3-37. Position for segmental bronchial drainage of lateral basal segments of lower lobes: feet elevated 30°, child lying on abdomen, rotated 1/4 turn upward with upper leg flexed and supported by pillow. Therapist claps over uppermost portion of lower ribs. (Reverse position for opposite lung) (modified from Waring). [87]

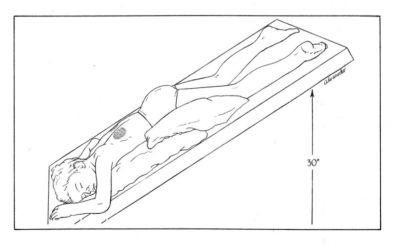

Fig. 3-38. Position for segmental bronchial drainage of posterior basal segments of lower lobes: feet elevated 30°, child prone with hips supported by pillow. Therapist claps over lower ribs to each side of spine (modified from Waring). [87]

Therapy is most likely to be effective if administered at the onset of symptoms. Parents should be taught to start treatment when coughing begins if it is known this will be followed by wheezing. In children in whom symptoms of allergic rhinitis usually precede exacerbations of asthma early administration of bronchodilators may minimize or prevent chest symptoms. The regular use of oral bronchodilators at 6-8 hour intervals should continue for 3 days after any overt wheezing has subsided for continued treatment of the airway obstruction which persists. Children in whom wheezing recurs 2-3 days each week often benefit from continual treatment with oral bronchodilators. Gravity-assisted segmental bronchial drainage with clapping with the cupped hand facilitates mobilization of secretions and is usually well tolerated except when severe airway obstruction is present.

Failure of moderate or severe wheezing to improve within 30-60 minutes after administration of an oral bronchodilator indicates a need for prompt further therapy. Treatment with 1:1,000 aqueous epinephrine administered by subcutaneous injection in appropriate doses is usually effective in affording relief. Bronchospasm may not recur as soon as the pharmacological action of epinephrine has abated, but when airway obstruction has been relieved by aqueous epinephrine, it is safest to follow this 30 minutes later with administration of a longer acting preparation such as Sus-Phrine to assure sustained bronchodilation for several hours. Use of oral bronchodilators should also then be resumed.

Failure of wheezing to respond satisfactorily to adequate treatment with 1:1000 aqueous epinephrine would establish the need for hospitalization for treatment of status asthmaticus (see below).

Inhalation of isoproterenol, isoetharine, metaproterenol, or terbutaline is often an effective alternative to administration of epinephrine. Home use of such drugs should usually be supervised by parents to minimize the likelihood of overuse, and children should be observed for possible side effects. Delivery by inhalation avoids the hazard of inadvertent intravascular injection and may therefore sometimes be preferable to injection of epinephrine by a parent. When parental supervision is uncertain the possibility of overuse of isoproterenol delivered by inhalation can be minimized by use of a nebulizer driven by an air compressor or a hand nebulizer rather than a Freon selfpropelled nebulizer. There is no published evidence that delivery of bronchodilators by intermittent positive pressure offers any substantial advantage over these other methods. Inhalation of metaproterenol or terbutaline has the added advantage of a much longer duration of action.

Frequently recurrent nocturnal asthmatic attacks are often preventable by the administration of a long acting bronchodilator at bedtime.

TREATMENT OF EXERCISE-INDUCED ASTHMA

Exercise-induced asthma probably occurs in most asthmatics if exercise is sufficiently prolonged and strenuous, but the ease with which it can be induced is variable. Susceptibility to exercise-induced asthma can be determined by obtaining a careful history and measurement of pulmonary function before, during and after exercise.

Physical activity should not be restricted unnecessarily in those asthmatics in whom exercise is not followed by clinically significant airway obstruction.

Asthmatic children in whom exercise provokes airway obstruction and in whom nasal breathing is impractical or insufficient to afford protection should be advised to prevent or to minimize this response by use of an oral bronchodilator 30-60 minutes before anticipated exercise, or an inhaled bronchodilator 15-20 minutes before exercise, or by inhalation of a single dose of cromolyn 15-60 minutes before exercise. [242]

For those children in whom 1-2 minutes of exercise is followed by bronchodilation while more prolonged exercise provokes airway obstruction, activities requiring only intermittent, brief intervals of exercise are likely to be better tolerated than those requiring sustained exercise. Such children may tolerate baseball more readily than basketball. Asthmatics subject to exercise induced asthma usually tolerate swimming better than any other form of exercise. [262]

There is a dearth of objective evidence of improvement of pulmonary function in asthmatic children participating in programs of general physical conditioning, but there is general agreement that such programs are beneficial psychologically. [263] With careful management it is probably possible for almost all asthmatic children to participate safely in most forms of physical exercise despite the potential adverse effect of exercise.

TREATMENT OF STATUS ASTHMATICUS

Status asthmaticus is a medical emergency requiring immediate treatment (Table 3.15). Its diagnosis is established by lack of satisfactory improvement in wheezing due to asthma following three adequate doses of 1:1000 aqueous epinephrine or two doses of terbutaline administered at 20 minute intervals (0.01 ml/Kg, maximum 0.3 ml for epinephrine, maximum 0.25

ml for terbutaline). Therapy should be started as soon as possible after the initial clinical assessment and submission of specimens for laboratory evaluations (see above).

HYDRATION

Dehydration should be corrected by administration of intravenous fluids. Administration of 360-400 ml/M^2 body surface area of a solution containing one-third normal saline in 5 or 10% glucose or 5% glucose in normal saline during the first 45-60 minutes has been recommended.[86,264] After renal flow has been established a polyionic, hypotonic solution containing potassium can be administered at rates of 2400-3000 ml/M^2/24 hours with moderate or severe dehydration.[264] If there is no dehydration 1500 ml/M^2/24 hours is adequate. Subsequent needs are indicated by frequent clinical evaluation and measurement of blood chemistries. Evidence of increased rates of secretion of antidiuretic hormone during status asthmaticus indicates the need for caution to avoid water intoxication.[189] On the other hand sufficient fluids must be infused to prevent hypovolemia and peripheral vascular collapse, and it is likely that dehydration may contribute to inspissation of tracheobronchial secretions.

AMINOPHYLLINE

Intravenous aminophylline is the drug of choice for the treatment of status asthmaticus. Plasma concentrations of at least 5-10 μ g/ml are usually necessary for effective bronchodilation, and concentrations greater than 20 μ g/ml are usually associated with signs or symptoms of toxicity (see page 124). If doses of previously administered xanthines have not been excessive and at least 6 hours have elapsed since the last retained oral dose (8-12 hours for sustained release preparations, 12 hours since the last rectal dose), aminophylline can usually be safely administered intravenously at a dose of 5 mg/Kg even if the plasma concentration is unknown. A longer interval may be necessary for patients who have been receiving continual treatment with a sustained release preparation, and it is safest to determine the serum theophylline concentration before administering more theophylline to these or other patients when there is uncertainty about the adequacy of the interval since the last dose. This loading dose should be diluted to 10-50 ml and infused over 20-30 minutes. This dose can usually be repeated safely at 8 hour intervals, but administration of a constant infusion at a rate expected to maintain the serum concentration at 10-20 μ g/ml is more effective (Table 3.16). Recommended initial infusion rates must be adjusted as indicated by the

TABLE 3.15   MANAGEMENT OF STATUS ASTHMATICUS

1. Hospitalization

2. History and Physical Examination
   State of hydration, evidence of infection, cause of exacerbation and known allergies, adequacy of ventilation, possible complications.

3. Laboratory studies
   Complete blood count; urinalysis; arterial blood gases and pH; serum sodium, potassium, and chloride; blood urea nitrogen; chest roentgenogram; sputum smear, culture, and sensitivities.

4. Intravenous fluids
   360-400 ml/M^2 during first hour; then 1500-3000 ml/M^2 /24 hrs when dehydration present.

5. Aminophylline
   5 mg/Kg diluted and infused intravenously over 20 minutes. Follow with constant infusion of 0.5-1.1 mg/Kg/h to maintain serum concentration at 10-20 μg/ml.

6. Oxygen
   Maintain arterial PO_2 >65 mm Hg and < 100 mm Hg.

7. Sodium bicarbonate
   1.5-2 mEq/Kg diluted and infused intravenously over 10-20 minutes when metabolic acidosis present.
   Same dose may be infused over next 45 minutes and repeated each hour if arterial pH remains less than 7.25 and serum sodium less than 145 mEq/L.

8. Aqueous epinephrine, 1:1000
   0.01 ml/Kg (maximum 0.3 ml) by subcutaneous injection. (Responsiveness may have been restored by improvement in hydration and acid-base balance).
   If epinephrine elicits improvement, Sus-Phrine can be administered 30 minutes later (0.005 ml/Kg, maximum 0.3 ml).

9. Isoproterenol, 1:200, or Bronkosol
   0.01 ml/Kg (maximum 0.5 ml) diluted to 1.5-9 ml with sterile saline, nebulized and inhaled.
   May repeat q4h.
   Avoid use within 1-2 hours of epinephrine administration.

Table 3.15 (cont'd.)

10. Adrenal corticosteroids
    Hydrocortisone, 4 mg/Kg, or methyl prednisolone, 0.8
    mg/Kg, q4h by intravenous injection if insufficient
    response to first intravenous dose of aminophylline.
    Administer immediately with history of recent previous
    treatment with adrenal corticosteroids.

11. Antibiotics
    As indicated for treatment of infection

12. Endotracheal intubation and controlled ventilation for pro-
    gression to respiratory failure despite above measures.

SEDATIVES, TRANQUILIZERS, MORPHINE, AND ANTIHISTA-
MINES CONTRAINDICATED.

---

serum theophylline concentration found 1 hour after the infusion
has been started if response is inadequate or whenever signs or
symptoms of toxicity occur. The volume of distribution of theophylline varies from 0.3-0.7 L/Kg, so administration of each
additional dose of 2mg/Kg is expected to increase the serum
concentration by 4 μg/ml if given within 20-30 minutes. Cal-
culation of loading doses such as these are usually based upon
total body weight even for obese children, but it is recommended that maintenance dosage be based initially upon ideal body
weight for obese children. [181]
    In some children in whom theophylline may be metabolized
especially rapidly larger doses may be necessary, but it is safest for the size and frequency of larger doses or the rate of
constant infusions to be guided by determination of plasma theophylline concentrations. Infants may be especially likely to
develop potentially toxic plasma concentrations from doses of
theophylline not associated with toxicity in older children. [266]
Any child receiving treatment with theophylline should be observed for signs and symptoms of toxicity.

OXYGEN

    Sufficient oxygen should be administered to maintain the
arterial PO_2 between 65 mm Hg and 100 mm Hg. The oxygen
must be fully humidified to prevent irritation of the bronchial
mucosa. Other complications of prolonged administration of
oxygen in high concentrations include capillary congestion, interstitial edema, fibrin deposition, hemorrhage, atelectasis
and later capillary proliferation and pulmonary fibrosis. [267]
Hypoventilation may follow administration of oxygen to subjects

with hypercapnia probably because of elimination of the hypoxic drive to ventilation.[268] This complication requires immediate artificial ventilation and continued oxygen therapy.

Oxygen can be delivered by nasal cannula, open face tent, or Venturi mask. In children who may tolerate none of these methods well, use of a tent may be necessary, but it is difficult to maintain satisfactory oxygen concentrations in tents and these should be monitored frequently.

MIST

Mist is probably not beneficial[184] and potentially harmful. Inhalation of nebulized saline can provoke bronchospasm in asthmatic children,[186] and inhalation of air at 95% relative humidity has been followed by increased airway obstruction in asthmatics.[269]

SODIUM BICARBONATE

Correction of acidosis with sodium bicarbonate may restore responsiveness to epinephrine if there has not been a satisfactory response to intravenous aminophylline. The dose of 1.5-2 mEq/Kg can be given by intravenous infusion over 15-20 minutes, repeated more slowly over the next 45 minutes, and repeated each hour thereafter if hourly determinations show the arterial pH to remain less than 7.30 due to metabolic acidosis

TABLE 3.16　INITIAL THEOPHYLLINE INFUSION RATE FOLLOWING LOADING DOSE[265]

PATIENT	INFUSION RATE* (mg/Kg/h)
Children < 9 years old	0.85
Children > 9 years old & healthy adult smokers	0.75
Healthy adult nonsmokers	0.5
Heart failure	0.3
Liver dysfunction	0.2
Liver dysfunction and heart failure	0.1

* Increase by 25% to convert to aminophylline

with plasma bicarbonate less than 20 mEq/L and if the serum sodium concentration remains less than 145 mEq/L. [85] It may be most reasonable to limit use of bicarbonate to those patients with arterial pH less than 7.25.

SYMPATHOMIMETICS

After unresponsiveness to epinephrine has been established, its continued use can only be expected to elicit side effects so it should be discontinued. After restoration of normal hydration and acid base balance, however, responsiveness to epinephrine may also be restored. If satisfactory improvement then follows injection of 1:1000 aqueous epinephrine, Sus-Phrine can be administered 30 minutes later for a more sustained effect.

Inhalation of an isoproterenol aerosol or Bronkosol often elicits bronchodilation even in children found to be unresponsive to epinephrine administered by subcutaneous injection. Isoproterenol, 1:200, or Bronkosol can be administered at a dose of 0.01 ml/Kg (maximum 0.5 ml), diluted with 1.5-8.5 ml sterile saline, at 4 hour intervals if necessary. Isoproterenol should be temporarily discontinued if the heart rate exceeds 180/minute. Administration by an oxygen-powered nebulizer minimizes the risk of associated decreases in arterial P_{O2}. [137] Delivery with intermittent positive pressure should be avoided because of evidence that this may cause increased airway resistance[270] and to minimize the risk of pneumomediastinum or pneumothorax. [94] It is prudent to avoid use of isoproterenol or Bronkosol within 2 hours of administration of epinephrine because of the possibility of an increased risk of cardiac arrhythmias.

Inhalation of terbutaline or albuterol may prove to be safer and more effective than isoproterenol for the treatment of status asthmaticus. [271]

ADRENAL CORTICOSTEROIDS

Administration of an adrenal corticosteroid is indicated if there has not been prompt improvement following intravenous administration of aminophylline. Immediate use of a steroid is essential in any child who has received steroid therapy at least within the previous 9 months because of possible adrenal insufficiency. [216]

Intravenous hydrocortisone is preferable to use of a steroic with a longer duration of action, because it minimizes adrenal suppression through permitting treatment for the shortest time necessary for satisfactory control of the asthma. Methylprednisolone, which causes less sodium retention, may be substituted, however.

There is evidence that clinical improvement is associated with intravenous administration of hydrocortisone when plasma cortisol concentrations of at least 100 μ g/dl are maintained in asthmatics. [209] Such levels are usually maintained for 4 hours after intravenous administration of hydrocortisone at a dose of 4 mg/Kg. [272] The corresponding dose of methylprednisolone is 0.8 mg/Kg. The corticosteroid should be discontinued as soon as permitted by the child's clinical state.

Delays of 6-12 hours before recognition of clinical response following corticosteroid administration have been generally accepted, but there has been evidence of significant clinical improvement and changes in pulmonary function within 1 hour after intravenous administration of hydrocortisone or prednisolone. [209, 273] Steroids are not as rapidly effective as bronchodilators and must not be relied upon for an immediate effect.

ANTIBIOTICS

Although bacterial infections only very rarely provoke asthmatic attacks, [12-15] as many as half of children who have died in status asthmaticus have been found to have evidence of bacterial pulmonary infection at postmortem examination. [121-123] Even if chest roentgenograms disclose no evidence of infection it is wise to consider this possibility in a child who has responded poorly to treatment of status asthmaticus.

SEDATIVES

The administration of sedatives, tranquilizers, and morphine or other opiates is contraindicated in status asthmaticus because of their depressant effect upon the respiratory center. [84, 86] Restlessness and agitation are signs of hypoxemis which should be treated with oxygen rather than sedatives which can not only aggravate hypoxemia but also obscure these indications of increasing ventilatory impairment. Deaths during status asthmaticus have often followed administration of such agents. [121-123]

In the very rare child for whom sedation may become necessary, it should be administered only when frequent blood gas determinations assure adequate monitoring of ventilation and with facilities for mechanical control of ventilation immediately available. Chloral hydrate, 15 mg/Kg every 8 hours by mouth or by rectum, has been recommended for use when these safeguards are available. [85]

ANTIHISTAMINES

Antihistamines are contraindicated in status asthmaticus because of their potential inspissating effect upon tracheobronchial secretions as well as their sedative effect.

POSTURAL DRAINAGE

Gravity-assisted postural drainage with clapping with the cupped hand facilitates removal of tracheobronchial secretions after the child has improved and only mild or moderate airway obstruction is still evident (see page 144). It is not tolerated well when severe airway obstruction is present and should be discontinued immediately until further improvement has occurred if it aggravates wheezing or causes increased dyspnea.

CONTROLLED VENTILATION

Rarely a child with status asthmaticus does not respond to these measures. Use of a formal scoring system can facilitate detection of impending respiratory failure (see Table 3.8), [86], [127] and the basis of the diagnosis of respiratory failure has already been indicated. Respiratory failure, coma, apnea, or cardiorespiratory arrest due to status asthmaticus are indications for endotracheal intubation and mechanical ventilation. [128]

Controlled, mechanical ventilation often permits rapid restoration of normal acid-base balance through increased removal of carbon dioxide by more effective ventilation. This is facilitated by a decreased inspiratory flow rate with sustained pressure at peak inspiratory pressure and a relatively slow respiratory rate with a long expiratory pause and the addition of a slight expiratory resistance to help prevent airway collapse. [274] The work of breathing is assumed by the ventilator, decreasing oxygen utilization. Mechanical ventilation also permits more efficient administration of aerosol therapy.

If the child is apneic or gasping ventilatory assistance should be supplied immediately by administration of 100% oxygen (humidified) by bag and mask while preparations are being made for mechanical ventilation (Table 3.17). Sedation is no longer contraindicated when mechanical ventilation is imminent and should be instituted to facilitate intubation and to afford amnesia unless the child is unconscious. Nasotracheal intubation should be completed by an anesthesiologist initially consulted when impending respiratory failure was recognized.

Use of a volume-cycled ventilator is usually necessary because of the increased airway resistance which would otherwise prevent delivery of adequate tidal volumes. A nomogram can

TABLE 3.17 CONTROLLED VENTILATION FOR
RESPIRATORY FAILURE DUE TO STATUS
ASTHMATICUS[128, 275, 276]

A. INDUCTION

1. Manual assistance of ventilation with 100% oxygen (humidified) by bag and mask.
2. Sedation if patient is conscious: sodium pentobarbital, 1 mg/Kg, I.V.
3. Nasotracheal intubation under direct vision laryngoscopy.
4. Administration of oxygen.
5. Aspiration of tracheal secretions with sterile catheter. (must be completed within a few seconds).
6. Connection of endotracheal tube to volume-cycled ventilator. Apply slight expiratory resistance and set for moderate hyperventilation.
7. Chest roentgenogram to verify proper placement of endotracheal tube.

B. MAINTENANCE

1. Continuous muscle paralysis. (Pancuronium bromide, 60-100 μg/Kg followed by 15 μg/Kg q 25-60 minutes as needed).
2. Maintenance of light sleep or sedation with pentobarbitol, 1-2 mg/Kg q3-6h.
3. Monitoring with continuous ECG, rectal temperature, ventilator pressures and volumes, and frequent blood gas determinations.
4. Continual nursing attendance with observation of skin color, breath sounds, pulse, blood pressure, muscle tone, and ventilator function at least q15 min.
5. Aseptic aspiration of trachea q30-60 min. after instillation of 2-5 ml sterile saline.
6. Frequent readjustment of ventilator as dictated by blood gas determinations and clinical state. (Maintain arterial Pco_2 near 30 mm Hg and $Po_2 > 65$ and < 100 mm Hg).
7. Full humidification of inspired gases with heated micronebulizer.
8. Manual hyperventilation for 5-10 breaths q30 minutes unless ventilator supplies automatic deep breaths periodically to help prevent atelectasis.

Table 3.17 (cont'd.)

C. DISCONTINUATION

1. After sufficient improvement and restoration of normal acid-base balance (usually within 24-48h) discontinuation of muscle relaxant.
2. Setting of ventilator to assist when adequate spontaneous ventilation has recurred.
3. Disconnection of ventilator if blood gases have remained normal and clinical state satisfactory.
4. Connection of source of heated, humidified oxygen to endotracheal tube.
5. Extubation after tracheal aspiration if condition has remained satisfactory and effective cough reflex has returned.

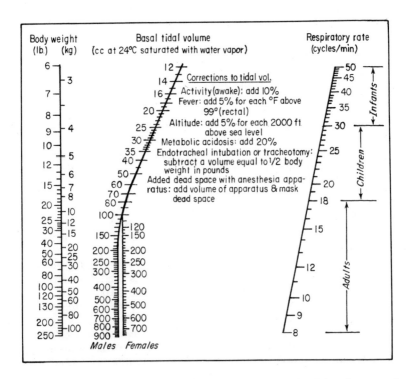

Fig. 3-39. Nomogram for estimation of initial tidal volume and respiratory rate by weight and sex for mechanical ventilation. 277

be used initially to estimate tidal volume and respiratory rate or an initial tidal volume of 10 ml/Kg body weight can be used, [278] but subsequent changes should be based upon the child's clinical state and frequent determination of arterial blood gases (Fig. 3.39).

After mechanical ventilation has started, a chest roentgenogram should be obtained to verify that the endotracheal tube does not extend past the carina into one of the mainstem bronchi.

Continual muscle paralysis facilitates optimal ventilation and lessens the possibility of the development of a pneumothorax which can occur from coughing against the inspiratory phase of the ventilator. [128] Although tubocurarine can cause histamine release, it has been used in asthmatic patients for this purpose without any evident complications. [128,276] Gallamine triethiodide is also effective, but recurrent or prolonged paralysis has followed its use in patients with renal failure. [279] Either tubocurarine or gallamine triethiodide is more satisfactory than succinylcholine because of their longer action and reversibility with prostigmine or edrophonium chloride when required. Pancuronium bromide has also been reported effective, and it does not cause histamine release. [280]

With restoration of normal acid-base balance and clinical improvement, extubation is usually possible within 24-48 hours.

Complications of endotracheal intubation and mechanical ventilation for status asthmaticus include unrecognized hypoventilation, impairment of venous return causing arterial hypotension, tension pneumothorax or pneumomediastinum, iatrogenic pulmonary infection, and subglottic edema following extubation. Convulsions can occur from hypoxemia (especially likely during the intubation procedure) or a sudden decrease in arterial P_{CO2} with an increase in pH from overventilation. With frequent determination of blood gases, careful observation of the child, scrupulous aseptic technique in aspiration of secretions, continuation of other forms of therapy for status asthmaticus, and extubation as soon as clinically indicated these complications can often be avoided or at least detected early enough to minimize their effects.

INTRAVENOUS ISOPROTERENOL

Because of the complications of treatment of status asthmaticus with mechanical ventilation other possible forms of therapy have been sought. Intravenous administration of isoproterenol as a slow, constant infusion has been reported to obviate the need for mechanical ventilation in some asthmatics with respiratory failure. [278,281,282] This form of therapy has been recommended only for use in asthmatics with respiratory failure or impending respiratory failure who have failed to respond to the usual medical management of status asthmaticus (see Table 3.14). Some have also failed to respond to intravenous isoproterenol and have required mechanical ventilation.

Use of intravenous isoproterenol (Table 3.18) necessitates continuous electrocardiographic monitoring of the patient with chest electrodes and an oscilloscope and administration of the isoproterenol with a slow infusion pump (Holter, Harvard, or Sigma). The initial dose of 0.1 μ g/Kg/min. has been increased by 0.1 μ g/Kg/min. every 15 minutes until arterial P_{CO2} has begun to decrease or pulse rate has increased to 200/min. or a persistent cardiac arrhythmia has occurred. Constant observation by the physician is recommended while the dose is being increased. The required maximum dose has varied from 0.10-1.70 μ g/Kg/min.[282] After clinical improvement and restoration of acid-base balance, the dose has been decreased by 0.1 μ g/Kg/min. at 1-2 hour intervals if blood gases have remained normal. Treatment with intravenous isoproterenol for at least 36 hours has usually been necessary, but treatment for as long as 143 hours has been reported.[282]

Sudden death has occurred in asthmatics receiving isoproterenol intravenously, and myocardial ischemia has been reported in a 14-year-old boy who received as little as 0.11 μg/Kg/minute.[283, 284]

Intravenous administration of sympathomimetics with less cardiac activity than isoproterenol might be safer. Intravenous injection of albuterol has been reported effective in the treatment of asthma, but nebulization and administration of such an agent by inhalation may be even more effective and safer.[285]

MORTALITY

Data from the Bureau of Vital Statistics indicate a decrease in the frequency of death from asthma in children between 1950 and 1976 not entirely accounted for by the two revisions of the code for the International Classification of Diseases which tended to decrease the number of deaths ascribed to asthma (Fig. 3.40). Nevertheless, approximately 60 children continue to die from asthma each year in the United States. Most of these probably die during status asthmaticus.

Postmortem examinations of children who have died during status asthmaticus has usually disclosed occlusion of airways with thick, tenacious, mucoid secretions found by microscopic examination to contain epithelial cells, eosinophils, and sometimes Charcot-Leyden crystals. Eosinophilic infiltration of the bronchial mucosa, basement membrane thickening, bronchiolar muscular hypertrophy, and mucous glandular hyperplasia are the other characteristic findings.[121-123]

TABLE 3.18	SUMMARY OF REPORTED TREATMENT OF RESPIRATORY FAILURE WITH INTRAVENOUS ISOPROTERENOL[278, 281, 282]

1. Used only with respiratory failure or impending respiratory failure despite intravenous fluids, aminophylline, sodium bicarbonate, and hydrocortisone in optimal amounts.
2. Continuous ECG with chest electrodes and oscilloscope to monitor heart rate and rhythm.
3. Radial artery cannulation with 20 gauge plastic cannula to monitor arterial pulse and pressure with a strain gauge and to serve as source of specimens for blood gas determinations. Cannula flushed constantly with heparin solution (1 unit/ml) delivered by constant infusion pump.
4. Intravenous infusion site for delivery of isoproterenol separate from that through which maintenance fluids infused.
5. Addition of 0.5 mg isoproterenol to 50 ml fluid in infusion reservoir before intravenous tubing filled (10 μ g isoproterenol/ml).
6. Delivery of isoproterenol with slow infusion pump.

   Initial dose: 0.1 μ g/Kg/min.

7. Blood gas determinations every 15-30 min. initially; every 2-4h after satisfactory response to therapy.
8. Increase in rate of delivery of isoproterenol by 0.1 μ g/Kg/min every 15 min until arterial PCO2 has begun to fall or persistent arrhythmia has occurred or heart rate has increased to 200/min.
9. After clinical improvement has occurred and arterial blood gases restored to normal, reduction in dose of isoproterenol by 0.1 μ g/Kg/min every 1-2 hours if blood gases remain normal. Treatment for at least 36 hours usually necessary.

Factors incriminated as possible causes of death have included infection, oversedation, aminophylline and sympathomimetic toxicity, inadequate provision of supplemental adrenal corticosteroids in patients previously treated with long-term corticosteroids, and failure to institute adequate therapy early enough in the course of the asthmatic attack.[121-123] Parents must be taught to recognize asthmatic attacks, to begin appropriate treatment at the onset of symptoms, and to seek more intensive treatment at the physician's office or hospital if moderate or severe airway obstruction is not relieved within 30-60 minutes after administration of an oral bronchodilator.

Physicians who treat asthmatic children must prescribe optimal therapy, including safe, effective drugs in appropriate doses. Infants and children less than five years old should be recognized as those with the highest mortality rate from asthma (see Fig. 3.40, Table 3.19); they should be observed very closely and treated with great care.

Exposure to offending allergens must be eliminated or minimized (see Chapters IX and XII), and factors known to trigger asthmatic attacks avoided or their effects modified as indicated previously.

Compliance with prescribed drug regimens and precautions recommended to minimize exposure to allergens is fostered by a genuine interest in the patient and his family as well as the disease. The entire family must understand the nature of the problem and its management. Restrictions upon activity and life style can be reduced through optimal control of symptoms,

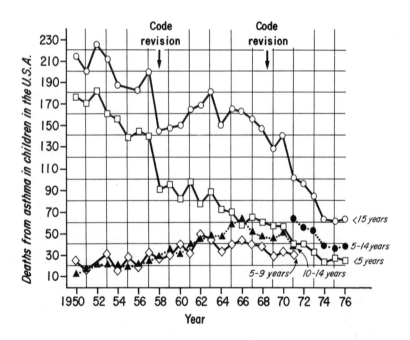

Fig. 3-40. Deaths from asthma in children in the United States, 1950-1976, by age group, with years of revisions of code for the International Classification of Diseases indicated. Each revision decreased the number of deaths ascribed to asthma.

TABLE 3.19   DEATH RATES IN CHILDREN FROM ASTHMA
                PER 100,000 POPULATION IN EACH AGE
                GROUP IN THE UNITED STATES, 1960-1977

Year	Age (Years) 1	1-4	5-9	10-14
1960	0.6	0.4	0.2	0.2
1961	0.9	0.4	0.2	0.2
1962	0.5	0.3	0.2	0.3
1963	0.6	0.4	0.2	0.3
1964	0.4	0.3	0.1	0.3
1965	0.5	0.3	0.2	0.3
1966	0.5	0.2	0.2	0.3
1967	0.5	0.3	0.2	0.3
1968	0.3	0.3	0.2	0.2
1969	0.5	0.3	0.1	0.2
1970	0.4	0.3	0.2	0.2
1971	0.4	0.2	0.2	0.2
1972	0.3	0.2	0.1	0.1
1973	0.4	0.1	0.1	0.1
1974	0.1	0.2	0.1	0.1
1975	0.2	0.1	0.1	0.1
1976	0.1	0.2	0.1	0.1
1977	0.1	0.1	0.1	0.1

Ages 5-9 and 10-14 grouped after 1970.
Apparent large changes in some years are due to rounding of
figures.

but avocational and vocational guidance may sometimes become
necessary. A comprehensive approach such as this is most
likely to counteract effectively fears of the disease and medications, guilt concerning extra attention received and necessary
restrictions upon the rest of the family, envy of the free life
styles of siblings and peers, and anger at what is perceived as
the insensitivity of physicians reported often by children with
chronic asthma.[286]

PROGNOSIS

Available information about the natural history of asthma
is based largely upon retrospective studies. Several of these
have indicated that approximately half of asthmatic children no

longer continue to have episodes of wheezing 10-20 years after the initial diagnosis, [287, 288] and as many as 68% of asthmatic children have been reported free of wheezing by 10 years of age. [289] Only 5-10% of children with asthma have continued to have frequent or severe exacerbations 10-20 years later. [287, 288] Those children with the onset of recurrent wheezing during the first two years of life have been reported to have a less favorable prognosis for freedom of symptoms within a few years, [288, 289] although some data do not agree with this. [290] Antecedent or concurrent atopic dermatitis or allergic rhinitis has also been associated with a greater likelihood of persistence of asthma. [288, 290] Nevertheless it is impossible to predict the future course of asthma in any particular child.

Evidence that therapy has a favorable effect upon prognosis, [291] the observation that allergic rhinitis often persists even in those asthmatics whose recurrent wheezing subsides, [287] and frequent later recurrences of asthma in patients previously free of symptoms for more than one year[292] emphasize the value of early, intensive treatment of asthma and the risk of deferring therapy in the hope that the child may "outgrow it".

REFERENCES

1. Siegel, S. C. , et al.: "Bronchial asthma", in Kelly, V. C. (ed.): Practice of Pediatrics, Harper & Row, Hagerstown, Md. , 1974, Vol. II, Chapter 63.
2. Nadel, J. A. : Mechanisms of airway response to inhaled substances. Arch Env Health 16:171, 1968.
3. Boat, T. F. , and Doershuk, C. F. : "Defense mechanisms of the respiratory tract", in Lough, M. D. , Doershuk, C. F. , and Stern, R. C. (ed.): Pediatric Respiratory Therapy, Year Book Med Pub, Chicago, 1974, p19.
4. Wilson, A. F. , et al.: Deposition of inhaled pollen and pollen extract in human airways. NEJM 288:1056, 1974.
5. Wilson, A. F. , et al.: Fate of inhaled whole pollen in asthmatics. J All 47:107, 1971.
6. Novey, H. S. , et al.: Early ventilation-perfusion changes in asthma. J All 46:221, 1970.
7. Busse, W. W. , et al.: Where is the allergic reaction in ragweed asthma? J All Clin Imm 50:289, 1972.
8. Woolcock, A. J. : Surfactant. Med J Austr 1:900, 1973.
9. Reinberg, A. , et al.: Nocturnal asthma attacks: their relationship to the circadian adrenal cycle. J All 34:323, 1963.
10. Karki, N. T. : The urinary excretion of noradrenalin and adrenalin in different age groups, its diurnal variation and the effect of muscular work on it. Acta Physiolog Scand 39, Suppl 132, 1956.
11. Deamer, W. C. : Pediatric allergy: some impressions gained over a 37-year period. Ped 48:930, 1971.
12. Berkovich, S. , et al.: The association of viral and mycoplasma infections with recurrence of wheezing in the asthmatic child. Ann All 28:43, 1970.
13. McIntosh, K. , et al.: The association of viral and bacterial respiratory infections with exacerbations of wheezing in young asthmatic children. J Ped 82:578, 1973.
14. Horn, E. C. , and Gregg, I. : Role of viral infection and host factors in acute episodes of asthma and chronic bronchitis. Chest 63:44s, 1973.
15. Minor, T. E. , et al.: Viruses as precipitants of asthmatic attacks in children. JAMA 227:292, 1974.
16. Mitchell, I. , Inglis, J. M. , and Simpson, H. : Viral infection as a precipitant of wheeze in children. Arch Dis Childh 53:106, 1978.
17. Ouellette, J. J. , and Reed, C. E. : Increased response of asthmatic subjects to methacholine after influenza vaccine. J All 36:558, 1965.

18. Kumar, L., et al.: Effect of live measles vaccine on bronchial sensitivity of asthmatic children to methacholine. J All 45:104, 1970.
19. Frick, O. L., German, D. F., and Mills, J.: Development of allergy in children I. Association with virus infections. J All Clin Immunol 63:228, 1979.
20. Friday, W. W., et al.: Airways function during mild viral respiratory illnesses. The effect of rhinovirus infection in cigarette smokers. Ann Int Med 80:150, 1974.
21. Ida, S., Hooks, J. J., Siraganian, R. P., and Notkins, A. L.: Enhancement of Ig-E mediated histamine release from human basophils by viruses: role of interferon. J Exp Med 145:892, 1977.
22. Minor, T. E., et al.: Greater frequency of viral respiratory infections in asthmatic children as compared with their nonasthmatic siblings. J Ped 85:472, 1974.
23. Flaherty, D. K., Martin, J. M., Storms, W. W., Kriz, R. J., Surfus, J. E., and Reed, C. E.: Antibody-dependent cellular cytotoxicity in asthmatics. J All Clin Immunol 59:48, 1977.
24. Phipatanakul, C. S., and Slavin, R. G.: Bronchial asthma produced by paranasal sinusitis. Arch Otolaryngol 100: 109, 1974.
25. Kiviloog, J.: Bronchial reactivity to exercise and methacholine in bronchial asthma. Scand J Resp Dis 54:347, 1973.
26. Patel, K. R., et al.: The effect of thymoxamine and cromolyn sodium on postexercise bronchoconstriction in asthma. J All Clin Imm 57:285, 1976.
27. Sly, R. M., et al.: Exercise-induced bronchospasm: effect of adrenergic or cholinergic blockade. J Allerg 40:93, 1967.
28. James, L., et al.: Effect of treadmill exercise on asthmatic children. J All Clin Imm, 57:408, 1976.
29. Bar-Or, O., Neuman, I., and Dotan, R.: Effects of dry and humid climates on exercise-induced asthma in children and preadolescents. J All Clin Immunol 60:163, 1977.
30. Shturman-Ellstein, R., Zeballos, R. J., Buckley, J. M., and Souhrada, J. F.: The beneficial effect of nasal breathing on exercise-induced bronchoconstriction. Am Rev Resp Dis 118:65, 1978.
31. Deal, E. C., Jr., McFadden, E. R., Jr., Ingram, R. H., Jr., Strauss, R. H., and Jaeger, J. J.: Role of respiratory heat exchange in production of exercise-induced asthma. J Appl Physiol 46:467, 1979.
32. Sly, R. M.: Effect of β-adrenoreceptor stimulants on exercise induced asthma. Pediatrics 56:910, 1975.

33. Air pollution in Donora, Pennsylvania: Epidemiology of the unusual smog episode of October, 1948. Pub Health Bull 306, 1949.

34. Ministry of Health: Mortality and morbidity during the London fog of December, 1952. Reports on Public Health and Related Subjects, No 95, London, 1954.

35. Spotnitz, M.: The significance of Yokohama asthma. Am Rev Resp Dis 92:371, 1965

36. Douglas, J. W. B., and Waller, R. E.: Air pollution and respiratory infection in children. Brit J Prev Soc Med 20: 1, 1966.

37. Colley, J. R. T.: Respiratory symptoms in children and parental smoking and phlegm production. Brit Med J 2:201, 1974.

38. Cammeron, Paul: The presence of pets and smoking as correlates of perceived disease. J All 40:12, 1967.

39. Bolin, J. F., Dahms, T. E., and Slavin, R. G.: Effects of passive smoking on asthma. J All Clin Immunol 63:151, 1979.

40. Purcell, K., et al.: The effect on asthma in children of experimental separation from the family. Psychosomat Med 31:144, 1969.

41. Stevenson, I.: Variations in the secretion of bronchial mucus during periods of life stress. Proc Assn Res Nerv Ment Dis 29:596, 1950

42. Stevenson, I., and Ripley, H. S.: Variations in respiration and in respiratory symptoms during changes in emotion. Psychosomat Med 14:476, 1952.

43. Freeman, E. H., et al.: Psychological variables in allergic disorders: a review. Psychosomat Med 26:543, 1964.

44. Falliers, C. J., et al.: Growth rate of children with intractable asthma. J All 32:420, 1961.

45. Falliers, C. J., et al.: Childhood asthma and steroid therapy as influences on growth. Am J Dis Chil 105:127, 1963.

46. Iliff, A., and Lee, V. A.: Pulse rate, respiratory rate, and body temperature of children between two months and eighteen years of age. Child Devel 23:237, 1952.

47. Miller, H. C.: Clinical evaluation of respiratory function in newborn infants. Ped Cl N A, Feb, 1957, p17

48. Waring, W. W.: "The history and physical examination," in Kendig, E. L., Jr. (ed.): Disorders of the Respiratory Tract in Children, 3rd edition, W. B. Saunders Co., Philadelphia, 1977, p77.

49. Azcuy, A., et al.: Experimentally induced barrel deformity of the chest in dogs. Am Rev Resp Dis 84:680, 1961.

50. Meredith, H.V.: The rhythm of physical growth. A study of eighteen anthropometric measurements on Iowa City white males ranging in age between birth and eighteen years. University of Iowa Studies. Studies in Child Welfare 11: 128, 1935.

51. Boynton, B.: The physical growth of girls. A study of the rhythm of physical growth from anthropometric measurements on girls between birth and eighteen years. University of Iowa Studies. Studies in Child Welfare 12:105, 1936.

52. Howatt, W.F., and DeMuth, G.R.: Configuration of the chest. Ped 35:177, 1965.

53. Adams, F. (translator): The genuine works of Hippocrates. 1:206, William Wood & Co., New York, 1891.

54. Sly, R.M., et al.: Objective assessment of minimal digital clubbing in asthmatic children. Ann All 30:575, 1972.

55. Waring, W.W., et al.: Quantitation of digital clubbing in children. Am Rev Resp Dis 104:166, 1971.

56. Laennec, R.T.H.: A treatise on the diseases of the chest and mediate auscultation. Translated by Forbes, J., 3rd ed., Thomas and Underwood, London, 1829.

57. Cammann, G.P., Self-adjusting stethoscope. N Y Med Times 4:140, 1855.

58. Alison, S.S.: Physical examination of the chest in pulmonary consumption. John Churchill, London, 1861.

59. Druger, G.: The Chest: Its signs and sounds. Humetrics Corporation, Los Angeles, 1973.

60. Rebuck, A.S., and Pengelly, L.D.: Development of pulsus paradoxus in the presence of airways obstruction. NEJM 288:66, 1973.

61. Knowles, G.K., and Clark, T.J.H.: Pulsus paradoxus as a valuable sign indicating severity of asthma. Lancet 2: 1356, 1973.

62. Lukens, J.N.: Eosinophilia in children. Ped Cl N A 19: 969, 1972.

63. Strang, L.B.: Eosinophilia in children with asthma and bronchiectasis. Brit Med J 1:167, 1960.

64. Lowell, F.C.: Clinical aspects of eosinophilia in atopic disease. JAMA 202:875, 1967.

65. Horn, B.R., et al.: Total eosinophil counts in the management of bronchial asthma. NEJM 292:1152, 1975.

66. Honsinger, R.W., Jr., et al.: The eosinophil and allergy. Why? J All Clin Imm 49:142, 1972.

67. Ohman, J.L., Jr., et al.: Effect of propranolol on the isoproterenol, responses of cortisol, isoproterenol, and aminophylline. J All Clin Imm 50:151, 1972.

68. Reed, C. E. , et al.: Reduced effect of epinephrine on circulating eosinophils in asthma and after beta-adrenergic
blockade or Bordetella pertussis vaccine. J All 46:90, 1970.
69. Epstein, R. L.: Constituents of sputum: a simple method.
Ann Int Med 77:259, 1972.
70. Dunnill, M. S.: The pathology of asthma, with special reference to changes in the bronchial mucosa. J Clin Path
13:27, 1960.
71. Pierce, C. H. , and Knox, A. W.: Ciliocytophthoria in sputum from patients with adenovirus infections. Proc Soc
Exp Biol Med 104:492, 1960.
72. Polgar, G. , and Promadhat, V.: Pulmonary function testing in children: techniques and standards. W. B. Saunders
Co. , Philadelphia, 1971.
73. Chai, H. , et al.: Therapeutic and investigational evaluation of asthmatic children. J All 41:23, 1968.
74. Comroe, J. H. , Jr. , Forster, R. E. , II, Du Bois, A. B. ,
Briscoe, W. A. , and Carlsen, E.: The lung, 2nd ed. ,
Year Book Med Pub, Inc. , Chicago, 1962.
75. Newball, H. H.: The unreliability of the maximal midex-
piratory flow as an index of acute airway changes. Chest
67:311, 1975.
76. Landau, L. I. , et al.: Factors determining the shape of
maximum expiratory flow-volume curves in childhood asthma. Aust N Z J Med 3:557, 1973.
77. Abboud, R. T. , and Morton, J. W.: Comparison of maximal mid-expiratory flow, flow volume curves, and nitrogen
closing volumes in patients with mild airway obstruction.
Am Rev Resp Dis 111:405, 1975.
78. Zapletal, A. , et al.: Maximum expiratory flow-volume
curves and airway conductance in children and adolescents.
J Appl Physiol 26:308, 1969.
79. Landau, L. I. , et al.: Contribution of inhomogeneity of
lung units to the maximal expiratory flow-volume curve in
children with asthma and cystic fibrosis. Am Rev Resp
Dis 111:725, 1975.
80. McFadden, E. R. , Jr.: The chronicity of acute attacks of
asthma-mechanical and therapeutic implications. J All
Clin Imm 56:18, 1975.
81. Posey, W. C. , and Tinkelman, D. G.: Dose response
characteristics of nebulized isoproterenol in asthmatic
children. J All Clin Immunol 63:258, 1979.
82. McFadden, E. R. , Jr. , et al.: Acute effects of inhaled isoproterenol on the mechanical characteristics of the lungs in
normal man. J Clin Invest 49:779, 1970.

83. Parker, C. D. , et al.: Methacholine aerosol as test for bronchial asthma. Arch Int Med 115:452, 1965.
84. Richards, W. , et al.: Status asthmaticus in children. JAMA 201:75, 1967.
85. Mansmann, H. C. , Jr.: Management of the child with bronchial asthma. Ped Cl N A 15:357, 1968.
86. Bierman, C. W. , and Pierson, W. E. : The pharmacologic management of status asthmaticus in children. Ped 54:245, 1974.
87. Waring, W. W. : "Diagnostic and therapeutic procedures, " in Kendig, E. L. , Jr. (ed): Disorders of the respiratory tract in children, 3rd edition, W. B. Saunders Co. , Philadelphia, 1977, p105.
88. Davis, R. H. , et al.: Capillary pH and blood gas determinations in asthmatic children. J All Clin Imm 56:33, 1975.
89. Siggaard-Andersen, O. : Blood acid-base alignment nomogram. Scand J Clin Lab Invest 15:211, 1963.
90. Filley, G. F. : Acid-base and blood gas regulation. Lea and Febiger, Philadelphia, 1971.
91. Simon, G. , et al.: Radiological abnormalities in children with asthma and their relation to the clinical findings and some respiratory function tests. Thorax 28:115, 1973.
92. Eggleston, P. A. , et al.: Radiographic abnormalities in acute asthma in children. Ped 54:442, 1974.
93. Felson, B.: Chest Roentgenology, W. B. Saunders Co. , Philadelphia, 1973.
94. Bierman, C. W. : Pneumomediastinum and pneumothorax complicating asthma in children. Am J Dis Chil 114:42, 1967.
95. Glass, W. M. , and Goodman, M. : Unsuspected foreign bodies in the young child's esophagus presenting with respiratory symptoms. Laryngoscope 76:605, 1966.
96. Hyde, J. S. , and Saed, A. M. : Acute bronchiolitis and the asthmatic child. J Asthma Res 4:137, 1966.
97. Phelan, P. D. , and Williams, H. E. : Sympathomimetic drugs in acute viral bronchiolitis. Ped 44:493, 1969.
98. McQuillan, J. , et al.: The use of cough/nasal swabs in the rapid diagnosis of respiratory syncitial virus infection by its fluorescent antibody technique. J Hyg 68:283, 1970.
99. Wittig, H. J. , et al.: The relationship between bronchiolitis and childhood asthma. J All 30:19, 1959.
100. Simon, G. , and Jordan, W. S. : Infections and allergic aspects of bronchiolitis. J Ped 70:533, 1967.
101. Rooney, J. C. , and Williams, H. E. : The relationship between proved viral bronchiolitis and subsequent wheezing. J Ped 79:744, 1971.

102. Moller, K. L.: The prognosis of bronchitis asthmatoides during the first year of life. Acta Paed 44:399, 1955.

103. Freeman, G. L., and Todd, R. H.: The role of allergy in viral respiratory tract infections. Am J Dis Child 104: 330, 1962.

104. Foucard, T., et al.: Virus serology and serum IgE levels in children with asthmatoid bronchitis. Acta Paed Scand 60:621, 1971.

105. Schwachman, H.: "Cystic fibrosis," in Kendig, E. L., Jr. (ed.): Disorders of the respiratory tract in children, 3rd edition, W. B. Saunders Co., Philadelphia, 1977, p760.

106. Gibson, L. E., and Cooke, R. E.: A test for concentration of electrolytes in sweat in cystic fibrosis of the pancreas utilizing pilocarpine by iontophoresis. Ped 23:545, 1959.

107. Patterson, R., et al.: Serum immunoglobulin levels in pulmonary allergic aspergillosis and certain other lung diseases, with special reference to immunoglobulin E. Am J Med 54:16, 1973.

108. Weiss, W. I., et al.: Hypersensitivity pneumonitis due to contamination of a home humidifier. J All 47:113, 1971.

109. Hodges, G. R., et al.: Hypersensitivity pneumonitis caused by a contaminated cool-mist vaporizer. Ann Int Med 80:501, 1974.

110. Fink, J. N.: Hypersensitivity pneumonitis: A case of mistaken identity. Hosp Pract 9:119, 1974.

111. Stiehm, E. R., and Fudenberg, H. H.: Serum levels of immune globulins in health and disease: A survey. Ped 37:715, 1966.

112. Talner, N. S.: Congestive heart failure in the infant. Ped Cl N A 18:1011, 1971.

113. Kueppers, F., and Black, L. F.: α_1 -antitrypsin and its deficiency. Am Rev Resp Dis 110:176, 1974.

114. Glasgow, J. F. T., et al.: Alpha$_1$ antitrypsin deficiency in association with both cirrhosis and chronic obstructive lung disease in two sibs. Am J Med 54:181, 1973.

115. Mathis, R. K., et al.: Alpha$_1$ -antitrypsin in the respiratory-distress syndrome. NEJM 288:59, 1973.

116. Euler, A. R., Byrne, W. J., Ament, M. E., Fonkalsrud, E. W., Strobel, C. T., Siegel, S. C., Katz, R. M., and Rachelefsky, G. S.: Recurrent pulmonary disease in children: a complication of gastroesophageal reflux. Ped 63:47, 1979.

117. Stein, M. R., Weber, R. W., and Towner, T. G.: The effect of theophylline on the lower esophageal sphincter pressure. J All Clin Immunol 61:137, 1978.

118. Mansfield, L. E., and Stein, M. R.: Gastroesophageal reflux and asthma: a possible reflex mechanism. Ann All 41:224, 1978.

119. Lecks, H. I., et al.: Newer concepts in occurrence of segmental atelectasis in acute bronchial asthma and status asthmaticus in children. J Asthma Res 4:65, 1966.

120. Lee, F. A., et al.: Unexpected chest radiograph findings in not acutely ill allergic children, quoted by Kravis, L. P.: The complications of acute asthma in children. Clin Ped 12:538, 1973.

121. Richards, W., and Patrick, J. R.: Death from asthma in children. Am J Dis Child 110:4, 1965.

122. Palm, C. R., et al.: A review of asthma admissions and deaths at Children's Hospital of Pittsburgh from 1935 to 1968. J All 46:257, 1970.

123. Buranakul, B., et al.: Causes of death during acute asthma in children. Am J Dis Child 128:343, 1974.

124. Ushinski, S. C., et al.: The effect of acidosis on the response of tracheal smooth muscle to aminophylline and acetylcholine. Pharmacologist 11:277, 1969.

125. Van Metre, T. E., Jr.: Adverse effects of inhalation of excessive amounts of nebulized isoproterenol in status asthmaticus. J All 43:101, 1969.

126. Conolly, M. E., et al.: Resistance to β -adrenoreceptor stimulants (a possible explanation for the rise in asthma deaths). Brit J Pharmacol 43:389, 1971.

127. Wood, D. W., et al.: A clinical scoring system for the diagnosis of respiratory failure. Am J Dis Child 123:227, 1972.

128. Wood, D. W., et al.: The management of respiratory failure in childhood status asthmaticus. Experience with 30 episodes and evaluation of a technique. J All 42:261, 1968.

129. Ahlquist, R. P.: A study of the adrenotropic receptors. Am J Physiol 153:586, 1948.

130. Lands, A. M., et al.: Differentiation of receptor systems activated by sympathomimetic amines. Nature 214:597, 1967.

131. Goodman, L. S., and Gilman, A.: The pharmacological basis of therapeutics, 3rd ed, MacMillan, New York, 1965.

132. Nelson, H. S.: The effect of ephedrine on the response to epinephrine in normal men. J All Clin Imm 51:191, 1973.

133. Tinkelman, D. G., and Avner, S. E.: Ephedrine therapy in asthmatic children. JAMA 237:553, 1977.

134. Conolly, M. E. , et al. : Metabolism of isoprenaline in dog and man. Brit J Pharmacol 46:458, 1972.
135. Keighley, J. F. : Iatrogenic asthma associated with adrenergic aerosols. Ann Int Med 65:985, 1966.
136. Reisman, R. E. : Asthma induced by adrenergic aerosols. J All 46:162, 1970.
137. Gazioglu, K. , et al. : Effect of isoproterenol on gas exchange during air and oxygen breathing in patients with asthma. Am J Med 50:185, 1971.
138. Murray, A. B. , et al. : Effect of isoproterenol and salbutamol aerosols in asthmatic children. J All Clin Imm 53:83, 1974.
139. Davis, C. , and Conolly, M. E. : Beta agonist resistance in human bronchial muscle. Clin Sci Mol Med 52:28p, 1977.
140. Galant, S. P. , Duriseti, L. , Underwood, S. , and Insel, P. A. : Decreased beta-adrenergic receptors on polymorphonuclear leukocytes after adrenergic therapy. New Eng J Med 299:933, 1978.
141. Jenne, J. W. , Chick, T. W. , Strickland, R. D. , and Wall, F. J. : Subsensitivity of beta responses during therapy with a long-acting beta-2 preparation. J All Clin Immunol 59:383, 1977.
142. Nelson, H. S. , Raine, D. , Jr. , Doner, H. C. , and Posey, W. C. : Subsensitivity to the bronchodilator action of albuterol produced by chronic administration. Am Rev Resp Dis 116:871, 1977.
143. Larsson, S. , et al. : Lack of bronchial beta adrenoreceptor resistance in asthmatics during long-term treatment with terbutaline. J All Clin Immunol 59:93, 1977.
144. Sackner, M. A. , Silva, G. , Zucker, C. , and Marks, M. B. : Long-term effects of metaproterenol in asthmatic children. Am Rev Resp Dis 115:945, 1978.
145. Fraser, P. M., et al. : The circumstances preceding death from asthma in young people in 1968 to 1969. Brit J Dis Chest 65:71, 1971.
146. Greenberg, M. J. : Isoprenaline in myocardial failure. Lancet ii:442, 1965.
147. Collins, J. M. , et al. : The cardio-toxicity of isoprenaline during hypoxia. Brit J Pharmacol 36:35, 1969.
148. Galant, S. P. , Groncy, C. E. , Duriseti, S. , and Strick, L. : The effect of metaproterenol in chronic asthmatic children receiving therapeutic doses of theophylline. J All Clin Immunol 61:73, 1978.
149. Arner, B. : A comparative clinical trial of different subcutaneous doses of terbutaline and orciprenaline in bronchial asthma. Acta Med Scand Suppl 512:45, 1970.

150. Formgren, H.: Clinical comparison of inhaled terbutaline and orciprenaline in asthmatic patients. Scand J Resp Dis 51:203, 1970.

151. Formgren, H.: A clinical comparison of the effect of oral terbutaline and orciprenaline. Scand J Resp Dis 51:195, 1970.

152. Weber, R. W. , Petty, W. E. , and Nelson, H. S.: Aerosolized terbutaline in asthmatics. J All Clin Immunol 63:116, 1979

153. Sly, R. M. , et al.: Comparison of subcutaneous terbutaline with epinephrine in the treatment of asthma in children. J All Clin Imm 59:128, 1977.

154. Leegaard, J. , and Fjulsrud, S.: Terbutaline in children with asthma. Arch Dis Childh 48:229, 1973.

155. Wolfe, J. D. , Tashkin, D. P. , Calvarese, B. , and Simmons, M.: Bronchodilator effects of terbutaline and aminophylline alone and in combination in asthmatic patients. New Eng J Med 298:363, 1978.

156. Walker, S. R. , et al.: The clinical pharmacology of oral and inhaled salbutamol. Clin Pharm Ther 13:861, 1972.

157. Harris, L.: Comparison of cardiorespiratory effects of terbutaline and salbutamol aerosols in patients with reversible airways obstruction. Thorax 28:592, 1973.

158. Holten, K.: Bronchodilator effect and effect on blood gases after subcutaneous injection and inhalation of terbutaline. Brit J Dis Chest 68:111, 1974.

159. Murray, A. B., et al.: The effects of pressurized isoproterenol and salbutamol in asthmatic children. Ped 54: 746, 1974.

160. Ritchie, J. M.: "Central nervous system stimulants. The xanthines", in Goodman, L. S. , and Gilman, A. (ed): The pharmacological basis of therapeutics, 5th ed. , MacMillan Pub Co. , New York, 1975.

161. Ellis, E. F. , and Eddy, E. D.: Anhydrous theophylline equivalence of commercial theophylline formulations. All Clin Imm 53:116, 1974.

162. Flora, A. R.: Comparison of theophylline blood levels. tablet vs. liquids. Curr Ther Res 12:611, 1970.

163. Koyosooko, R. , et al.: Effect of ethanol on theophylline absorption in humans. J Pharmaceut Sci 64:299, 1975.

164. Cohen, A. , et al.: A rapidly dissolving theophylline tablet. Curr Ther Res 17:497, 1975.

165. Yunginger, J. W. , et al.: Serum theophylline levels and control of asthma following rectal theophylline. Ann All 24:469, 1966.

166. Armand, J. , et al.: La toxicite de la theophylline chez l'enfant. Lyon Med 229:485, 1973.

167. Ellis, E. F. , et al. : Pharmacokinetics of theophylline in asthmatic children. J All Clin Imm 53:79, 1974.
168. Jenne, J. W. , et al. : Effect of congestive heart failure on the elimination of theophylline. J All Clin Imm 53:80, 1974.
169. Mangione, A. , et al. : Pharmacokinetics of theophylline in hepatic disease. Chest 73:616, 1978.
170. Vallner, J. J. , et al. : Effect of pH on the binding of theophylline to serum proteins. Am Rev Resp Dis 120:83, 1979.
171. Chang, K. C. , et al. : Altered theophylline pharmacokinetics during acute respiratory viral illness. Lancet 1: 1132, 1978.
172. Weinberger, M. , et al. : Inhibition of theophylline clearance by troleandomycin. J All Clin Immunol 59: 228, 1977.
173. Kozak, P. P. , Jr. , et al. : Administration of erythromycin to patients on theophylline. J All Clin Immunol 60: 149, 1977.
174. Powell, J. R. , et al. : The influence of cigarette smoking and sex on theophylline disposition. Am Rev Resp Dis 116:17, 1977.
175. Kappas, A. , et al. : Effect of charcoal-broiled beef on antipyrine and theophylline metabolism. Clin Pharm Ther 23:445, 1978.
176. Conney, A. H. , et al. : Nutrition and chemical biotransformation in man. Clin Pharm Ther 22:707, 1977.
177. Landay, R. A. , et al. : Effect of phenobarbital on theophylline disposition. J All Clin Immunol 62:27, 1978.
178. Piafsky, K. M. , et al. : Effect of phenobarbital on the disposition of intravenous theophylline. Clin Pharm Ther 22:336, 1977.
179. Sheen, A. E. , et al. : Comparison of serum theophylline concentrations measured by high pressure liquid chromatography and quantitative enzyme-multiplied immunoassay technique. Ann All 42:77, 1979.
180. Wyatt, R. , et al. : Oral theophylline dosage for the management of chronic asthma. J Ped 92:125, 1978.
181. Gal, P. , et al. : Theophylline disposition in obesity. Clin Pharm Ther 23:438, 1978.
182. Hendeles, L. , et al. : Guide to oral theophylline therapy for the treatment of chronic asthma. Am J Dis Child 132: 876, 1978.
183. Sheen, A. , and Sly, R. M. : Serum theophylline concentrations in asthmatic children. Ann All 41:327, 1978.

184. Hein, E., et al.: Simultaneous use of rapidly absorbed and sustained release theophylline preparations in children. Ann All 43:217, 1979.
185. Taylor, W. F., et al.: Ephedrine and theophylline in asthmatic children: quantitative observations on the combination and ephedrine tachyphylaxis. Ann All 23:437, 1965.
186. Badiei, B., et al.: Effect of theophylline, ephedrine and their combination upon exercise-induced airway obstruction. Ann All 35:32, 1975.
187. Boat, T. F., and Doershuk, C. F.: "Defense mechanisms of the respiratory tract," in Lough, M. D., Doershuk, C. F., and Stern, R. C.: Pediatric respiratory therapy. Year Book Med Pub., Chicago, 1974, p 19.
188. Blanshard, G.: The viscometry of sputum. Arch Middlesex Hosp 5:222, 1955.
189. Baker, J. W., et al.: Elevated antidiuretic hormone levels during status asthmaticus. J All Clin Imm 53:101, 1974.
190. Cambar, P. J., and Aviado, D. M.: Bronchopulmonary effects of paraquat and expectorants. Arch Environ Health 20:488, 1970.
191. Falliers, C. J., et al.: Controlled study of iodotherapy for childhood asthma. J All 38:183, 1966.
192. Siegal, S.: The asthma-suppressive action of potassium iodide. J All 35:252, 1964.
193. Bernecker, C.: Intermittent therapy with potassium iodide in chronic obstructive disease of the airways. Acta Allergol 24:216, 1969.
194. Dolan, T. F., Jr., and Gibson, L. E.: Complication of iodide therapy in patients with cystic fibrosis. J Ped 79:684, 1971.
195. Vagenakis, A. G., et al.: Control of thyroid hormone secretion in normal subjects receiving iodides. J Clin Invest 52:528, 1973.
196. Block, S. H.: Goiter complicating therapy with iodinated glycerol (Organidin). J Ped 83:84, 1973.
197. Hirsch, S. R., et al.: Sputum liquefying agents: A comparative in vitro evaluation. J Lab Clin Med 74:346, 1969.
198. Webb, W. R., and Degerli, I. V.: Acetylcysteine as a mucolytic agent in clinical practice. Clin Med 71:1531, 1964.
199. Morrow, P. E.: Aerosol characterization and deposition. Am Rev Resp Dis 110:88, 1974.
200. Baxter, J. D., and Forsham, P. H.: Tissue effects of glucocorticoids. Am J Med 53:573, 1972.
201. Schayer, R. W., et al.: Inhibition by cortisone of the binding of new histamine in rat tissues. Proc Soc Exper Biol Med 87:590, 1954.

202. Logsdon, P. J., et al.: Stimulation of leukocyte adenyl cyclase by hydrocortisone and isoproterenol in asthmatic and nonasthmatic subjects. J All Clin Imm 50:45, 1972.

203. Coffey, R. G., et al.: Increased adenosine triphosphatase activity in leukocytes of asthmatic children. J Clin Invest 54:138, 1974.

204. Mano, K., et al.: The effect of hydrocortisone on beta adrenergic receptors in lung tissue. J All Clin Immunol 63:147, 1979.

205. Ignarro, L. J., and Cech, S. Y.: Lysosomal enzyme secretion from human neutrophils mediated by cyclic GMP: inhibition of cyclic GMP accumulation and neutrophil function by glucocorticosteroids. J Cyclic Nucleotide Res 1: 283, 1975.

206. Morris, H. G.: "Corticosteroids in asthma", in Frazier, C. A., (ed): Annual Review of allergy 1972. Med. Exam. Pub. Co., Inc., Flushing, N. Y., 1973, p 104.

207. Peterson, R. E., et al.: The physiological disposition and metabolic fate of hydrocortisone in man. J Clin Invest 34:1779, 1955.

208. Morris, H. G., et al.: Effect of oral prednisone on the measurement of plasma steroid concentrations by the competitive protein-binding radioassay. J Ped 85:248, 1974.

209. Dwyer, J., et al.: A study of cortisol metabolism in patients with chronic asthma. Austr Ann Med 16:297, 1967.

210. Siegel, S. C.: ACTH and the corticosteroids in the management of allergic disorders in children. J Ped 66:927, 1965.

211. Lieberman, P., et al.: Complication of long-term steroid therapy for asthma. J All Clin Imm 49:329, 1972.

212. Siegel, S. C., et al.: Adrenal function in allergy. III. Effect of prolonged intermittent steroid therapy in allergic children. Ped 24:434, 1959.

213. Boss, N., et al.: Quantitative assay of the suppressive effect of synthetic corticoids in man. Evaluation of the circadian rhythm of serum cortisol after single oral dose of fluocortolone and prednisolone. Acta Endocrinol 67: 508, 1971.

214. Morris, H. G., and Jorgensen, J. R.: Recovery of endogenous pituitary-adrenal function in corticosteroid-treated children. J Ped 79:480, 1971.

215. Hayes, M. A., and Kushlan, S. D.: Influence of hormonal treatment for ulcerative colitis upon the course of surgical treatment. Gastroent 30:75, 1956.

216. Graber, A. L., et al.: Natural history of pituitary-adrenal recovery following long-term suppression with corticosteroids. J Clin Endocrinol 25:11, 1965.

217. Plumpton, F. S. , and Besser, G. M. : The adrenocortical response to surgery and insulin-induced hypoglycemia in corticosteroid-treated and normal subjects. Brit J Surg 56:216, 1969.

218. Liddle, G. W. , et al. : Clinical application of a new test of pituitary reserve. J Clin Endocrinol Metab 19:875, 1959.

219. Zachmann, M. : Long term corticosteroid treatment and growth. Resp Suppl 27:244, 1970.

220. Reimer, L. G. , et al. : Growth of asthmatic children during treatment with alternate-day steroids. J All Clin Imm 55:224, 1975.

221. Friedman, M. , and Strang, L. B. : Effect of long-term corticosteroids and corticotrophin on the growth of children. Lancet ii:568, 1966.

222. Wright, W. C. , et al. : Effects of synthetic ACTH on cortocosteroid-induced growth suppression. J All Clin Imm 53:52, 1974.

223. Daly, J. R. , and Glass, D. : Corticosteroid and growth-hormone response to hypoglycemia in patients on long-term treatment with corticotrophin. Lancet 1:476, 1971.

224. Svedmyr, N. , et al. : Relaxing effect of ACTH on human bronchial muscle in vitro. Scand J Resp Dis 51:171, 1970.

225. Rosenblum, A. H. , and Rosenblum, P. : Anaphylactic reactions to adrenocorticotropic hormone in children. J Ped 64:387, 1964.

226. Mendelson, L. M. , et al. : Anaphylaxis-like reactions to corticosteroid therapy. J All Clin Imm 54:125, 1974.

227. El-Shaboury, A. H. : Effect of a synthetic corticotropic polypeptide on adrenal function in hypersensitive asthmatics. Lancet 1:298, 1965.

228. Easton, J. G. , et al. : Effect of alternate-day steroid administration on adrenal function in allergic children. J All Clin Imm 48:355, 1971.

229. Kumar, L. , et al. : Plasma 17-OH corticosteroid concentrations in children with asthma. J Ped 79:955, 1971.

230. Morris, H. G. , et al. : Plasma steroid concentrations during alternate-day treatment with prednisone. J All Clin Imm 54:350, 1974.

231. Siegel, S. C. , et al. : Adrenal function in allergy. IV. Effect of dexamethasone aerosols in asthmatic children. Ped. 33:245, 1964.

232. Klein, R. , et al. : Treatment of chronic childhood asthma with beclomethasone dipropionate aerosol: I. A double-blind crossover trial in nonsteroid-dependent patients. Ped 60:7, 1977.

233. Sly, R. M. , et al.: Treatment of asthma in children with triamcinolone acetonide aerosol. J All Clin Immunol 62: 76, 1978.

234. Gaddie, J. , et al.: Aerosol beclomethasone dipropionate: a dose-response study in chronic bronchial asthma. Lancet ii:280, 1973.

235. Wyatt, R. , et al.: Effects of inhaled beclomethasone dipropionate and alternate day prednisone on pituitary-adrenal function in children with chronic asthma. New Eng J Med 299:1387, 1978.

236. Mellis, C. M. , and Phelan, P. D.: Asthma deaths in children - a continuing problem. Thorax 32:29, 1977.

237. Andersson, E. , and Smidt, C. M.: An investigation of the bronchial mucous membrane after long-term treatment with beclomethasone dipropionate (Becotide). Acta Allergol 29:354, 1974.

238. Altounyan, R. E. C.: Inhibition of experimental asthma by a new compound, disodium cromoglycate, Intal. Acta Allergol 22:487, 1967.

239. Cox, J. S. G.: Disodium cromoglycate (FPL-670) ("Intal") A specific inhibitor of reaginic antibody-antigen mechanisms. Nature 216:1328, 1967.

240. Blair, A. M. J. N. , and Woods, A.: The effects of isoprenaline, atropine and disodium cromoglycate on ciliary motility and mucous flow measured in vivo in cats. Brit J Pharmacol 35:379, 1969.

241. Clarke, P. S.: Effect of disodium cromoglycate on exacerbations of asthma produced by hyperventilation. Brit Med J i:317, 1971.

242. Sly, R. M.: Effect of cromolyn sodium on exercise-induced airway obstruction in asthmatic children. Ann Allergy 29:362, 1971.

243. Breslin, A. B. X. , and Pepys, J.: Effect of sodium cromoglycate on asthmatic reactions to environmental temperature changes. Clin All 5:325, 1975.

244. Pepys, J. , et al.: Inhibitory effects of disodium cromoglycate on allergen-inhalation tests. Lancet 2:137, 1968.

245. Woenne, R. , et al.: Sodium cromoglycate-induced changes in the dose-response curve of inhaled methacholine and histamine in asthmatic children. Am Rev Resp Dis 119: 927, 1979.

246. Cox, J. S. G.: Administration of disodium cromoglycate. Brit Med J ii:634, 1969.

247. Cox, J. S. G.: Disodium cromoglycate. Brit Med J iii: 177, 1969.

248. Marks, M. B.: Cromolyn sodium prophylaxis in asthmatic children under five. Ann All 39:306, 1977.

249. Hiller, E. J. , et al.: Nebulized sodium cromoglycate in young asthmatic children. Arch Dis Childhood 52:875, 1977.
250. Dahl, R. , and Henriksen, J. M.: Inhibition of exercise-induced bronchoconstriction by nebulized sodium cromoglycate in patients with bronchial asthma. Scand J Resp Dis 60:51, 1979.
251. Lobel, H. , et al.: Pulmonary infiltrates with eosinophilia in asthmatic patient treated with disodium cromoglycate. Lancet ii:1032, 1972.
252. Levin, S. J.: β -dimethylaminoethyl benzhydryl ether hydrochloride (Benadryl). Its use in allergic diseases. J All 17:145, 1946.
253. Hawkins, D. F.: Bronchoconstrictor and bronchodilator actions of antihistamine drugs. Brit J Pharmacol 10:230, 1955.
254. Bidwell, S. M. R. , and Boyd, E. M.: Diphenhydramine hydrochloride, U. S. P. XIV, and respiratory tract fluid. J Pharmacol Exper Ther 104:224, 1952.
255. Booij-Noord, H. , et al.: Protection tests on bronchial allergen challenge with disodium cromoglycate and thiazinamium. J All 46:1, 1970.
256. Karlin, J. M.: The use of antihistamines in asthma. Ann All 30:342, 1972.
257. Karlin, J. M.: The use of antihistamines in allergic disease. Ped Cl N A 22:157, 1975.
258. Lorin, M. I. , and Denning, C. R.: Evaluation of postural drainage by measurement of sputum volume and consistency. Am J Phys Med 50:215, 1971.
259. Motoyama, E. K.: "Assessment of lower airway obstruction in cystic fibrosis", in Mangos, J. A. , and Talamo, R. C. (ed): Fundamental problems in cystic fibrosis and related diseases, Intercontinental Med Book Corp. , New York, 1973, p 335.
260. Huber, A. L. , et al.: Effect of chest physiotherapy on asthmatic children. J All Clin Imm 53:109, 1974.
261. Feldman, J. , et al.: Maximal expiratory flows after postural drainage. Am Rev Resp Dis 119:239, 1979.
262. Fitch, K. D. , and Morton, A. R.: Specificity of exercise in exercise-induced asthma. Brit Med J 4:577, 1971.
263. Sly, R. M. , et al.: The effect of physical conditioning upon asthmatic children. Ann All 30:86, 1972.
264. Siegel, S. C. , and Richards, W.: Status asthmaticus in children. Int Anesthesiol Cl 9:99, 1971.
265. Hendeles, L. , et al.: Monitoring serum theophylline levels. Clin Pharmacolinetics 3:294, 1978.

266. Shannon, D. C. , et al.: Prevention of apnea and bradycardia in low-birth weight infants. Ped 55:589, 1975.
267. Winter, P. M. , and Smith, G. : The toxicity of oxygen.
Anesthesiol 37:210, 1972.
268. Arnold, W. H. , Jr. , and Grant, J. L. : Oxygen-induced
hypoventilation. Am Rev Resp Dis 95:255, 1967.
269. Melville, G. N. , and Ward, E. E. : Variation in forced
expiratory volume curves of asthmatic patients with increased water content. Rev All 25:506, 1971.
270. Moore, R. B. , et al.: The effect of intermittent positive
pressure breathing on airway resistance in normal and
asthmatic children. J All Clin Imm 49:137, 1972.
271. Streeton, J. A. , and Morgan, E. B. : Salbutamol in status
asthmaticus and severe chronic obstructive bronchitis.
Postgrad Med J Suppl 47:125, 1971.
272. Collins, J. V. , et al.: Intravenous corticosteroids in
treatment of acute bronchial asthma. Lancet ii:1047, 1970.
273. Ellul-Micallef, R. , and Fenech, F. F. : Intravenous prednisolone in chronic bronchial asthma. Thorax 30:312, 1975.
274. Beam, L. R. , et al.: Medically irreversible status
asthmaticus in children. JAMA 194:968, 1965.
275. Downes, J. J. , and Wood, D. W. : "Mechanical ventilation
in the management of status asthmaticus in children", in
Eckenhoff, J. E. (ed): Science and practice in anesthesia,
J. B. Lippincott Co. , Philadelphia, 1965, p 141.
276. Mansmann, H. C. , Jr. , et al.: Controlled ventilation
with muscle paralysis in status asthmaticus. Ann All 25:
11, 1967.
277. Radford, E. P. , Jr. , et al.: Clinical use of a nomogram
to estimate proper ventilation during artificial respiration.
NEJM 251:877, 1954.
278. Cotton, E. K. , and Parry, W. : Treatment of status asthmaticus and respiratory failure. Ped Cl N A 22:163, 1975.
279. McLaughlin, A. P. , III, et al.: Hazards of gallamine administration in patients with renal failure. J Urol 108:
515, 1972.
280. Levin, N. , and Dillon, J. B. : Status asthmaticus and pancuronium bromide. JAMA 222:1265, 1972.
281. Wood, D. W. , et al.: Intravenous isoproterenol in the
management of respiratory failure in childhood status
asthmaticus. J All Clin Imm 50:75, 1972.
282. Wood, D. W. , and Downes, J. J. : Intravenous isoproterenol
in the treatment of respiratory failure in childhood status
asthmaticus. Ann All 31:607, 1973.
283. Kurland, G. , et al.: Fatal myocardial toxicity during
continuous infusion intravenous isoproterenol therapy of
asthma. J All Clin Immunol 63:407, 1979.

284. Matson, J. R. , et al.: Myocardial ischemia complicating the use of isoproterenol in asthmatic children. J Ped 92: 776, 1978.
285. Bloomfield, P. , et al.: Comparison of salbutamol given intravenously and by intermittent positive-pressure breathing in life threatening asthma. Brit Med J 1:848, 1979.
286. Tinkelman, D. G. , et al.: The impact of chronic asthma on the developing child: Observations made in a group setting. Ann All 37:174, 1976.
287. Rackemann, F. M. , and Edwards, M. C.: Asthma in children: A follow-up study of 688 patients after an interval of 20 years. NEJM 246:815, 1952.
288. Buffum, W. P. , and Settipane, G. A.: Prognosis of asthma in childhood. Am J Dis Child 112:214, 1966.
289. Williams, H., and McNicol, K. N.: Prevalence, natural history, and relationship of wheezy bronchitis and asthma in children. An epidemiological study. Brit Med J 4:321, 1969.
290. Johnstone, D. E.: A study of the natural history of bronchial asthma in children. Am J Dis Child 115:213, 1968.
291. Johnstone, D. E., and Crump, L.: Value of hyposensitization therapy for perennial bronchial asthma in children. Ped 27:39, 1961.
292. Ryssing, E.: Continued follow-up investigation concerning the fate of 298 asthmatic children. Acta Paediat 48: 255, 1959.

CHAPTER IV | ALLERGIC RHINITIS

In the second century, A. D., Galen observed that some individuals always sneezed in the presence of certain plants, and the Persian physician, Rhazes, described seasonal rhinitis in the tenth century.[1] John Bostock, a London physician, established seasonal allergic rhinitis as a clinical entity in 1819 with a description of his own symptoms,[2] and in 1828 he introduced the term 'hay fever'.[3]

'Hay fever' remains the commonest term used for seasonal allergic rhinitis; other terms include summer or autumnal catarrh, rose fever, and pollinosis. Since it is rarely caused by hay and fever is not one of its signs, seasonal allergic rhinitis is a better term to distinguish it from perennial allergic rhinitis.

PATHOGENESIS

Sensitization of subjects genetically predisposed to atopy follows ingestion or inhalation of antigen. With reexposure antigen reacts with specific IgE antibody fixed to the surface of mast cells, which are found in abundance just beneath the nasal epithelium. This sets up a chain of biochemical events leading to the release of the chemical mediators of Type I anaphylactic reactions (see Chapter II). Histamine may be the most important of these for eliciting signs and symptoms of allergic rhinitis because exogenous histamine is known to cause the local vascular dilatation and edema typical of allergic rhinitis and antihistamines are effective in the treatment of allergic rhinitis. Increased kinin-like activity has been found in nasal secretions of subjects with allergic rhinitis and may also contribute to the vasodilation and increased capillary permeability.[4] Release of eosinophil chemotactic factor of anaphylaxis probably accounts for the characteristic nasal eosinophilia.

Submucosal edema and infiltration by eosinophils and fewer neutrophils are the changes usually evident in biopsy specimens obtained during exacerbations of allergic rhinitis.[5] Changes in staining properties of the mucopolysaccharide ground substance and basement membrane which are related to the duration and severity of the allergic reaction have been ascribed to changes in the colloidal state due to increases in tissue water.[6]

Repeated inhalation of an allergen, such as that which occurs during a pollen season, has been found to have a priming effect upon the nasal mucosa of subjects with allergic rhinitis, decreasing the threshold at which a challenge dose elicits nasal congestion. The effect may persist several weeks beyond the end of a pollen season and seems to be nonspecific, lowering the threshold for unrelated allergens which otherwise would elicit no symptoms.[7]

SYMPTOMATOLOGY
AND MEDICAL HISTORY

Symptoms of allergic rhinitis include nasal congestion, nasal discharge, sneezing, and nasal itching. The nasal discharge is usually clear and watery unless superimposed infection is present, but an unusually extreme abundance of eosinophils can also cause discoloration. Headache or pain over the paranasal sinuses may be present. Some children complain of itching of the throat or soft palate, and parents may complain that the child makes a clicking sound in his throat to relieve this itching. Drainage of the nasal discharge into the pharynx may cause frequent attempts to clear the throat or a dry cough or hoarseness due to laryngeal irritation. Aspiration of copious secretions may cause a loose cough, productive of mucus which is usually swallowed. Vomiting of mucoid material may follow swallowing of copious amounts of mucus.

Symptoms of allergic conjunctivitis are often associated with those of allergic rhinitis, especially when due to allergy to pollen. These include conjunctival itching and injection, excessive lacrimation, and edema of the eyelids and periorbital tissues.

Parents or others often ascribe the symptoms of allergic rhinitis to frequent or "constant colds", but the history of frequent or repetitive sneezing and nasal itching or associated symptoms of allergic conjunctivitis identify the basic problem as allergy rather than infection.

Frequent nasal obstruction may foster habitual mouth breathing, and there is evidence that temporary interruption of nasal ventilation is itself a cause of nasal obstruction, especially in subjects with allergic rhinitis.[8]

Patients sometimes report that assuming the recumbent position or chilling has aggravated nasal obstruction, and these responses are also known to be more extreme than normal in subjects with allergic rhinitis. [8]

In different children the symptoms vary in number, intensity, duration and pattern, depending upon the degree of hypersensitivity and extent of exposure to the offending allergen (see Chapters IX and XII).

PHYSICAL FINDINGS

Abnormal physical findings are restricted to the nose and face in uncomplicated allergic rhinitis (Figs. 4.1 A-G)

The nasal mucosa usually appears pale or blue, although soon after the onset of the allergic reaction it may appear red. The nasal turbinates are often enlarged, and the obstruction due to the engorged turbinates may alternate from one nostril to the other within hours or minutes, tending to involve the dependent nostril when the subject is lying on one side. Submucosal edema may cause a more or less prominent swelling at the floor of the nostril, the fourth turbinate, recognized by Rosenbaum as a sign of allergic rhinitis (Fig. 4.1 A). The turbinates may glisten with the clear discharge covering their surfaces, or a more profuse watery or mucoid discharge may be present. Mouth breathing may be due to enlarged adenoids even when nasal turbinates do not completely obstruct the airway. Tonsils are also often enlarged.

A blue or black discoloration may be evident in the orbito-palpebral grooves beneath the lower eyelids - 'allergic shiners' (Fig. 4.1 F). This has been ascribed to venous stasis due either to communication of veins draining the tissues beneath the lower eyelids with veins in the nasal cavity which can be partially obstructed by mucosal edema or to spasm of the musculus tarsalis in the lower lid. [9] Edema of the lower lids may also occur from severe, prolonged edema of the nasal mucosa. Through similar mechanisms it has been suggested that impairment of venous drainage and arterial blood flow may cause underdevelopment of sinuses, zygoma, and the nasal process of the maxilla, resulting in the flat face which results from chronic perennial allergic rhinitis. [9] It has been suggested that malocclusion and a high, arched, V-shaped palate may also be consequences of chronic edema of the nasal mucosa in infancy with venous stasis causing local tissue changes in the alveolar and palatal bones and adjacent muscles (Fig. 4.1 D). [10]

Gingival hyperplasia can result from chronic mouth breathing in children with perennial allergic rhinitis. [11]

A wrinkle just beneath the lower lids present from early infancy has been associated with the presence of allergic rhinitis, asthma, and atopic dermatitis (Dennie's line) (Fig. 4.1 E). [12]

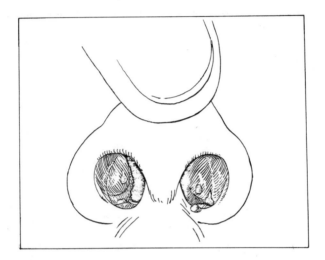

Fig. 4-1A. The allergic facies and signs of allergic rhinitis. Enlarged inferior turbinates with muco-serous discharge and 'fourth turinates' at floor of nostrils.

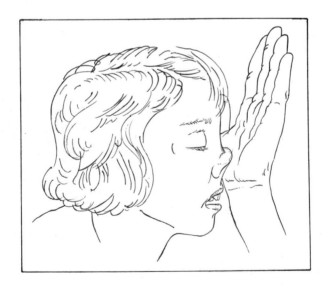

Fig. 4-1B. The allergic facies and signs of allergic rhinitis. Allergic salute.

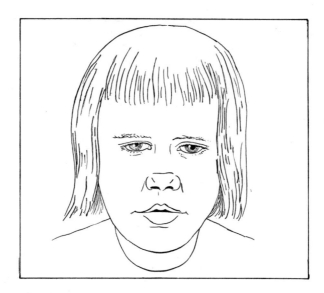

Fig. 4-1C. The allergic facies and signs of allergic rhinitis. Transverse nasal crease.

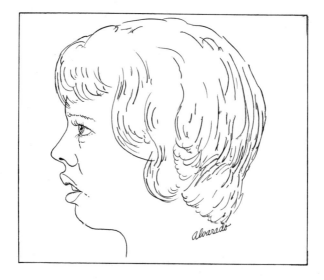

Fig. 4-1D. The allergic facies and signs of allergic rhinitis. Mouth breathing and malocclusion.

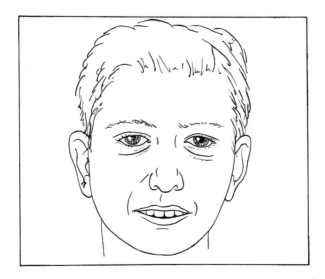

Fig. 4-1E. The allergic facies and signs of allergic
rhinitis. Dennie's lines beneath lower eyelids.

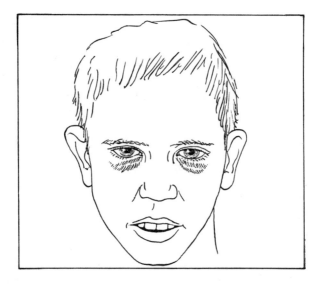

Fig. 4-1F. The allergic facies and signs of allergic
rhinitis. Allergic shiners.

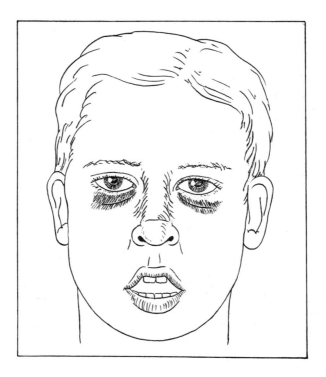

Fig. 4-1G. The allergic facies and signs of allergic rhinitis.

Nasal itching causes grimacing, nose wrinkling, and the allergic salute, an efficient maneuver in which the palm or heel of the hand is used to push the tip of the nose upward and backwards, temporarily improving the airway, relieving the itching, and wiping away the nasal discharge. After the allergic salute has been practiced regularly for about 2 years a transverse nasal crease may become evident at the juncture of the bulbous tip of the nose and the more rigid bridge (Fig. 4.1 C).13 Initially present only as a crease, it can later become a horizontal hypopigmented or hyperpigmented groove. This transverse nasal crease is pathognomonic of allergic rhinitis, but must be differentiated from the familial transverse nasal groove, inherited as a mendelian dominant and unrelated to allergy.14 The hereditary groove is not obliterated by downward pressure on the tip of the nose, unlike the acquired crease or groove.

Conjunctival injection or edema may also be present.

LABORATORY FINDINGS

EOSINOPHILIA

Mild or moderate peripheral eosinophilia can occur in subjects with seasonal allergic rhinitis during the offending pollen season, but total eosinophil counts rarely exceed 800 per cubic mm. and may remain entirely normal.[15] For normal values and other causes of eosinophilia see Chapter III. Mild peripheral eosinophilia has been reported in normal infants during their first 1 1/2 months (mean 521 per cubic mm at 6-7 weeks), but this returns to normal by 2-3 months of age.[16]

NASAL SECRETION CYTOLOGY

The presence of more than 3-10% eosinophils in nasal secretions is reported in both allergic rhinitis and "nonallergic rhinitis," a clinically similar condition in which specific allergens cannot be implicated. As many as 30% of normal newborns have been found to have nasal eosinophilia, and although this usually subsides by 3 months of age, in rare infants it has continued at least until 10 months of age.[16,17] Examination of nasal smears is especially helpful in differentiating allergic rhinitis from upper respiratory infections because nasal secretions may appear purulent due to an abundance of either eosinophils or neutrophils.[15]

A specimen of nasal secretions suitable for examination can be obtained by asking a cooperative child to sneeze or to blow his nose on waxed paper or cellophane. If a specimen cannot be obtained in this way, a cotton-tipped applicator can be used to swab the nasal mucosa or secretions can be obtained by aspiration with a small, rubber bulb syringe or feeding tube. The specimen is transferred to a glass slide, gently teased out to facilitate staining and examination, and dried. The smear is covered with Hansel's stain* and allowed to stand 20-30 seconds. Distilled water is than added for 30 seconds. The stain is then poured off, and the slide is flooded with distilled water to remove excess stain. The slide is then flooded with 95% ethyl or methyl alcohol, drained, and dried.

Wright stain is suitable for identification of eosinophils in peripheral blood but not for nasal smears.

Eosinophils with their red staining granules are readily distinguished from blue-stained neutrophils. Since the specimen is not uniform the entire slide should be scanned initially, and

* Lide Laboratories, Inc., 515 Timberwyck, St. Louis, Missouri 63131.

the presence of clumps of eosinophils reported. If the numbers of eosinophils and neutrophils in 10 representative fields are reported an estimate of the proportion of eosinophils can be made. The presence of clumps or more than 3-10% eosinophils usually indicates allergic rhinitis. During periods of intense exposure to allergen most of the cells are often eosinophils.

Absence of eosinophils in the nasal smear does not rule out allergic rhinitis. During upper respiratory infections in children with allergic rhinitis neutrophils predominate in nasal smears and eosinophils may be absent. Eosinophils are also present when there has been no recent exposure to the offending allergen. Although nasal eosinophilia has been reported in most children with allergic rhinitis due to hypersensitivity to inhalant allergens, it may occur much less frequently in those with allergic rhinitis due only to food allergy.[18]

ROENTGENOGRAMS
OF PARANASAL SINUSES

Radiographs may show some increased density over maxillary antra and ethmoid sinuses due to edema of the mucous membranes such as that seen in the nose itself.

PULMONARY FUNCTION
TESTING

Most routine pulmonary function tests are normal in subjects with uncomplicated allergic rhinitis, but inhalation of methacholine can be followed by increases in airway obstruction less extreme than those seen in asthmatics and involving especially the small, peripheral airways.[19] Exercise has also been found to elicit airway obstruction in some children with allergic rhinitis, changes which are again less extreme than those observed in asthmatics following similar exercise (see Chapter III).[20] It is possible that such responses may prove useful in identifying those patients at risk for the development of asthma.

Significantly increased airway resistance has been reported in nonasthmatic subjects with allergic rhinitis.[21]

IMMUNOGLOBULIN E

Total serum IgE concentrations are usually normal in children with uncomplicated allergic rhinitis. See Chapter XIII for the significance of identification of specific allergens by the radioallergosorbent test.

ALLERGY SKIN TESTING

Specific allergens can be identified by allergy skin testing. Techniques, interpretation and limitations are discussed in Chapter XIII.

DIFFERENTIAL DIAGNOSIS

The diagnosis of allergic rhinitis is usually easily established from the typical history and physical findings and confirmed by the presence of nasal eosinophilia. When symptoms are not seasonal and not clearly related to exposure to a common allergen other possible diagnoses must be considered.

INFECTIOUS RHINITIS

Upper respiratory tract infection is the commonest condition which must be differentiated from allergic rhinitis, and infections can be superimposed upon allergic rhinitis. Features which tend to lessen the likelihood of infection include absence of fever, absence of illness in the rest of the family or other contacts, absence of a purulent nasal discharge after the first few days and absence of cervical lymphadenopathy. Other characteristics favoring the diagnosis of allergic rhinitis include a family history of atopic diseases; seasonal exacerbations or symptoms which have been persistent or recurrent with more than 6 exacerbations each year, each more than 7-10 days or less than 3 days in duration; nasal itching and repetitive sneezing; pale rather than red nasal mucosa and a transverse nasal crease; nasal eosinophilia; and relief following use of antihistamines.

NONALLERGIC RHINITIS

"Nonallergic rhinitis" is a term applied to patients in whom no specific allergen can be implicated despite other findings consistent with perennial allergic rhinitis. It is much more common in adults than children. Nasal eosinophilia is usually found. Immunotherapy is ineffective, but symptoms usually respond to antihistamines.

SINUSITIS

Acute, suppurative sinusitis is characterized by fever, nasal congestion, purulent discharge draining into the middle meatus or from above the middle turbinate, pain and tenderness over the involved sinuses, usually starting 3-5 days after an upper respiratory infection. Acute suppurative sinusitis almost always responds to treatment with a topical vasoconstrictor and an appropriate systemic antibiotic.

Recurrent or chronic sinusitis may be more difficult to differentiate from perennial allergic rhinitis and can occur as a complication of allergic rhinitis. Symptoms include nasal obstruction, rhinorrhea, postnasal drip, sore throats, cough, recurrent fever, anorexia, malaise, headache (frontal, parietal, or vertex), and epistaxis. There may be adenoidal and tonsillar hypertrophy. Transillumination is helpful if frontal or antral sinuses are sufficiently developed. Roentgenograms may disclose haziness or opacification of involved sinuses. Most of these features, including the roentgenographic findings, can be due to allergic rhinitis. Many of the same features helpful in differentiating allergic rhinitis from infectious rhinitis are equally applicable here.

RHINITIS MEDICAMENTOSA

Overuse of topical vasoconstrictor nose drops and sprays can elicit a "rebound" phenomenon characterized by increased nasal congestion and edema and responsive only to their discontinuation. The diagnosis is usually apparent from the history.

FOREIGN BODY

A nasal foreign body with consequent infection should be suspected if there is a history of sudden onset of a chronic, purulent, unilateral nasal discharge.

NASAL POLYPOSIS

Nasal polyps present as pale pink, gray, or white, grape-like masses arising from the surface of the middle turbinate or the ostia of the ethmoid or maxillary sinus and causing nasal obstruction. Widening of the bridge of the nose may be evident. Secondary infection is often present so the nasal discharge may be either mucoid or mucopurulent. Nasal polyps are very rare in children except for their occurrence in more than 6% of children with cystic fibrosis. [22] Nasal polyps occasionally occur as a complication of allergic rhinitis. The diagnosis is established by physical examination, but application of a topical vasoconstrictor may be necessary to permit adequate examination.

VASOMOTOR RHINITIS

Vasomotor rhinitis is a poorly understood entity with symptoms which are the same as those of allergic rhinitis except that symptoms are not elicited by exposure to any specific allergen. Allergy skin tests are negative. Nasal smears disclose an abundance of neither eosinophils nor neutrophils. Symptoms are thought to be mediated by an autonomic nervous system response to nonspecific stimuli and irritants such as changes in temperature or humidity, smoke, dust, and emotional factors. The diagnosis is one of exclusion.

COMPLICATIONS

Complications of allergic rhinitis include superimposed infection, hypertrophy of tonsils and adenoids, secretory otitis media, alveolar hypoventilation with cor pulmonale, nasal polyposis, epistaxis, and orofacial dental deformities.

INFECTION

Obstruction of the nasal airway and ostia of the paranasal sinuses may predispose the child to the development of infectious rhinitis and acute or chronic sinusitis. When due to bacterial agents infection should be treated with antimicrobials and decongestants. Long term response is largely dependent upon adequacy of management of the basic allergy.

HYPERTROPHY OF TONSILS AND ADENOIDS

Tonsillar and adenoidal hypertrophy is so commonly associated with allergic rhinitis in children that its presence in youngsters less than 4 years old has been considered an indication of the presence of allergy until proved otherwise.[13] Surgical removal of these tissues has often been followed by regrowth when there has been inadequate management of the allergy, and some children with allergic rhinitis have had two or three tonsillectomies or adenoidectomies. With adequate allergy management, on the other hand, signs and symptoms sometimes considered indications for surgery often subside. Surgery is probably rarely indicated, and when allergic rhinitis is present a trial of allergy management should usually be undertaken before surgery is considered.

SECRETORY OTITIS MEDIA

Secretory otitis media can occur as a complication of allergic rhinitis or in association with it. Details of pathogenesis, diagnosis, and treatment are found in Chapter VII. Improvement has often followed institution of appropriate treatment of the associated allergy.

COR PULMONALE DUE TO ALVEOLAR HYPOVENTILATION

Chronic upper airway obstruction can cause hypoxemia, hypercapnia, and acidosis with pulmonary hypertension and cor pulmonale. [23] Stridor usually due to enlarged tonsils and adenoids is present, and somnolence and cyanosis may be evident. Accentuation and fixed splitting of the pulmonic second sound may be heard by auscultation, and there may be right heart failure. Chest roentgenograms disclose cardiomegaly, usually with prominence of the pulmonary artery. Electrocardiograms almost always reveal right atrial and right ventricular hypertrophy, and T wave inversion may be seen in precordial leads. Administration of oxygen can further suppress ventilation, causing further dangerous increases in arterial Pco_2. The diagnosis can be confirmed by cardiac catheterization. Digitalization may be necessary. Relief of the upper airway obstruction is followed by restoration of normal acid-base balance and relief of pulmonary hypertension, and this is one of the few well established indications for tonsillectomy and adenoidectomy.

NASAL POLYPOSIS

Nasal polyposis occasionally occurs in children as a complication of allergic rhinitis, but more often occurs without associated allergy, especially as a complication of cystic fibrosis[22] and must be considered in the differential diagnosis (see above).

EPISTAXIS

Recurrent epistaxis due to rubbing, scratching, and picking at the congested nasal mucosa is especially common at night in children with allergic rhinitis. Bleeding is usually minimal and easily controlled by application of sustained pressure. Epistaxis often decreases in frequency after institution of allergy treatment. Application of vaseline within the nostrils at bedtime may be helpful, but if used at all it must be used sparingly to prevent its aspiration by a child who may be sniffing frequently.

OROFACIAL DENTAL DEFORMITIES

Malocclusion, a high, arched, V-shaped palate, and underdevelopment of maxillary sinuses, zygoma, and the nasal process of the maxilla have been ascribed to chronic perennial allergic rhinitis. [9,10] It has been suggested that local tissue hypoxia and acidosis may follow venous stasis and arterial obstruction due to edema of the nasal mucosa, resulting in or contributing to improper development.

TREATMENT

As with other allergic diseases, the most effective form of treatment is elimination of exposure to the offending allergen (see Chapters IX and XII). When allergens such as pollens and atmospheric molds, which cannot be avoided, are identified, immunotherapy is often beneficial (see Chapter XIV). Use of pharmacologic agents is often necessary for the treatment of acute exacerbations or while awaiting response to other forms of therapy.

ANTIHISTAMINES

Antihistamines are the most commonly prescribed drugs for the treatment of allergic rhinitis. The ethylamine moiety of antihistamines which block H_1-receptors, competes with histamine for receptor sites, inhibiting the increased capillary permeability and smooth muscle activity of histamine (see Chapter II). They are effective in the control of rhinorrhea and sneezing and sometimes relieve conjunctival itching and lacrimation. They are most effective if administered before allergenic exposure and histamine release.

The chief limitation to the use of antihistamines is the frequent occurrence of side effects. Sedation is the commonest side effect. Others include excitation, nervousness, insomnia, dizziness, tinnitus, incoordination, blurred vision, and diplopia. Gastrointestinal side effects such as anorexia, nausea, vomiting, constipation, or diarrhea are sometimes prevented by administration of the drug with meals. Other side effects include dryness of the mouth, urinary frequency and dysuria, palpitation and headache. Mild drowsiness and other side effects may subside after a few days with continued treatment, but there may also be some loss of therapeutic effectiveness with prolonged therapy. When this occurs, effectiveness is usually restored by interrupting use of that antihistamine for a few days or weeks.

Different individuals vary widely in their suspectibility to side effects and in their therapeutic response to different antihistamines. An effective dose for one subject may cause intolerable side effects in another, and the same dose may be ineffective and cause no side effects in a third subject. Patients must be cautioned to reduce the dosage if clinically significant side effects occur, but in the absence of both side effects and the desired clinical response, a gradual increase in dosage to as much as double the usually recommended dose of diphenhydramine or chlorpheniramine is often well tolerated and may afford more effective symptomatic control,[24] and even larger doses have occasionally been recommended.[25] If adequate symptomatic relief without intolerable side effects occurs at no dose of a particular antihistamine which can be found, an antihistamine of a different chemical class should be selected for the next trial (Table 4.1).[26]

It is apparently safe to prescribe some antihistamines (diphenhydramine, tripelennamine, chlorpheniramine) for the treatment of allergic rhinitis in children who also have asthma, [24] but their use during status asthmaticus is contraindicated because of the potential inspissating effect upon tracheobronchial secretions.

SYMPATHOMIMETICS

Sympathomimetics with alpha-adrenergic activity cause vasoconstriction and are therefore effective decongestants (Table 4.2). In patients in whom rhinorrhea can be controlled with an antihistamine but nasal congestion remains, concurrent use of a decongestant may be helpful. The chief limitation of the numerous preparations containing both an antihistamine and a decongestant is the inability to vary the dose of the antihistamine without changing the dose of the decongestant, but some of these preparations are suitable for certain patients. Side effects associated with oral administration include tachycardia, increases in blood pressure, insomnia, nervousness, irritability, headache, nausea, vomiting, and epigastric pain. Topical therapy with nasal drops or sprays at effective doses does not elicit the side effects which follow oral administration (Table 4.3), but prolonged administration may be followed by increased nasal congestion after the initial immediate improvement, and finally rhinitis medicamentosa may supervene. Consequently use of topical vasoconstrictors should be restricted to not more than a few days in succession. For best results drops should be instilled into the dependent nostril with the child supine and his head held backwards and turned to one side. This position should be maintained for 30-60 seconds. Nasal sprays are administered in the erect position with the head tilted slightly forward. The spray should be sniffed during its administration. Only one person should be treated from the same container.

CROMOLYN SODIUM

Nasal insufflation of cromolyn sodium (10 mg.) or instillation of a 2% cromolyn spray has been found effective in preventing nasal symptoms of allergic rhinitis following subsequent experimental[27] or natural exposure to allergens.[28] Treatment at 3-4 hour intervals has been found suitable in subjects with

TABLE 4.1 CLASSIFICATION AND USUALLY RECOMMENDED DOSAGE OF ORAL H_1-BLOCKING ANTIHISTAMINES

CLASS	DRUG	DOSAGE (mg/Kg/day)/doses/day	PREPARATIONS mg/tab or cap	mg/5ml	SIDE EFFECTS
Ethanolamines	Diphen- hydramine (Benadryl)	5/4	25, 50	12.5	Extreme sedation
	Doxylamine (Decapryn)	2/4-6	12.5, 25	6.25	Anticholinergic activity
	Carbinoxamine (Clistin)	0.4/3-4	4(8, 12SA)	4	
Ethylenediamines	Tripelennamine (Pyribenzamine)	5/4-6	25, 50(50, 100 SA)	25	Moderate sedation
	Methapyrilene (Histadyl)	5/4-6	25, 50	20	Gastrointestianl side effects
Alkylamines	Chlorpheniramine (Chlortrimeton and others)	0.33/4	4(8, 12SA)	2.5	Mild sedation
	Bromphenir- amine (Dimetane)	0.5/3-4	4(8, 12SA)	2	Occasional CNS stimulation

Class	Drug				Side Effects
	Dexchlorphenira-mine (Polaramine)	0.15/4	2(4, 6SA)	2	
	Triprolidine (Actidil)	0.125/2-3	2.5	1.25	
	Dimethindene (Forhistal)	0.1/1-3	1(2.5SA)	1 (drops: 0.5 mg/0.6 ml)	Safe dosage not established for children 6 y.o.
Cyclizines	Hydroxyzine (Atarax, Vistaril)	2/4	10, 25, 50, 100	10, 25	Sedation
Phenothiazines	Promethazine (Phenergan)	0.5 mg/Kg hs & ¼ dose in A. M.	12.5, 25, 50	6.25, 25	Extreme sedation
	Methdilazine (Tacaryl)	0.3-2/3	8 (3.6 chew-able)	4	
Other	Cyproheptadine (Periactin)	0.25/3-4	4	2	Sedation
	Azatadine (Optimine)	1-2 mg q12h	1		Sedation Not recommended for children 12 y.o.

TABLE 4.2   NASAL DECONGESTANTS FOR ORAL
             ADMINISTRATION

DRUG	DOSAGE mg/Kg/day/ doses/day	PREPARATIONS mg/tab or cap	mg/ 5 ml
Ephedrine	3-4/4-6	25, 50 (15, 30 60SA)	11, 15, 20
Phenylephrine	1/6		5
Pseudoephedrine	4/4	30, 60	30

either perennial or seasonal allergic rhinitis.[28, 29] Occasional
complaints of associated nasal irritation, sore throat, or headache have rarely necessitated discontinuation of therapy.   The
low frequency of serious side effects is an important advantage
over treatment with antihistamines, but some patients with allergic rhinitis have failed to improve during treatment with
cromolyn.   The drug is most effective if administered before
exposure to allergen because it acts through preventing release
of chemical mediators from mast cells following the antigen-
antibody reaction (see Chapter II).

ADRENAL CORTICOSTEROIDS

Systemic adrenal corticosteroids are known to be very effective in controlling symptoms of allergic rhinitis although
their precise mechanisms of action are unknown (see Chapter
III).   Their use for the treatment of allergic rhinitis is rarely
if ever indicated because of the numerous possible side effects,
including adrenal suppression (see Chapter III).

Dexamethasone nasal spray has been found effective in
relieving symptoms of allergic rhinitis,[30] and in shrinking nasal polyps, [31] but it also can cause adrenal suppression at therapeutic doses.[32] Intranasal administration of beclomethasone
dipropionate aerosol, $50\mu g$ to each nostril t. i. d. -q. i. d. , has
also been found highly effective in the treatment of seasonal or
perennial allergic rhinitis, and available evidence indicates no
adrenal suppression at these doses.[33, 34]

TABLE 4.3   TOPICAL NASAL DECONGESTANTS

DRUG	PREPARATIONS (%)		DOSE (for each nostril)	PRECAUTIONS
	Solution	Spray		
Oxymetazoline (Afrin)	0.05	0.05	2-4 gtt or 2-3 squeezes b.i.d.-q.i.d. Not recommended for children < 6 years old	Caution with hypertension, hyperthyroidism, diabetes mellitus, or use of MAO inhibitors
Phenylephrine (Neosynephrine)	0.125, 0.25, 0.5, 1.0	0.25, 0.5	<12 mo: 2-4gtt/0.125 q6h >12 mo: 2-4gtt or 1-2 squeezes/0.25 q4-6h	
Xylometazoline (Otrivin)	0.05, 0.1	0.05, 0.1	< 6 mo: 1gtt/0.05% q6h< 12 yrs: 2-3gtt 0.05% or 1 squeeze q4-6h> 12 yrs: 2-3 gtt or 1-2 squeezes /0.1% q4-6h	

PROGNOSIS

Little is known about the natural history of allergic rhinitis. Prospective and retrospective studies have indicated complete disappearance of symptoms of allergic rhinitis during childhood in not more than 7-9% of affected children.[35] Improvement or remission is more likely in those with less severe symptoms. Spontaneous remissions occur occasionally, but improvement is probably much more often related to treatment, including avoidance of allergens.

REFERENCES

1. Rhazes: Trois traites d'anatomie arabes. Traduction de P. de Koning. Brill, Leyden, 1903.
2. Bostock, J.: Case of a periodical affection of the eyes and chest. Med-Chir Trans 10:161, 1819.
3. Bostock, J.: Of the catarrhus aestivus, or summer catarrh. Med-Chir Trans 14:437, 1828.
4. Dolovich, J., et al.: Kinin-like activity in nasal secretions of allergic patients. Int Arch Allergol 38:337, 1970.
5. Bohrod, M. G.: Histology of allergic and related lesions. Progr Allergy 4:31, 1954.
6. Rappaport, B. Z., et al.: The mucoproteins of the nasal mucosa of allergic patients before and after treatment with corticotropin. J All 24:35, 1953.
7. Connell, J. T.: Quantitative intranasal pollen challenges. III The priming effect in allergic rhinitis. J All 43:33, 1969.
8. Solomon, W. R.: Comparative effects of transient body surface cooling, recumbency, and induced obstruction in allergic rhinitis and control subjects. J All 37:216, 1966.
9. Marks, M. B.: Significance of discoloration in the lower orbitopalpebral grooves in allergic children (allergic shiners). Ann All 21:26, 1963.
10. Marks, M. B.: Allergy in relation to orofacial dental deformities in children: A review. J All 36:293, 1965.

11. Marks, M. B.: Unusual signs of respiratory tract allergy. Ann All 31:611, 1973.
12. Morgan, D. B.: A suggestive sign of allergy. Arch Dermat 57:1050, 1948.
13. Myers, W. A.: The "nasal crease", a physical sign of allergic rhinitis. JAMA 174:1204, 1960.
14. Anderson, P. C.: Familial transverse nasal groove. Arch Dermat 84:316, 1961.
15. Lowell, F. C.: Clinical aspects of eosinophilia in atopic disease. JAMA 202:875, 1967.
16. Matheson, A., et al.: Local tissue and blood eosinophils in newborn infants. J Ped 51:502, 1957.
17. Crawford, L. V.: A study of the nasal cytology in infants with eczemoid dermatitis. Ann All 18:59, 1960.
18. Murray, A. B.: Nasal secretion eosinophilia in children with allergic rhinitis. Ann All 28:142, 1970.
19. Townley, R. G., et al.: Comparative action of acetylbeta-methylcholine, histamine, and pollen antigens in subjects with hay fever and patients with bronchial asthma. J All 36:121, 1965.
20. Konig, P., and Godfrey, S.: Prevalence of exercise-induced bronchial lability in families of children with asthma. Arch Dis Childhood 48:513, 1973.
21. Fairshter, R. D., Novey, H. S., Marchioli, L. E., and Wilson, A. F.: Large airway constriction in allergic rhinitis: Response to inhalation of helium-oxygen. J All Clin Immunol 63:39, 1979.
22. Schwachman, H., et al.: Nasal polyposis in patients with cystic fibrosis. Ped 30:389, 1962.
23. Macartney, F. J., et al.: Cor pulmonale as a result of chronic nasopharyngeal obstruction due to hypertrophied tonsils and adenoids. Arch Dis Childhood 44:585, 1969.
24. Karlin, J. M.: The use of antihistamines in allergic disease. Ped Cl N A 22:157, 1975.
25. Hyde, J. S., and Lourdes, D. F.: Theophylline and chlorpheniramine in childhood asthma. Dose requirements for children 6 to 12 years (therapeutic orphans) and young adults 13 to 18 years of age receiving cromolyn sodium prophylaxis. Ann All 32:73, 1974.
26. Harris, M. C., et al.: Asthmalytic and antihistamine compounds. Dis Chest 48:106, 1965.
27. Engstrom, I.: The effect of disodium cromoglycate on nasal provocation tests in children with seasonal allergic rhinitis. Acta Allergol 26:101, 1971.
28. Blair, H., and Viner, A. S.: A double blind trial of a 2% solution of sodium cromoglycate in perennial rhinitis. Clin All 5:139, 1975.

29. Holopainen, E., et al.: Effect of disodium cromoglycate on seasonal allergic rhinitis. Lancet i:55, 1971.
30. Norman, P. S., and Winkenwerder, W. L.: Suppression of hay fever symptoms with intranasal dexamethasone aerosol. J All 36:284, 1965.
31. Smith, R. E.: Dexamethasone nasal aerosol in nasal polyps and hypertrophic allergic rhinitis. Ann All 23:273, 1965.
32. Norman, P. S., et al.: Adrenal function during the use of dexamethasone aerosols in the treatment of ragweed hay fever. J All 40:57, 1967.
33. Harris, D. M., et al.: The effect of intranasal beclomethasone dipropionate on adrenal function. Clin All 4:291, 1974.
34. Gibson, G. J., et al.: Double-blind cross-over trial comparing intranasal beclomethasone dipropionate and placebo in perennial rhinitis. Brit Med J iv:503, 1974.
35. Smith, J. M.: A five-year prospective survey of rural children with asthma and hay fever. J All 47:23, 1971.

CHAPTER V | ATOPIC DERMATITIS

Atopic dermatitis is a cutaneous eruption which usually begins in infancy as a very pruritic, erythematous, exudative, papulovesicular eruption and in its more chronic phases is characterized by scaling and lichenification. It was described as early as 1892 by Besnier, who called it prurigo diathesique,[1] but it has subsequently also been known as prurigo Besnier, disseminated neurodermatitis, flexural eczema, and infantile eczema. Because of certain similarities and the frequent clinical association with atopic respiratory disease, it was spoken of as atopic dermatitis[2] soon after Coca had introduced the concept of atopy (see Chapter I). This continues to be the commonest term in use in the United States, although the pathogenesis is less well established than that of the atopic respiratory diseases.

INCIDENCE

The true incidence of atopic dermatitis is unknown. Estimates of 1.1-3.1% of general populations reported from Great Britain have been based upon retrospective studies.[3,4] Estimates based upon data collected in the United States have ranged from 1.6-2.9%.[5,6] In a prospective study of 1753 infants followed by pediatricians in Dallas, Texas, for periods varying from 6 months to 7 years the incidence of atopic dermatitis was 4.3%.[7]

Atopic dermatitis has been found to occur more commonly in well developed countries among some populations. Children of Chinese families moved from Taiwan to Honolulu or San Francisco have been reported to have atopic dermatitis seven times as often (22-27%) as Chinese children in Taiwan (3.8%).[8] Children of Chinese families with the highest incomes seemed most likely to have atopic dermatitis. An increased frequency has also been reported in children of Jamaican families moved to London as compared with Jamaican children in Jamaica.[9]

PATHOGENESIS

In approximately two thirds of children with atopic dermatitis there is a family history of atopic dermatitis, allergic rhinitis, or asthma. [10] Furthermore, atopic dermatitis is reported to have been followed by asthma in 45-53% of cases [11, 12] and by allergic rhinitis or asthma in 50-80% of cases. [11, 13, 14] These clinical associations, the frequent incrimination of specific allergens by allergy skin testing, and observations of improvement following avoidance of implicated foods led to the hypothesis that atopic dermatitis was due to a Type I hypersensitivity reaction occurring in the skin. This possibility is also favored by the demonstration of increased serum concentrations of IgE reported in as many as 77-82% of subjects with atopic dermatitis [15, 16] and extreme decreases in these elevated concentrations within 2 years of remission or healing of atopic dermatitis. [17] Although serum IgE concentrations often correlate with the extent and severity of atopic dermatitis, [16, 18] many subjects with atopic dermatitis have serum IgE concentrations within ranges usually accepted as normal, and exclusion of patients who also have allergic rhinitis or asthma may decrease somewhat the frequency with which elevated serum IgE levels are associated with atopic dermatitis. [18]

Peripheral eosinophilia has been found in subjects with atopic dermatitis and good correlation with activity of the dermatitis has been reported. [19] Nasal eosinophilia in infants and young children with atopic dermatitis who lack signs or symptoms of respiratory tract allergy apparently often precedes the development of allergic rhinitis or asthma, [20] however, and some data suggest that peripheral eosinophilia in infants with atopic dermatitis may also herald the development of respiratory allergy. [21]

Although specific allergens sometimes are identified by allergy skin testing in patients with atopic dermatitis, the results of testing are more often negative or fail to correlate with the history. Although allergens identified by skin testing may aggravate existing atopic dermatitis, [22] they are reported rarely if ever to cause new lesions of atopic dermatitis even when they cause urticaria. [23] Observations such as these, the absence of an abundance of eosinophils in affected skin, [22] and the occurrence of atopic dermatitis or a very similar dermatitis in subjects with congenital, sex-linked hypogammaglobulinemia [24] have suggested the condition may not be entirely due to Type I hypersensitivity.

The importance of self-inflicted trauma to the development of lesions of atopic dermatitis has been clearly established by the absence of lesions in areas protected from trauma following allergen challenge. [25] Pruritus resulting from the release of chemical mediators in the skin due to the reaginic antibody-antigen reaction may cause the scratching which elicits the lesions of atopic dermatitis.

There is evidence of suppression of delayed hypersensitivity in patients with atopic dermatitis and in some asthmatics as well. Reported abnormalities associated with atopic dermatitis have included anergy to <u>Candida albicans</u> and streptokinase-streptodornase as well as other antigens demonstrated by skin testing for delayed hypersensitivity; depressed responsiveness of lymphocytes to stimulation by concanavalin A, pokeweed, and phytohemagglutinin; inability to develop hypersensitivity to dinitrochlorobenzene or rhus oleoresin; and decreased numbers of thymus-derived lymphocytes circulating in the peripheral blood as determined by spontaneous sheep erythrocyte or T cell rosette formation. [26] An increase in the number of B lymphocytes carrying IgE has also been reported. [27] The correlation of severity of the dermatitis with both serum IgE concentration and cutaneous anergy to agents which commonly induce delayed hypersensitivity has suggested the possibility of defective T cell regulation of IgE production. [26]

PHYSIOLOGY AND PHARMACOLOGY

Several abnormalities of cutaneous physiology and pharmacology are commonly found in subjects with atopic dermatitis. One of these abnormalities is the white dermographism evident after the skin has been stroked firmly with a blunt instrument. [28] This maneuver normally elicits a red line which appears within a few seconds, becomes maximal within 30-50 seconds and is due to capillary and venular dilatation. A bright red flare, spreading for variable distances beyond the area to which pressure was applied and evident 20-60 seconds after a firm stroke, has been ascribed to reflex dilatation of arterioles. [29] A wheal often observed 1-3 minutes after the stroke and maximal 3-5 minutes after the stroke results from transudation of fluid due to increased vascular permeability possibly in response to nonspecific release of histamine or other chemical mediators.

Firm stroking of the skin of more than 80% of patients with atopic dermatitis, on the other hand, has been found to elicit white dermographism. [30,31] The usual red line appears within 15 seconds, but in another 5-15 seconds it is replaced by a slightly larger line of pallor. This blanching persists 2-5 minutes and may be surrounded by a red flare. [28] Whealing does not occur. The phenomenon may not be demonstrable during remissions of atopic dermatitis[30] and is usually evident only in areas of skin affected by the disease. [32] It is probably due to vasoconstriction, but more specific details of the mechanism are unknown. White dermographism has been reported in 10% of subjects with atopic respiratory disease who did not have atopic dermatitis, [31] and it has also been found in subjects with several other skin diseases. [33]

An abnormal response to the intradermal injection of 0.1 ml of a 1:1000 dilution of acetylcholine has also been found in 60-70% of patients with atopic dermatitis in most reports and in more than 20% of patients with atopic respiratory disease who have not had atopic dermatitis. [34] In the normal subject such an injection in followed by a flare of arteriolar dilatation within 5-10 seconds. This persists for 3-10 minutes and is accompanied by sweating and piloerection. This initial response, ascribed to an axon reflex, is followed by a more slowly developing longer lasting erythema appearing in 5-10 minutes and sometimes persisting another 20 minutes, also accompanied by sweating. [35] This later response has been attributed to direct action of the acetylcholine on blood vessels and sweat glands.

In subjects with atopic dermatitis the normal axon reflex flare is often followed, usually within 3 minutes, by the development of an area of blanching, rather than erythema. This blanch may persist for 15-30 minutes and occasionally has been evident for more than 60 minutes. The abnormal response has usually been restricted to portions of skin involved with atopic dermatitis.

One group of normal infants has been studied for the possible value of this phenomenon in predicting those subject to subsequent development of atopic diseases. A delayed blanch followed intradermal injection of methacholine in 37% in infancy, but reevaluation five years later failed to reveal any correlation with the appearance of signs or symptoms of atopic diseases although responses to retesting with methacholine usually resembled the initial responses. [36]

The delayed blanch is apparently due to edema rather than to vasoconstriction. [34]

Other abnormal cutaneous responses associated with atopic dermatitis include the blanching which follows application of nicotinic acid esters to the skin instead of the normal erythematous response; blanching and absence of the flare which normally follows intradermal injection of histamine; absence of the flare which normally follows intradermal injection of serotonin; and blanching instead of the erythema which normally follows intradermal injection of bradykinin. [34]

There is evidence of an abnormal increase in binding of norepinephrine in skin affected by atopic dermatitis, [37] and increased skin concentrations of acetylcholine have been reported in subjects with atopic dermatitis. [34]

The abnormally low skin temperature over the fingers and toes of patients with atopic dermatitis and their increased sensitivity to cooling may be further evidence of a tendency for peripheral vasoconstriction,[28,38] although some data dispute this.[39] Skin over the antecubital and popliteal spaces differs from that over the digits, however, in that these flexural areas cool less rapidly and rewarm faster than those in normal subjects. These same phenomena have been observed in subjects with atopic respiratory disease who lack atopic dermatitis.[28] Intramuscular administration of histamine has been reported to cause greater elevations of cheek and flexural skin temperature in subjects with atopic dermatitis than in normal subjects.[40]

A decrease in skin blood flow in patients with atopic dermatitis has been measured by capacitance plethysmography.[41] This could be accounted for by peripheral vasoconstriction or a decrease in blood pressure. Subnormal blood pressures have occasionally been reported in association with atopic dermatitis,[28] but others have found normal blood pressure in such subjects.[39]

The dryness of the skin so typical of atopic dermatitis has been ascribed to sweat retention,[42] but an abnormally increased rate of sweating has followed intradermal injection of acetylcholine in patients with atopic dermatitis.[43] The xerosis has also been ascribed to the decrease in skin lipid content and sebaceous gland activity associated with atopic dermatitis.[44]

A decrease in the itch threshold which has been demonstrated by application of trypsin to antecubital spaces of subjects with atopic dermatitis and the abnormally long duration of itching which follows application of trypsin even to uninvolved skin in such patients may be related to increased numbers or heightened sensitivity to mediating nerves.[45]

CLINICAL MANIFESTATIONS

Atopic dermatitis usually begins within the first year of life with a peak age of onset at 2 1/2 months, but it can start at anytime during childhood, and occasionally has its onset after childhood.[11,22,46]

The distribution of the lesions is somewhat dependent upon the age of the child. In infancy the cheeks are usually involved and localized patches may be present over the extensor aspects of the extremities. Involvement of the forehead and scalp may also occur in infants and there may also be extension to the trunk. Between 9 and 18 months of age more generalized involvement of the extremities occurs, and the predilection for antecubital and popliteal spaces seen in older children becomes evident. Involvement of the back of the neck is also more common after 18 months of age.

The initial lesion is a patch of erythema or a maculopapular eruption with tiny vesicles at the tips of the papules. The vesicles may coalesce and rupture, causing a weeping, oozing, moist dermatitis. Crusting may occur, especially if pustules have formed due to superimposed infection. As vesicles dry, fine scales may become evident. The intense pruritus causes rubbing and scratching of the lesions after 2 months of age, and the excoriations contribute further to oozing and may cause infection. Pruritus also causes irritability and restlessness.

In older children chronic atopic dermatitis is characterized by lichenification - a brown or grey thickening of the skin with exaggeration of the normal skin furrows. Hypopigmentation may be evident in healed areas.

LABORATORY FINDINGS

EOSINOPHILIA

Total eosinophil counts in peripheral blood are usually but not always elevated, and good correlation with activity of the dermatitis has sometimes been found.[19] Nasal eosinophilia may precede the appearance of signs and symptoms of respiratory allergy.[20]

IMMUNOGLOBULIN E

Abnormally increased concentrations of serum IgE are usually present in children with atopic dermatitis and may be helpful in establishing the diagnosis in the rare patient in whom the clinical features may not be entirely typical. Details regarding the measurement of total serum IgE and the identification of specific allergens by the radioallergosorbent test will be found in Chapter XIII.

ALLERGY SKIN TESTING

Allergy skin testing has usually been reported to have disclosed positive reactions in 50-80% of subjects with atopic dermatitis, with positive reactions to foods especially frequent in children less than 2 years of age and egg white the single antigen most commonly implicated.[22, 47] Challenge with foods incriminated by allergy skin testing has often elicited allergic symptoms although these have consisted of urticaria or vomiting more often than atopic dermatitis.[47] Techniques, interpretation, and limitations of allergy skin testing are discussed in Chapter XIII.

DIFFERENTIAL DIAGNOSIS

The diagnosis of atopic dermatitis is usually easily established, but in early infancy it may be difficult to distinguish it from seborrheic dermatitis, and seborrheic dermatitis may precede the development of atopic dermatitis or both may be present at the same time although there is no evidence of any etiologic relationship.

SEBORRHEIC DERMATITIS

Seborrheic dermatitis is a recurrent inflammatory condition of unknown etiology characterized by the presence of dry or greasy scales over the areas of the body where sebaceous glands are most plentiful, including the scalp, forehead, perioral and postauricular areas, axillae, periumbilical, inguinal and perianal areas, and skin over the sternum and spine. The onset is usually within the first two months with involvement of the scalp, forehead, and postauricular areas. The lesions are usually yellow or reddish-yellow and well demarcated. Pruritus is common in older children but not as intense as that of atopic dermatitis. Other characteristics useful in differentiating it from atopic dermatitis are indicated in Table 5.1.

LEINER'S DISEASE

Leiner's disease, erythroderma desquamativum, is a generalized seborrheic dermatitis associated with intractable diarrhea, recurrent infection, and progressive wasting due to a familial deficiency of opsonin activity related to dysfunction of C5.[48] The condition was often fatal before infusion of fresh plasma was found to be effective in its treatment. Surviving infants usually have recovered completely within several months.

SCABIES

Scabies is an intensely pruritic dermatosis due to the presence of the mite, Sarcoptes scabiei, and characterized by the presence of papules, vesiculopapules, and pustules over the palms and soles of infants and burrows and linear excoriations due to scratching. It is highly contagious, and other family members are often affected. Other areas of predilection include axillae, areas between fingers and toes, flexor aspects of forearms, ulnar aspects of wrists, buttocks, and external genitalia. Mites or ova can be demonstrated in scrapings of vesicles. Response to a therapeutic trial of gamma benzene hexachloride can also establish the diagnosis.

LETTERER-SIWE DISEASE

Letterer-Siwe disease, a form of histiocytosis X, is a fatal disorder of the reticuloendothelial system occurring in infancy and characterized by hepatosplenomegaly, pulmonary infiltration, lymphadenopathy, failure to thrive, and a maculo-papular, petechial eruption involving predominantly the scalp and trunk. Superimposed infection is common. The diagnosis is established by biopsy, but the condition is easily differentia-ted from atopic dermatitis by physical examination.

CONTACT DERMATITIS

Contact dermatitis is a papulovesicular or erythematous eruption due to type IV hypersensitivity to a contactant. It is usually easily differentiated from atopic dermatitis by morphol-ogy and distribution. Other features helpful in diagnosis are indicated in Table 5.1.

RITTER'S DISEASE

Ritter's disease or dermatitis exfoliativa neonatorum, is a form of toxic epidermal necrolysis (scalded skin syndrome) occurring in infants and children and usually due to infection with phage group 2 staphylococci.[49] It usually occurs during the first two weeks of life as generalized erythema followed by the appearance of large bullae or generalized exfoliation. The condition is often fatal despite treatment with antibiotics.

METABOLIC DISORDERS

Cutaneous eruptions resembling atopic dermatitis have been reported in as many as one third of children with phenylketon-uria,[50] and similar eruptions have been associated with ahis-tidinemia as well as gluten-induced enteropathy.[51]

IMMUNODEFICIENCY DISORDERS

Atopic dermatitis or a very similar eruption occurs in the Wiskott-Aldrich syndrome, a sex-linked recessive disorder in which the dermatitis is associated with thrombocytopenia, re-current infections, impairment of formation of antibodies to polysaccharide antigens, and a progressive depletion of thymus dependent lymphocytes.[52] Similar eruptions have occasionally been reported in association with congenital sex linked hypo-gammaglobulinemia[24] and ataxia telangiectasia.[53]

TABLE 5.1 DIFFERENTIAL DIAGNOSIS OF ATOPIC DERMATITIS, SEBORRHEIC DERMATITIS AND CONTACT DERMATITIS

	Atopic Dermatitis	Seborrheic Dermatitis	Contact Dermatitis
Age of Onset	Usually infancy	First 3 months or late childhood	Late childhood or later
Family History of Atopic Respiratory Disease	Usually positive	Usually negative	Usually negative
Family History of Seborrhea	Usually negative	Often positive (acne, oily skin, baldness, dandruff)	Usually negative
Personal History of Atopic Respiratory Disease	Usually positive	Usually negative	Usually negative
Distribution of Lesions	Predilection for face, neck, antecubital and popliteal spaces; may be generalized	Predilection for scalp, forehead, nasolabial folds, behind ears, over sternum	Exposed areas

Table 5.1 (cont'd.)

	Atopic Dermatitis	Seborrheic Dermatitis	Contact Dermatitis
Character of Lesions	Erythematous, papular or papulovescular, weeping, crusting, or dry with fine scales. Lichenification after infancy. Poorly demarcated. Intense pruritus.	Mild or moderately erythematous. Scales often large and greasy. Central clearing of flexural lesions. Well demarcated. Little or no pruritus.	Erythematous, papulovescular. Poorly demarcated. Moderate pruritus.
Character of Uninvolved Skin	Dry and thick	Normal or oily	Normal or thin and moist
Total eosinophil Count	Usually elevated	Normal	Normal
Serum Total IgE	Usually elevated	Normal	Normal
Allergy Skin Testing	Usually positive to scratch or intracutaneous (immediate wheal and flare)	Normal	Usually positive to patch or contact (24-48 hours)

Atopic dermatitis has also been found to be associated with depressed in vivo cellular immunity or impairment of neutrophil chemotaxis and susceptibility to infection in children with extreme increases in serum IgE.[54, 55]

OTHER CONDITIONS

Other disorders which are usually easily differentiated from atopic dermatitis by morphology, distribution, culture, or microscopic examination of skin scrapings include cutaneous candidiasis, trichophyton infections, ammoniacal diaper dermatitis, and icthyosis.

COMPLICATIONS

BACTERIAL INFECTION

Superimposed bacterial infection is the commonest complication of atopic dermatitis. Crusting is usually more extreme than that which may be evident without secondary infection, and pustules and tenderness may be present. The commonest cause is Staphylococcus aureus, but beta hemolytic streptococci also often cause superimposed infection. Systemic treatment with antibiotics is indicated because it is more effective than topical treatment and topical therapy carries an added risk of inducing hypersensitivity to antibiotics.

Bacterial infection is probably a common complication because of frequent loss of the integrity of the skin as a protective barrier due to the rubbing and scratching which follow pruritus, but there is also evidence of decreased capacity for the phagocytosis of yeast particles by neutrophils of subjects with severe atopic dermatitis.[56]

VIRAL INFECTION

Increased susceptibility to vaccinia, herpes simplex, molluscum contagiosum, and occasionally other viruses[57] is apparently due not only to the presence of damaged skin but also to the suppression of cellular immunity,[26] because the increased susceptibility is seen even when the dermatitis is in remission.

Kaposi's varicelliform eruption is also known as eczema vaccinatum when due to vaccinia virus and eczema herpeticum when caused by herpes simplex virus. It begins with multiple vesicular-pustular lesions, most numerous over the face and in areas involved with atopic dermatitis, but also over intact skin. The lesions increase in size to 10-15 mm and then become umbilicated.[58] New crops of vesicles may continue to appear for 7-10 days. Facial edema is common. In eczema vaccinatum, which usually begins within a few days or up to 3 weeks after exposure, regional lymphadenopathy is usually present, and there may be hepatosplenomegaly. Fever is present. The diagnosis can be confirmed by the appearance of specific neutralizing antibodies.

Treatment of eczema vaccinatum includes administration of vaccinia immune globulin, and administration of methisazone has been reported effective.[59] Available therapy of Kaposi's varicelliform eruption otherwise consists only of supportive measures. The mortality has been reported to be as high as 6%.[60]

Atopic dermatitis or the presence of another type of dermatitis is a contraindication to smallpox vaccination, and contact with others who have been vaccinated must be avoided until the vaccination is well healed. It is estimated that 9% of patients with atopic dermatitis who are vaccinated may develop eczema vaccinatum if no special precautions are observed.[61] When travel was necessary to an area where smallpox was endemic, vaccination could be followed by administration of vaccinia immune globulin, 0.3 ml/Kg, by intramuscular injection at another site.[62] Eradication of smallpox has eliminated this complication.

Molluscum contagiosum is a mildly contagious disease characterized by discrete, waxy, umbilicated papules of varying size from which a cheesy material can be extracted. Treatment consists of incision and curettage followed by application of an escharotic agent such as podophyllin, 7% tincture of iodine, or 10% salicyclic acid.[63]

OCULAR COMPLICATIONS

Cataracts are reported to have been found to have developed, usually in adolescence or early adult life, in as many as 5% of subjects with atopic dermatitis. Keratoconus, possibly representing a thickening of the cornea in response to rubbing of the eyelids, has been reported less frequently.[58]

TREATMENT

The most effective form of treatment for any allergic disease is elimination of exposure to the offending allergen (see Chapters IX and XII). Foods are sometimes implicated by history or allergy skin testing in infants or children with atopic dermatitis, and appropriate dietary restrictions may be followed by improvement. Satisfactory responses occur more often in infants in whom dietary restrictions have been imposed soon after the onset of the dermatitis. Older children with chronic atopic dermatitis are less likely to improve in response to institution of such measures.

There is no objective evidence that immunotherapy with food extracts is beneficial, but there is some evidence to suggest that immunotherapy may sometimes be helpful in the treatment of atopic dermatitis when specific inhalant allergens can be identified.[64] Immunotherapy can also aggravate atopic dermatitis, however, a response which may limit the dosage which can be reached in patients receiving treatment for allergic rhinitis or asthma (see Chapter XIV).

Other measures useful in the management of atopic dermatitis include control of scratching, avoidance of irritants, topical therapy, and systemic antibiotics when superimposed bacterial infection is present.

SCRATCHING

The evident lesions of atopic dermatitis are due to self inflicted trauma which follows pruritus.[25] Fingernails must be clipped short to minimize the extent to which the skin can be damaged. Elbow splints made from cardboard or magazines are useful in preventing an infant from reaching his face. Rough bedding and clothing should be avoided and contact with wool should be avoided. Soft, undyed, unstarched cotton clothing is safest. Cotton diapers are recommended, and a dacron-stuffed pad between the sheet and plastic-covered crib mattress is useful in preventing overheating with consequent irritation of the skin. Room temperature should not exceed 74ºF. Avoidance of animal danders and sources of house dust is indicated not only because of their possible importance as inhalant allergens but also because they may be irritants.

Wrapping involved extremities with soft cotton cloths held in place with elastic bandages prevents scratching as well as contact with environmental irritants. In warm climates this may cause increased perspiration with consequent aggravation of pruritus, however.

BATHING

Regimens prohibiting or sharply restricting contact with soap and water have often been found very helpful in the treatment of atopic dermatitis.[65,66] Substitution of Cetaphil lotion for cleansing is thought to promote hydration of the dry skin, while water may remove lipids and hydrophilic materials from the skin causing its further dehydration. It is recommended that the entire skin surface be cleansed at least twice daily with Cetaphil lotion with rubbing until it foams. It is then wiped off gently with a soft cloth, leaving a film of lotion on the skin.

Water is permitted only for occasional cleaning of the diaper area; soap and water, only for cleansing of the scalp and hair with protection of the rest of the body with towels and for occasional cleansing of the hands.

Tub baths in clear water may be permitted once or twice each week but may aggravate the dermatitis. The water should be tepid, since hot water can aggravate the pruritus.

There is not complete agreement that avoidance of contact with water is important, and many children with atopic dermatitis tolerate swimming without any evident aggravation of the dermatitis.

Sebulex and similar shampoos containing sulfur and salicylic acid are useful for treating the crusting and scaling of the scalp whether due to atopic or seborrheic dermatitis.

ADRENAL CORTICOSTEROIDS

Adrenal corticosteroids are the most effective topical preparations available for the treatment of atopic dermatitis. Although much safer than systemic corticosteroids, some absorption can occur following topical application. The same side effects associated with systemic administration of corticosteroids, including adrenal suppression, are possible, especially if large amounts are applied over large areas of acutely inflamed skin or if occlusive dressings are applied over the steroids,[58, 67] but adrenal suppression due to topical steroids is probably rare.[68]

Water-washable creams are usually better tolerated than ointments, possibly because of increased warmth and pruritus caused by ointments,[65] but creams occasionally cause stinging. Hydrocortisone, 0.5%, is inexpensive and often effective. More effective preparations include 0.1% betamethasone valerate (Valisone), 0.25% desoximetasone (Topicort), 0.025% fluocinolone acetonide (Synemol), 0.05% flurandrenolone acetonide (Cordran), and 0.1% triamcinolone acetonide (Aristocort, Kenalog). Addition of urea to 1% hydrocortisone cream (Carmol HC) has been reported to increase the effectiveness of the steroid.[69] Fluocinolone acetonide, 0.01% in propylene glycol (Synalar solution) may be better tolerated than a cream and is more easily applied to large areas. These preparations are all free of parabens, but many other topical preparations contain parabens, and sensitization can occur following topical administration of parabens as well as neomycin and other antibiotics.

COMPRESSES

In the acute, exudative, weeping stage, compresses of clear tap water or aluminum acetate solution (Burow's solution) are indicated. The solution should not be warmer than room

temperature; ice cold solutions sometimes are helpful in relieving intense pruritus. Plain gauze or white, cotton handker-
chiefs or bed linens are suitable for wet dressings. After im-
mersion in the solution they are applied flat to the affected area.
When the cloth has begun to dry in 5-10 minutes it is again im-
mersed in the solution. Applications for 15 minutes three or
four times daily usually bring the oozing under control within
a few days. A fluorinated corticosteroid in propylene glycol
solution can be applied after the compresses are removed.

After weeping and crusting have subsided compresses can
be discontinued and topical treatment with a steroid lotion or
cream continued.

TARS

Coal tar preparations are less effective than topical corticosteroids and may induce photosensitization but are often
recommended for the treatment of subacute and chronic atopic
dermatitis. [22]

ANTIHISTAMINES

Antihistamines are generally considered beneficial when
used in doses large enough to cause sedation, thereby lessening self-inflicted damage to the skin. There is evidence that
antihistamines may increase itch thresholds and shorten the
duration of itching induced by the intracutaneous injection of
trypsin in some subjects with atopic dermatitis. [22] Initial dosage should be similar to that recommended for allergic rhinitis
(see Chapter IV), but larger doses may be necessary for sedation and whatever antipruritic effect may be possible.

ANTIBIOTICS

When secondary bacterial infection is present it must be
treated with an appropriate systemic antibiotic such as penicillin or erythromycin. Topical antimicrobial therapy is less effective and more likely to induce hypersensitivity.

PREVENTION

More than 40 years ago infants fed whole cow's milk were
reported to develop atopic dermatitis seven times as often as
breast-fed infants. [70] In a prospective study of children whose
parents or siblings had atopic dermatitis or atopic respiratory
disease, dietary avoidance of cow's milk in infancy for variable
intervals of up to 9 months was associated with a decreased frequency of the development of atopic dermatitis (7%) as compared with siblings who had received cow's milk (32%) and unrelated children with similar family histories of allergy who had
received cow's milk (29%). [71,72] Furthermore, subsequent

development of respiratory allergic diseases as well as atopic
dermatitis was also less frequent in the infants from whom
cow's milk had been withheld initially (15%) as compared with
the control children (52-64%).

A subsequent study also disclosed a much lower frequency
of the development of respiratory allergy in infants from whom
milk and milk products, beef, veal, chilken, egg, and wheat
were withheld for the first 7-9 months (15%) as compared with
controls (57%).[73] The frequency of the development of atopic
dermatitis was considered too low to permit conclusions regarding its association with diet (5% in the infants receiving the
hypoallergenic diet and 2% in the control group).

Other studies have failed to confirm that dietary elimination of cow's milk in infancy reduced the risk for development
of atopic diseases,[7] but egg, veal, beef, chicken, and wheat
were not restricted in these studies, milk was often eliminated
from the diet for only 6 months or even less, and the children
were often observed for only two years or even less. It is not
clear what effect these differences may have had upon the data.
The more intensive heat treatment applied during the processing of currently available proprietary cow's milk formulas has
also been suggested as an explanation of the differences in the
results of these studies, because this has reduced somewhat
the antigenicity of these preparations.[7]

For the infant at risk for the development of atopic diseases
because of his genetic background it still seems prudent to recommend dietary avoidance of cow's milk, beef, veal, egg,
chicken, and wheat for the first 9 months. Nursing throughout
this period can be recommended, but the mother should also
avoid excessive amounts of these foods in her diet to minimize
transmission of potential allergens by her milk. When the
mother cannot nurse the infant a soy bean formula is usually a
satisfactory substitute, but allergy to soy protein can also occur (see Chapter IX). Prophylactic precautions to minimize
exposure to household inhalant allergens also seem desirable
although there is no proof that these affect subsequent development of atopic diseases (see Chapter XII).

PROGNOSIS

The very few retrospective studies of the prognosis of atopic dermatitis which have been published suggest that in as many
as 35% of infants with moderate or severe atopic dermatitis it
may persist for at least 20 years.[4, 13, 14] The disease may
continue at least until 13 years of age in approximately 50% of
affected children,[4, 13] but resolves by 3 years of age in 25%.[13]

Subsequent development of atopic respiratory disease has
been reported in 50-80% of children with atopic dermatitis;[11,
13, 14] asthma, in as many as 45-53% in some series.[11, 12]

REFERENCES

1. Besnier, E. : Premiere note et observations preliminaires pour servir d'introduction a l'etude des prurigos diathesiques (dermatites multiformes prurigineuses chroniques exacerbantes et paroxystiques, du type du prurigo de Hebra). Ann derm syph 3:634, 1892.
2. Coca, A. F. , and Sulzberger, M. B. : Yearbook Derm Syph, p59, Year Book Pub. , Chicago, 1933.
3. Walker, R. B. , and Warin, R. P. : The incidence of eczema in early childhood. Brit J Derm 68:182, 1956.
4. Brereton, E. M. , et al. : The prevalence and prognosis of eczema and asthma in Cambridgeshire school children. Med Officer 102:317, 1959.
5. Service, W. C. : The incidence of major allergic diseases in Colorado Springs. JAMA 112:2034, 1939.
6. Freeman, G. L. , and Johnson, S. : Allergic diseases in adolescents. Am J Dis Child 107:549, 1964.
7. Halpern, S. R. , et al. : Development of childhood allergy in infants fed breast, soy, or cow milk. J All Clin Imm 51:139, 1973.
8. Worth, R. M. : Atopic dermatitis among Chinese infants in Honolulu and San Francisco. Hawaii Med J 22:31, 1962.
9. Davis, L. R. , et al.: Atopic eczema in European and Negro West Indian infants in London. Brit J Dermat 73:410, 1961.
10. Baer, R. L. : Atopic dermatitis. J. B. Lippincott Co. , Philadelphia, 1955.
11. Glaser, J. : Allergy in childhood. Chas. C. Thomas, Springfield, 1956.
12. Pasternack, B. : The prediction of asthma in infantile eczema. J Ped 66:164, 1965.
13. Vowles, M. , et al. : Infantile eczema: observations on natural history and prognosis. Brit J Dermat 67:53, 1955.
14. Stifler, W. C. , Jr. : A 21 year follow-up of infantile eczema. J Ped 66:166, 1965.
15. Juhlin, L. , et al. : Immunoglobulin E levels in atopic dermatitis, urticaria, and various dermatoses. Arch Derm 100:12, 1969.
16. Stone, S. P. , et al. : IgE levels in atopic dermatitis. Arch Derm 108:806, 1973.
17. Johansson, S. G. O. , and Juhlin, L. : Immunoglobulin E in "healed" atopic dermatitis and after treatment with corticosteroids and azathioprine. Brit J Derm 82:10, 1970.
18. Johnson, E. E. , et al.: Serum IgE concentration in atopic dermatitis. J All Clin Imm 54:94, 1974.

19. Hellerstrom, S., and Lidman, H.: Studies of Besnier's prurigo (atopic dermatitis). Acta Dermat vener 36:11, 1956.
20. Crawford, L. V.: A study of the nasal cytology in infants with eczemoid dermatitis, Ann All 18:59, 1960.
21. Voorhorst, R., et al.: Development of the atopic syndrome in a group of patients with (atopic) constitutional dermatitis. Acta Allergol 18:56, 1963.
22. Rajka, G.: Atopic dermatitis. W. B. Saunders Co., Philadelphia, 1975.
23. Cooke, R. A.: A consideration of some allergy problems. I. Allergic dermatitis (eczema). J All 15:203, 1944.
24. Peterson, R. D. A., et al.: Wheal and erythema allergy in patients with agammaglobulinemia. J All 33:406, 1962.
25. Engman, M. F., et al.: Eczema and environment. Med Cl N A 20:651, 1936.
26. McGready, S. J., and Buckley, R. H.: Depression of cell-mediated immunity in atopic eczema. J All Clin Imm 56: 393, 1975.
27. Carapeto, F. J., Winkelmann, R. K., and Jordon, R. E.: T and B lymphocytes in contact and atopic dermatitis. Arch Dermatol 112:1095, 1976.
28. Eyster, W. H., Jr., et al.: Studies on the peripheral vascular physiology of patients with atopic dermatitis. J Inv Dermat 18:37, 1952.
29. Muller, L. R.: Studien Uber den Dermographismus und dessen diagnostische Bedeutung. Deutsche Ztschr Nervenh 47-48:413, 1913.
30. Reed, W. B., et al.: Vascular reactions in chronically inflamed skin. Arch Dermat 77:91, 1958.
31. Rajka, G.: Prurigo Besnier (atopic dermatitis) with special reference to the role of allergic factors. I. The influence of atopic hereditary factors. Acta Dermat-vener 40:285, 1960.
32. Russell, B., and Last, S. L.: Besnier's Prurigo: Observations on abnormal cutaneous and central nervous reactions. Brit J Dermat 67:65, 1955.
33. Whitfield, A.: On the white reaction (white line) in dermatology. Brit J Dermat 50:71, 1938.
34. Sly, R. M., and Heimlich, E. M.: Physiologic abnormalities in the atopic state: a review. Ann All 25:192, 1967.
35. Scott, A.: The distribution and behavior of cutaneous nerves in normal and abnormal skin. Brit J Dermat 70:1, 1958.
36. Olive, J. T., Jr., et al.: Delayed blanch phenomenon in children: reevaluation of 5-year-old children originally tested as newborns. J Invest Dermatol 54:256, 1970.

37. Solomon, L. R., et al.: The physiological disposition of C14-norepinephrine in patients with atopic dermatitis and other dermatoses. J Inv Dermat 43:193, 1964.
38. Weber, R. G., et al.: Further contributions to the vascular physiology in atopic dermatitis. J Inv Dermat 24:19, 1955.
39. Varonier, H. S., and Hahn, W. W.: Cardiac and vascular reactivity in atopic and nonatopic children. J Allergy 38:352, 1966.
40. Williams, D. H.: Skin temperature reaction to histamine in atopic dermatitis. J Inv Dermat 1:119, 1938.
41. Bystryn, J. C., and Hyman, C.: Skin blood flow in atopic dermatitis. J Invest Derm 52:189, 1969.
42. Wheatley, V. R.: Secretions of the skin in eczema. J Ped 66:200, 1965.
43. Warndorff, J. A.: The response of the sweat glands to acetylcholine in atopic subjects. Brit J Dermatol 83:306, 1970.
44. Prose, P. H.: Pathologic changes in eczema. J Ped 66: 178, 1965.
45. Rajka, G.: Itch duration in the involved skin of atopic dermatitis (prurigo Besnier). Acta Derm vener 47:154, 1967.
46. Sedlis, E.: Natural history of infantile eczema: Its incidence and course. J Ped 66:158, 1965.
47. Stifler, W. C., Jr., et al.: Some challenge studies with foods. J Ped 66:235, 1965.
48. Jacobs, J. C., and Miller, M. E.: Fatal familial Leiner's disease: A deficiency of the opsonic activity of serum complement. Ped 49:225, 1972.
49. Melish, M. E., and Glasgow, L. A.: The staphylococcal scalded skin syndrome: development of an experimental model. NEJM 282:1114, 1970.
50. Knox, W. E.: "Phenylketonuria", in Stanbury, J. B., Wyngaarden, J. B., and Fredrickson, D. S. (ed): The metabolic basis of inherited disease, Second ed., McGraw-Hill, New York, 1966, p 258.
51. Rostenberg, A., Jr., and Solomon, L. M.: Infantile eczema and systemic disease. Arch Derm 98:41, 1968.
52. Buckley, R. H.: "Deficiencies in immunity", in Joklik, W. K., and Smith, D. T. (ed): Zinsser microbiology, 15th ed., Appleton, Century, Crofts, New York, 1972, p 311.
53. Reed, W. B., et al.: Cutaneous manifestations of ataxia telangiectasia. JAMA 195:746, 1966.
54. Buckley, R. H., et al.: Extreme hyperimmunoglobulinemia E and undue susceptibility to infection. Ped 49:59, 1972.
55. Hill, R. H., and Quie, P. G.: Raised serum IgE levels and defective neutrophil chemotaxis in three children with eczema and recurrent infections. Lancet 1:183, 1974.

56. Michaelsson, G.: Decreased phagocytic capacity of the neutrophil leukocytes in patients with atopic dermatitis. Acta Dermat vener 53:279, 1973.
57. Nahmias, A. J. , et al. : Generalized eruption in a child with eczema due to Coxsackie virus A16. Arch Derm 97: 147, 1968.
58. Norins, A. L.: Atopic dermatitis. Ped Cl N A 18:801, 1971.
59. Grosfield, J. C. M. , and van Ramshorst, A. G. S.: Eczema vaccinatum. Dermatologica 141:1, 1970.
60. Copeman, P. W. M. , and Wallace, H. J.: Eczema vaccinatum. Brit Med J 2:906, 1964.
61. Ericksson, G. , and Forsbeck, M.: The assessment, and the vaccination, of patients with cutaneous disorders. Acta Med Scand Suppl 464:147, 1966.
62. American Academy of Pediatrics: Report of the committee on infectious diseases, 17th ed. , 1974, p 163.
63. Keipert, J. A.: The association of molluscum contagiosum and infantile eczema. Med J Aust 1:267, 1971.
64. Kaufman, H. S. , and Roth, H. L.: Hyposensitization with alum precipitated extracts in atopic dermatitis: a placebo-controlled study. Ann All 32:321, 1974.
65. Scholtz, J. R.: Management of atopic dermatitis. Calif. Med 102:210, 1965.
66. Jacobs, A. H.: Management of children with atopic dermatitis. Cutis 10:585, 1972.
67. Keczkes, K. , et al.: The effect on adrenal function of treatment of eczema and psoriasis with triamcinolone acetonide. Brit J Derm 79:475, 1967.
68. Wilson, L. , et al.: Plasma corticosteroid levels in outpatients treated with topical steroids. Brit J Derm 88:373, 1973.
69. Roth, H. L. , and Gellin, G. A. : Atopic dermatitis: treatment with a urea-corticosteroid cream. Cutis 11:237, 1973.
70. Grulee, C. G. , and Sanford, H. N.: The influence of breast and artificial feeding on infantile eczema. J Ped 9:223, 1936.
71. Glaser, J. , and Johnstone, D. E.: Soy bean milk as a substitute for mammalian milk in early infancy. Ann All 10: 433, 1952.
72. Glaser, J. , and Johnstone, D. E.: Prophylaxis of allergic disease in the newborn. JAMA 153:620, 1953.
73. Johnstone, D. E. , and Dutton, A. M.: Dietary prophylaxis of allergic disease in children. NEJM 274:715, 1966.

CHAPTER VI | URTICARIA

Urticaria or hives is a cutaneous eruption characterized by frequently evanescent, erythematous or blanched wheals of various sizes and shapes usually associated with pruritus. Angioedema (angioneurotic edema or giant hives) is a more extensive area of edema of the deeper layers of skin and subcutaneous tissue.

INCIDENCE

The true incidence of urticaria is unknown because it is usually of short duration, subsiding without treatment, but 16% of college students have reported histories of urticaria.[1] Many subjects with urticaria have not had other manifestations of atopic diseases, but there is apparently an increased incidence of acute urticaria in atopic subjects.[2]

PATHOGENESIS

Urticaria and angioedema are due to localized vasodilation and transudation. These can result from the actions of specific mediators of Type I anaphylactic reactions (see Chapter II) released in response to immunologic or nonimmunologic stimuli. A variety of chemicals can cause histamine release. These include morphine, codeine, meperidine, d-tubocurarine, polymixin B, thiamine, and stilbamidine.[3]

Increased vascular permeability is also mediated by anaphylatoxins (C3a and C5a). Nonspecific factors which can aggravate urticaria by enhancing cutaneous vascular dilatation include heat, fever, exercise, emotional stress, ingestion of alcohol, and hyperthyroidism.

CLASSIFICATION AND CLINICAL MANIFESTATIONS

Specific mechanisms and manifestations vary, depending upon the type of urticaria (Table 6.1). Type I, Type II, and Type III hypersensitivity reactions have been implicated. Anaphylactoid reactions resemble anaphylactic reactions but do not follow immunologic reactions.

ANAPHYLACTIC REACTIONS

Urticaria may occur either as a manifestation of systemic anaphylaxis (see Chapter VIII) or as the only manifestation of Type I hypersensitivity. Drugs are the commonest cause, and any drug given by any route of administration can elicit urticaria. Penicillin has been implicated more frequently than any other single drug (see Chapter X).

Aspirin is not only a common primary cause of urticaria, but also a frequent cause of exacerbations of urticaria due to other agents. Subjects with aspirin sensitivity also often react to tartrazine and other azo dyes and benzoic acid derivatives, all of which are often added to foods and drugs (Table 6.2), and they may react to antipyrine and indomethacin as well as mefenamic acid.[4-6] Occasional patients with sensitivity to dyes or additives lack sensitivity to aspirin. The mechanism of aspirin sensitivity is unknown, but it is apparently not immunologic.[2] Alterations in arachidonic acid metabolism are implicated by similar reactions to indomethacin and mefenamic acid because

---

TABLE 6.1   CLASSIFICATION OF URTICARIA
             AND ANGIOEDEMA

I. IMMUNOLOGIC

   A. Anaphylactic
   B. Cytotoxic
   C. Toxic complex

II. POSSIBLY IMMUNOLOGIC

   A. Cold urticaria
   B. Solar urticaria
   C. Cholinergic urticaria
   D. Dermographism

III. ANAPHYLACTOID

   A. Chemical
   B. Hereditary angioneurotic
      edema

IV. CHRONIC IDIOPATHIC

TABLE 6.2   FOODS OFTEN CONTAINING
             AZO DYES OR BENZOIC ACIDS

AZO DYES

Candy: caramels, life savers, fruit drops, filled chocolates.
Soft drinks, fruit drinks, ades.
Jellies, jams, marmalade, fruit yogurts, ice cream, pie
     fillings, puddings (vanilla, butterscotch, chocolate),
     caramel custard, whips, dessert sauces, powdered
     cream.
Crackers, cheese puffs, chips, cake and cookie mixes,
     waffle and pancake mixes, some brands of macaroni and
     spaghetti, bakery goods except for plain rolls.
Mayonnaise, salad dressing, catsup (certain brands), mus-
     tard, remoulade, bearnaise and hollandaise sauces, other
     sauces.
Mashed rutabagas, purees, packaged soups and some canned
     soups.
Canned anchovies, herring, sardines, fish balls, caviar,
     cleaned shellfish.
Colored toothpastes.

BENZOIC ACID COMPOUNDS

Soft drinks, ciders, fruit drinks and ades.
Jellies, jams, marmalade, fruit gelatins, stewed fruit
     sauces.
Cheese, low calorie margarines, salad dressings, remou-
     lade, hollandaise, bearnaise and mustard sauces.
Refrigerated preserves of herring, sardines, anchovies,
     shellfish, and fish.

---

all three drugs inhibit synthesis of prostaglandins by the cyclo-
oxygenase pathway.

Other causes of urticaria due to Type I hypersensitivity include foods, parasitic infestations, insect bites and stings, and
rarely inhalants (Table 6.3).

Symptoms usually begin within minutes or hours after exposure to the offending allergen, but may persist for a few
weeks without evident reexposure. The response may be dose
related with urticaria only following ingestion of a large amount
of some food usually tolerated in smaller amounts, or in children with more severe hypersensitivity minimal exposure may
elicit a severe reaction.

TABLE 6.3   POSSIBLE CAUSES OF ACUTE
             OR CHRONIC URTICARIA

I. DRUGS

   A. Penicillin
   B. Aspirin
   C. Chemical liberators of histamine

codeine	amphetamine	chlortetracycline
meperidine	atropine	polymixin B
morphine	antazoline	quinine
d-tubocurarine	tolazoline	stilbamidine
thiamine	hydrallazine	dextran

   D. Others

II. FOODS

nuts	chocolate	cereal	peas
peanuts	egg	(including	beans
strawberries,	cow's milk	corn)	mushrooms
and other	and milk products	tomato	garlic
berries	citrus fruit	potato	yeast
fish	banana	beef	spices
shellfish		pork	

III. INHALANTS: Pollens, molds, animal danders, cosmetics

VI. INFECTION: Bacterial, mycotic, viral

V. PARASITIC INFESTATION: Enterobius, Ascaris, Schistosoma, Echinococcus, Trichinella, Toxocara, Trichomonas, Giardia lamblia, Entameoba histolytica

IV. INSECT BITES AND STINGS

VII. PHYSICAL AGENTS: Cold, heat, light, mechanical friction, water

VIII. CHOLINERGIC URTICARIA

IX. EMOTIONAL FACTORS

X. HEREDITARY ANGIONEUROTIC EDEMA

XI. URTICARIA PIGMENTOSA

XII. ASSOCIATED SYSTEMIC DISEASE: Systemic lupus erythematosus, periarteritis nodosa, malignant neoplasm.

Nonspecific histamine release can follow ingestion of strawberries, egg white, lobster, crayfish, and mussels or use of certain drugs (see Table 6.3).[2]

CYTOTOXIC REACTIONS

Urticaria may occur as a manifestation of Type II hypersensitivity probably in response to a byproduct of complement activation. Transfusion reactions due to interaction between IgG or IgM antibody and isoantigens on donor erythrocytes are examples of such reactions.

TOXIC COMPLEX REACTIONS

Serum sickness has been reported in 10% of patients treated with antisera made in animals. Signs and symptoms begin 7-12 days later and include fever, lymphadenopathy, splenomegaly, arthralgia, proteinuria, urticaria or angioedema, and pruritus and whealing at the injection site. Heterologous antisera are no longer used very frequently, but similar reactions can follow administration of drugs.

The urticarial prodrome reported in 10-20% of patients with type B viral hepatitis has been found to be associated with activation of both classic and alternative pathways of complement activation, circulating soluble complexes of hepatitis B surface antigen and antibody in relative antigen excess and necrotizing venulitis, implicating deposition of these complexes in the pathogenesis of the urticaria.[7] Decreased serum concentrations of total hemolytic complement, C3 and C4 are found.

COLD URTICARIA

Exposure to cold may cause localized or generalized urticaria or angioedema sometimes beginning only after subsequent rewarming. There may be associated headache, nausea, vomiting, tachycardia, or syncope. Ingestion of cold foods may cause laryngeal edema.

Familial cold urticaria is inherited as an autosomal dominant. Symptoms begin in infancy or early childhood. Erythema associated with a burning sensation is more common than wheals, and mucous membranes are not involved.[2]

Acquired, idiopathic cold urticaria, the commonest form, occurs more often in adults than children. The onset is usually sudden and may follow an infection, insect sting, penicillin injection, or emotional stress. A sudden decrease in temperature such as that associated with bathing or contact with a cold surface is followed by pruritus and whealing as rewarming occurs. The reaction usually subsides within one hour. Severe attacks may be associated with wheezing[8] or syncope which can cause death from drowning.[9]

Direct application of an ice cube or a test tube containing water at 10°C. to the skin for 2-10 minutes is usually followed by whealing as the skin rewarms. Occasionally cooling of an arm or the entire body or prolonged exposure to cold may be necessary to elicit the response.[2] Delayed reactions to cold are more rare.

In half of affected subjects the response can be passively transferred with serum to the skin of a normal recipient. In some cases this seems to be mediated by IgE,[8] but in others it is mediated by IgM.[10] There is evidence of associated mast cell degranulation, histamine release, and kinin activation.[2,11]

Cold urticaria has occasionally occurred in patients with syphilitic paroxysmal cold hemoglobinuria, multiple myeloma, and conditions associated with cryoglobulinemia.

SOLAR URTICARIA

Solar urticaria or actinic urticaria is also more frequent in adults than children. Intense pruritus, erythema, and whealing occur at the site of exposure to light within 3 minutes, peak within 10 minutes and usually subside within 3 hours. Occasionally a papular or vesicular eruption may appear 18-36 hours after exposure and subside 2-3 days later. The face and dorsa of the hands are often less sensitive than areas of skin which are not usually exposed. With sufficiently extensive reactions, dizziness, wheezing and collapse may occur.

The wavelength of light that elicits the response has usually been shorter than 370 m μ, but this varies from subject to subject, and patients sensitive to visible light have also been found. The activating wavelength can be determined by testing with a monochromator.[2] Sunlight or fluorescent light can also be used with appropriate filters. Solar urticaria due to wavelengths of 285-320 m μ have been passively transferred with serum, and mediation by a reaction between antibody and an antigen released or formed in irradiated skin has been suggested.[2,12] Urticaria due to wavelengths of 400-500 m μ has also been passively transferred but other longer wavelengths have not been transferable.[12]

Solar urticaria has sometimes been associated with systemic lupus erythematosus, porphyria, and treatment with drugs, including sulfonamides.[2]

DIRECT HEAT URTICARIA

Both immediate and delayed urticarial reactions have been reported following direct contact with heat in rare patients.[2,12] Attempts at passive transfer with serum have been unsuccessful. Activation of the alternative complement pathway has been implicated.[13]

CHOLINERGIC URTICARIA

Cholinergic urticaria is characterized by a generalized pruritic eruption of multiple 1-3 mm wheals surrounded by flares appearing within a few minutes following exercise, general heating, or emotional stress and subsiding usually within one hour. Sufficient exercise to cause perspiring is usually necessary to elicit cholinergic urticaria. Exacerbations have been associated with fever and the ingestion of hot or spicy foods.[2] Syncope may occur with severe attacks and association with vomiting, diarrhea, abdominal pain, excessive salivation, and headaches has been reported.[2] Wheezing has rarely occurred with cholinergic urticaria, and whealing has not been associated with the usual type of exercise induced asthma (see Chapter III). Exercise in an occlusive plastic suit, however, has been found to elicit small but significant obstructive pulmonary changes in all 7 adults with cholinergic urticaria who were studied.[39]

Localized whealing can be induced in susceptible subjects by intradermal injection of 0.05 ml of 0.02% methacholine chloride, 0.002% carbamoylcholine chloride, or even 3-6% saline, but the typical response may not occur during the refractory period after an exacerbation of cholinergic urticaria.[14] Exercise in a warm room while wearing warm clothing is also a reliable method for eliciting the response if the exercise is sufficiently prolonged and strenuous to provoke perspiring.

The response is thought to be mediated by cholinergic sympathetic fibers innervating sweat glands. Inhibition by antihistamines or pretreatment with histamine releasing agents indicates that the wheal itself is probably due to histamine release, and increased plasma concentrations of histamine have been detected in some patients during exacerbations of cholinergic urticaria induced by exercise.[15] The response can be passively transferred by serum.[2]

DERMOGRAPHISM

Dermographism, an abnormal tendency for the formation of wheals following mechanical stimulation of the skin, has usually been reported in 1-5% of general populations and may occur with an increased frequency in association with acute or chronic urticaria.[2] This condition may be present throughout most of the subject's life, but symptomatic dermographism associated with pruritus may subside somewhat after months or years. There have been occasional reports of delayed dermographism in which the initial response subsides within 20 minutes but whealing recurs 3-8 hours later and then persists for 24-48 hours.[2]

The mechanisms responsible for symptomatic dermographism are not completely understood, but there is evidence of mediation by histamine and kinins and the response can be passively transferred by serum, probably due to transfer of IgE.[16]

PRESSURE URTICARIA

Pressure urticaria, a phenomenon resembling delayed dermographism, is manifested by the development of deep, often painful edema 4-6 hours after application of pressure to the skin. The swelling usually persists for 8-24 hours.[17]

VIBRATORY ANGIOEDEMA

Vibratory angioedema is a condition transmitted as an autosomal dominant and characterized by localized erythema and edema following application of vibratory or frictional stimuli to the skin.[18] Intense, prolonged stimulation may also cause facial flushing and headache. Manifestations appear in early infancy and persist throughout the rest of the subject's life, although the severity may decrease with age. The response is not passively transferred with serum.

AQUAGENIC URTICARIA

Rare patients have been described in whom contact with water has elicited small wheals with flares resembling the lesions of cholinergic urticaria.[19] Brief contact with water may not elicit the response. Since exposure to water is often associated with other urticariogenic factors (cold, heat, exercise) other possible causes of urticaria must also be investigated.

HEREDITARY ANGIONEUROTIC EDEMA

Hereditary angioneurotic edema or hereditary angioedema is an autosomal dominant disorder of the biosynthesis of the serum α -2 globulin which inhibits the enzymatic activity of the first component of complement. This C1 esterase inhibitor may be absent, deficient, or nonfunctional. It is normally found in serum at a concentration of 18 mg% ($\pm$ 5 mg%).[20] Published data do not indicate whether there is any normal variation with age. In most affected subjects it is reduced to less than 25% of this normal concentration, but in 15% of patients with hereditary angioedema the nonfunctioning analogue is found at normal or increased concentrations. Determination of the serum concentration of C1 esterase inhibitor is not readily available in most laboratories, but the diagnosis can be suspected if decreased concentrations of C4, one of the substrates of C1, are found during an exacerbation. Serum C4 concentrations are usually decreased even when the patient is free of symptoms.

Although inherited as an autosomal dominant, occasional carriers have been free of symptoms for many years, and apparently new mutations have been frequent, so a positive family history is not necessary for the diagnosis.[2] Affected subjects are thought to be heterozygous; the homozygous state is probably incompatible with life.

The onset is usually in childhood with recurrent, subcutaneous or submucosal edema at irregular intervals of weeks, months or years often following trauma. Urticaria is not present. Lesions are not pruritic but may be mildly painful. Involvement of the gastrointestinal tract may cause nausea, vomiting, and severe abdominal pain. Laryngeal or pharyngeal edema has caused fatal asphyxia in 20-30% of affected subjects in some families, but in other kindreds the disease has seemed milder.

IDIOPATHIC

Chronic urticaria has been ascribed to bacterial or mycotic infections and sometimes has occurred in association with myeloproliferative diseases such as polycythemia vera, myeloid metaplasia, and myelogenous leukemia, especially when associated with the presence of increased numbers of basophils,[4] as well as viral hepatitis.

EMOTIONAL FACTORS

In many patients emotional tension has been found to be an aggravating factor, but psychogenic factors alone have not been shown to be sufficient causes of urticaria or angioedema.[2,4]

LABORATORY DATA

Routine laboratory procedures are not usually helpful in the diagnosis of urticaria. The history, morphology, and distribution of lesions may indicate a need for the previously described special tests for cholinergic urticaria, physical urticaria, or hereditary angioneurotic edema.

EOSINOPHILIA

Total eosinophil counts in peripheral blood are usually normal but occasionally are elevated. Peripheral eosinophilia with chronic urticaria does not necessarily indicate a parasitic infestation as the cause.

BASOPENIA

Temporary decreases in the numbers of circulating baso-phils have been associated with non-physical urticaria, but so few are normally present ($45/mm^3$) that this is not usually help-ful clinically. [2]

LEUKOCYTE COUNTS

Total leukocyte counts are usually normal, but leukocyto-sis may be helpful in indicating the presence of unrecognized infection.

STOOL EXAMINATIONS

Examination of several fresh stool specimens for ova, cysts, and parasites may be necessary to establish the presence of this cause of urticaria.

IMMUNOGLOBULINS

Serum IgE concentrations are usually normal, unless ele-vated due to the presence of a parasitic infestation. Children with chronic urticaria and recurrent infections have sometimes been found to have decreased serum concentrations of IgG, A, and M. [21] Serum immunoglobulin concentrations have been re-ported normal in adults with acute or chronic urticaria not as-sociated with infection, except for slight increases in IgG associated with chronic urticaria.

ALLERGY SKIN TESTING

Allergy skin testing is not usually helpful in determining the cause of urticaria except in the rare patient in whom an in-halant allergen is responsible or with hypersensitivity to peni-cillin (see Chapter X). It is occasionally helpful in implicating a food not previously suspected. Techniques, interpretation, and limitations are discussed in Chapter XIII.

COMPLEMENT

Serum complement concentrations are usually normal in patients with acute urticaria except when associated with viral hepatitis. Decreased concentrations of total hemolytic comple-ment (CH50), C3, C4, and other complement components have been found in many adults with chronic urticaria. [22, 23]

DIFFERENTIAL DIAGNOSIS OF URTICARIA

The diagnosis is usually easily established by history or physical examination, but "papular urticaria" due to insect bites, anaphylactoid purpura, and urticaria pigmentosa bear superficial similarities to urticaria.

PAPULAR URTICARIA

Although the term "papular urticaria" is contradictory in that an urticarial wheal is not a papule, the term is applied to the common, biphasic reaction which follows insect bites. [2] The immediate wheal is due to Type I hypersensitivity, while the delayed reaction is due to Type IV hypersensitivity. The diagnosis is usually apparent from the typical distribution of the pruritic lesions in groups over exposed portions of the body. Mosquitoes and fleas are most often responsible, but mites and other arthropods also cause similar lesions.

Hymenoptera stings can cause generalized urticaria, anaphylaxis or serum sickness (see Chapter XI).

ANAPHYLACTOID PURPURA

Anaphylactoid purpura (allergic vasculitis, Henoch-Schonlein purpura) is an acute, inflammatory process of unknown cause involving medium sized arterioles and venules of the skin, joints, intestines, and kidney. The cutaneous manifestations are usually easily differentiated from urticaria by the presence of purpura and the characteristic distribution over the lower extremities and buttocks, but urticarial lesions may also be present.

URTICARIA PIGMENTOSA

Urticaria pigmentosa is usually a localized disease due to solitary or multiple accumulations of mast cells in the skin evident as areas of increased pigmentation or nodules that develop wheals when rubbed or scratched (Darier's sign). Mastocytosis may also affect other organs. With extensive involvement flushing and other symptoms of histamine release may be induced by codeine and possibly other agents known to release histamine from mast cells.

DIFFERENTIAL DIAGNOSIS OF ANGIOEDEMA

Other causes of edema which must be differentiated from angioedema include infection, cardiac or renal failure, the

Melkersson Rosenthal syndrome, obstruction of the superior vena cava, and idiopathic scrotal edema

Most of these are readily differentiated from angioedema by associated clinical characteristics. Periorbital cellulitis or ethmoidal sinusitis may simulate periorbital angioedema, but the presence of erythema, tenderness, or other signs of infection may be helpful in establishing the diagnosis.

MELKERSSON ROSENTHAL SYNDROME

The Melkersson Rosenthal syndrome is a rare disorder characterized by recurrent weakness of the facial nerve with edema of the lips, eyelids, nose, or chin, and a fissured or scrotal tongue, beginning usually in childhood or adolescence.[24] It may manifest itself initially with recurrent edema of the lips. It is distinguished from angioedema by the tendency for each exacerbation to be followed by residual thickening of the tissues.

SUPERIOR VENA CAVA SYNDROME

The acute or gradual edema of the head, neck, upper extremities, and shoulders typical of obstruction of the superior vena cava may be confused with angioedema especially early in its development, when periorbital edema may be the only manifestation. Features useful in suggesting the diagnosis include jugular venous distention, the presence of pitting edema, and variation with position with a tendency for the edema to be most prominent in the morning. Determination of elevated venous pressure in the upper extremities as compared with the lower extremities establishes the diagnosis.

IDIOPATHIC SCROTAL EDEMA

Idiopathic scrotal edema of infants and children is an uncommon disorder manifested by acute unilateral or bilateral edema of the scrotum, sometimes also involving the penis, thighs, and lower abdomen. The scrotum usually appears bright pink. Pain is absent or minimal. It can be differentiated from testicular torsion, acute epididymo-orchitis, and inguinal hernia by physical examination. The cause is unknown, but hypersensitivity is suspected, and resolution may be accelerated by treatment with antihistamines.

ANGIOEDEMA WITH HYPOCOMPLEMENTEMIA

Rare patients have been reported to have recurrent erythematous, maculopapular cutaneous eruptions and angioedema associated with complement activation evident from decreased concentrations of C1q, C4, and C2.[25] These subjects have had normal serum concentrations of C1 esterase inhibitor.

COMPLICATIONS

Most of the serious complications of urticaria and angioedema have already been mentioned. These include airway obstruction due to laryngeal or pharyngeal edema (most common with hereditary angioneurotic edema or cold urticaria), syncope (potentially especially hazardous when occurring in a swimmer with cold urticaria), and hypotension or shock. Although electrocardiographic changes consistent with cardiac ischemia have been reported in association even with mild urticaria, such changes apparently occur only rarely with urticaria at least in children and young adults, although they might be expected in urticaria associated with airway obstruction or shock.[26]

TREATMENT

Indicated therapy and response to therapy depends upon the type of urticaria and its cause. Unfortunately, in a large number of cases the specific cause is not determined. When an ingestant, inhalant, or contactant is implicated, prevention of further exposure is the most important aspect of treatment, although this may be difficult with certain foods and food or drug dyes or other additives. When an infection or infestation is identified it must be eradicated if possible. When urticaria has followed hymenoptera stings, precautions should be observed to minimize the likelihood of reexposure and immunotherapy is presently considered indicated (see Chapter XI).

Aspirin has been found frequently to cause exacerbations in subjects with chronic urticaria, so it and other salicylates should be avoided by such patients (Table 6.4). It is prudent also to avoid ingestion of tartrazine and other azo dyes as well as benzoic acid derivatives, especially when aspirin has been implicated as a causative agent (see Table 6.2).[2]

SYMPATHOMIMETICS

Administration of 1:1000 aqueous epinephrine (0.01 ml/Kg, maximum 0.25 ml in children) by subcutaneous injection usually affords rapid relief of urticaria. This dose can be repeated

TABLE 6.4   PARTIAL LIST OF SOURCES OF
ASPIRIN AND OTHER SALICYLATES

DRUGS

Alka-Seltzer	Dasin	Measurin
Anacin	Decagesic	Midol
Anahist	Dolor	Pabirin
A. P. C.	Dristan	PAC
Ascriptin	Ecotrin	Percodan
Aspergum	Empirin	Persistin
Aspirin	Emprazil	Phenaphen
B-C Headache Powder	Equagesic	Phensal
Bufferin	Excedrin	Sal-Fayne
Cama	Fiorinal	Stanback
Coricidin	4-Way Cold Tablets	Trancogesic
Darvon	Liquiprin Tablet	Trigesic
		Vanquish

OTHER PREPARATIONS

Candy	Mint flavored foods
Food Preserva-tives	Mouthwash
	Teething powders
Gum	Toothpaste

twice at 20 minute intervals if necessary, or 1:200 epinephrine suspension (Sus-Phrine) can be administered for more sustained relief (0. 005 ml/Kg, maximum dose 0. 15 ml in children). Administration of epinephrine may be life-saving if laryngeal edema occurs[2], but if this fails to relieve the airway obstruction tracheostomy may be necessary.

Ephedrine is effective following oral administration and has a longer duration of action than 1:1000 aqueous epinephrine. Ephedrine can be administered at a dose of 0. 5-1. 0 mg/Kg t. i. d. -q. i. d. (maximum 50 mg. q. i. d.).

ANTIHISTAMINES

Antihistamines are often effective in the control of urticaria, but usually must be given very soon after the onset of symptoms for effective control of angioedema. [2] Hydroxyzine, an antihistamine that also has anticholinergic and antiserotonin properties, is one of the most effective drugs for the treatment of urticaria, especially physical urticaria. Because of individual variations in response, trials of antihistamines from several different chemical groups and gradual increases in dosage until the desired response or intolerable side effects supervene may be necessary (see Chapter IV). Chronic, intractable urticaria has been reported to respond to treatment with the H2 antagonist, cimetidine, or treatment with both cimetidine and cyproheptadine in some adults. [27] Cimetidine is not approved for this indication by the U. S. Food and Drug Administration.

ADRENAL CORTICOSTEROIDS

Adrenal corticosteroids are usually effective in controlling urticaria if administered in sufficiently large doses, but because of the numerous possible side effects (see Chapter VI), including suppression of the hypothalamic-pituitary-adrenal axis, they are rarely if ever indicated for the treatment of urticaria.

COLD URTICARIA

The most important aspects of management are prevention of contact with cold water, cold surfaces, and cold foods or beverages. Prolonged bathing under circumstances permitting cooling of the skin by evaporation should be avoided. Cold urticaria often responds to treatment with cyproheptadine or other antihistamines, but large doses may be necessary.

SOLAR URTICARIA

Avoidance of sunlight is desirable and topical preparations containing p-aminobenzoic acid are helpful in affording protection when the reaction is due to the shorter ultraviolet light wavelengths. Titanium dioxide combined with zinc oxide has been reported somewhat helpful as a sun screen against longer wavelengths. [28]

Gradual, progressive increases in exposure to sunlight may be associated with improved tolerance, probably due to increased pigmentation. [2]

Antihistamines are often effective.

CHOLINERGIC URTICARIA

It is reported that severe exacerbations of cholinergic urticaria can be prevented by rapid cooling soon after the onset of the attack. [2] Episodes of cholinergic urticaria are followed by refractory periods of a few hours up to 24 hours, depending upon the severity of the attack; thus, deliberate provocation of urticaria by exercise or a hot bath may permit subsequent exercise without urticaria on special occasions. [2]

Antihistamines are often helpful, and hydroxyzine may be especially effective.

VIBRATORY ANGIOEDEMA

Administration of isoproterenol has been reported to prevent vibratory angioedema, while epinephrine and diphenhydramine have modified this abnormal response. [29]

HEREDITARY
ANGIONEUROTIC EDEMA

Epsilon aminocaproic acid and trans-4-(aminomethyl) cyclohexane-1-carboxylic acid (tranexamic acid) have been found to decrease the severity and frequency of exacerbations of hereditary angioneurotic edema. These drugs inhibit plasminogen and plasmin and thus inhibit activation of C1 by plasmin. Epsilon aminocaproic acid has been found effective at a dose of 16-20 Gm daily (in 4-6 divided doses), but muscle weakness, fatigue, nasal congestion, and hypotension with syncope have occurred as side effects. [30] Temporary increases in dosage to 30 Gm daily for several days after the onset of an attack may lessen its severity. [31] Muscle necrosis has been associated with use of large doses. [32] Tranexamic acid, a more effective inhibitor of plasminogen activation, has prevented exacerbations when given at a dose of 1 Gm t. i. d. [33] Side effects included nausea, vomiting, and diarrhea. Thrombotic episodes have rarely been associated with one of these drugs, but since that is a potential hazard, any tendency to thromboembolic disorders has been considered a contraindication to their use.

Replacement therapy with fresh frozen plasma has been found effective in the treatment of acute episodes of edema and in the prevention of attacks in patients undergoing oral surgery. [34,35] Administration of 400-1500 ml to adults during attacks has been followed by improvement within 45 minutes after the infusion was started and almost complete recovery within 12 hours. [34] Administration of 2 units of fresh frozen plasma in acid-citrate-dextrose the day before dental procedures has been found to be effective prophylactic therapy in adults. [35]

Methyltestosterone, 20 mg. b. i. d. , has also been reported effective in preventing episodes of hereditary angioneurotic edema. [36] The mechanism is unknown. Side effects have included masculinization, hirsutism, and acne. Treatment with danazol, an androgen derivative, prevents attacks of angioedema and increases serum concentrations of C1 esterase inhibitor and C4, often to normal.[37] Amenorrhea has occurred in some women receiving the drug, but virilization has not been problematic in adults. Possible interference with normal sexual maturation may prevent its use in children, and the lack of knowledge of possible effects upon the fetus may contraindicate its use in pregnant women.

Response to treatment with epinephrine, antihistamines and adrenal corticosteroids has generally been poor, although it has been claimed that very large doses of epinephrine may be helpful.[38]

PROGNOSIS

Urticaria occurs most often as an acute, self-limited disorder which subsides within a few hours or days and may never recur even if the offending agent is not identified. Often the cause is easily recognized and recurrences can be prevented by avoidance.

In chronic urticaria, usually defined by persistence for 3-6 months, the cause may be established in as few as 30% of patients, and the prognosis accordingly is poor. It has been estimated that as many as 50% of patients with urticaria severe enough to have necessitated referral continue to have active disease 6 months after its onset, and 20% may still have intermittent urticaria at 10 years.[2] Of patients in whom urticaria has persisted for longer than 6 months 40% are likely still to be affected after 10 years, and urticaria has sometimes persisted as long as 50 years.

A mortality rate as high as 30% has been quoted for hereditary angioneurotic edema, but other forms of urticaria and angioedema are rarely life threatening unless associated with systemic anaphylaxis (see Chapter VIII).

REFERENCES

1. Sheldon, J. M., et al.: The vexing urticaria problem: present concepts of etiology and management. J All 25: 525, 1954.
2. Warin, R. P., and Champion, R. H.: Urticaria, W. B. Saunders Co., Philadelphia, 1974.
3. Paton, W. D. M.: Histamine release by compounds of simple chemical structure. Pharm Rev 9:269, 1957.
4. Lockey, S. D.: Reactions to hidden agents in foods, beverages, and drugs. Ann All 29:461, 1971.

5. Juhlin, L., et al.: Urticaria and asthma induced by food-and-drug additives in patients with aspirin hypersensitivity. J All Clin Imm 50:92, 1972.
6. Michaelsson, G., and Juhlin, L.: Urticaria induced by preservatives and dye additives in food and drugs. Brit J Derm 88:525, 1973.
7. Dienstag, J. L., Rhodes, A. R., Bhan, A. K., Dvorak, A. M., Mihm, M. C., Jr., and Wands, J. R.: Urticaria associated with acute viral hepatitis type B. Ann Int Med 89: 34, 1978.
8. Houser, D. D., et al.: Cold urticaria. Am J Med 49:23, 1970.
9. Horton, B. T., et al.: Hypersensitiveness to cold. JAMA 107:1263, 1936.
10. Wanderer, A. A., et al.: Immunologic characterization of serum factors responsible for cold urticaria. J All 48:13, 1971.
11. Beall, G. N.: Urticaria: a review of laboratory and clinical observations. Med 43:131, 1964.
12. Baer, R. L., and Harber, L. C.: "Reactions to light, heat, and trauma" in Samter, M. (ed): Immunological diseases, 2nd ed, Little, Brown, & Co., Boston, 1971, p 973.
13. Daman, L., Lieberman, P., Ganier, M., and Hashimoto, K.: Localized heat urticaria. J All Clin Immunol 61:273, 1978.
14. Lorincz, A. L.: The physical urticarias. Jap J Derm 76: 11, 1966.
15. Kaplan, A. P., et al.: In vivo studies of mediator release in cold urticaria and cholinergic urticaria. J All Clin Imm 55:394, 1975.
16. Newcomb, R. W., and Nelson, H.: Dermatographia mediated by immunoglobulin E. Am J Med 54:174, 1973.
17. Ryan, T. J., et al.: Delayed pressure urticaria. Brit J Derm 80:485, 1968.
18. Patterson, R., et al.: Vibratory angioedema: a hereditary type of physical hypersensitivity. J All Clin Imm 50: 174, 1972.
19. Tromovitch, T. A.: Urticaria from contact with water. Calif Med 106:400, 1967.
20. Rosen, F. S., et al.: Genetically determined heterogeneity of the C1 esterase inhibitor in patients with hereditary angioneurotic edema. J Clin Invest 50:2143, 1971.
21. Buckley, R. H., and Dees, S. C.: Serum immunoglobulins. III. Abnormalities associated with chronic urticaria in children. J All 40:294, 1967.
22. Mathison, D. A., Arroyave, C. M., Bhat, K. N., Hurewitz, D. S., and Marnell, D. J.: Hypocomplementemia in chronic idiopathic urticaria. Ann Int Med 86:534, 1977.

23. Laurell, A. B., Martensson, J., and Sjoholm, A. G.: Studies of C1 subcomponents in chronic urticaria and angioedema. Int Arch All Appl Immunol 54:434, 1977.
24. Kettel, K.: Melkersson's syndrome. Arch Otolaryngol 46: 341, 1947.
25. Sissons, J. G. P., et al.: Skin lesions, angio-edema, and hypocomplementemia. Lancet 2:1350, 1974.
26. Siegel, S. C., and Bergeron, J. G.: Urticaria and angioedema in children and young adults. Ann All 12:241, 1954.
27. Phanuphak, P., Schocket, A., and Kohler, P. F.: Treatment of chronic idiopathic urticaria with combined H1 and H2 blockers. Clin All 8:429, 1978.
28. Macleod, T. M., and Frain-Bell, W.: The study of the efficacy of some agents used for the protection of the skin from exposure to light. Brit J Derm 84:266, 1971.
29. Mellies, C. J., et al.: Clinical and pharmacologic studies of vibratory angioedema. J All Clin Imm 51:98, 1973.
30. Frank, M. M., et al.: Epsilon aminocaproic acid therapy of hereditary angioneurotic edema. A double blind study. NEJM 286:808, 1972.
31. Champion, R. H., and Lachmann, P. J.: Hereditary angioedema treated with E-aminocaproic acid. Brit J Derm 81: 763, 1969.
32. Korsan-Bengtsen, K., et al.: Extensive muscle necrosis after long-term treatment with aminocaproic acid (EACA) in a case of hereditary periodic edema. Acta Med Scand 185:341, 1969.
33. Sheffer, A. L., et al.: Tranexamic acid therapy in hereditary angioneurotic edema. NEJM 287:452, 1972.
34. Cohen, G., and Peterson, A.: Treatment of hereditary angioedema with frozen plasma. Ann All 30:690, 1972.
35. Jaffe, C. J., et al.: Hereditary angioedema: The use of fresh frozen plasma for prophylaxis in patients undergoing oral surgery. J All Clin Imm 55:386, 1975.
36. Spaulding, W. B.: Methyltestosterone therapy for hereditary episodic edema (hereditary angioneurotic edema). Ann Int Med 53:739, 1960.
37. Gelfand, J. A., Sherins, R. J., Alling, D. W., and Frank, M. M.: Treatment of hereditary andioedema with danazol. New Eng J Med 295:1444, 1976.
38. Roth, M., et al.: Adrenalin treatment for hereditary angioneurotic edema. Ann All 35:175, 1975.
39. Soter, N. A., Wasserman, S. I., Austen, K. F., and McFadden, E. R., Jr.: Release of mast-cell mediators and alterations in lung function in patients with cholinergic urticaria. New Eng J Med 302:604, 1980.

CHAPTER VII | OTOLOGIC ALLERGY

Although secretory otitis media is the commonest otologic problem in children for which allergy consultation is sought, allergic reactions can involve the external ear or inner ear as well as the middle ear.

EXTERNAL EAR

CONTACT DERMATITIS

Contact dermatitis may be due to hypersensitivity to metals such as nickel, chromium, silver, or gold, often used in earrings; chemicals found in cosmetics, nail polish, hair sprays, plastics, or soaps; drugs such as sulfonamides, antibiotics, or coal tar derivatives: rubber; leather; animal danders; and plants. The source of the contactant can sometimes be suspected from the distribution of the eruption. Postauricular dermatitis may be due to contact with the frames of glasses or hair sprays, while involvement of the external auditory canal suggests hypersensitivity to medication introduced as ear drops.

Common complaints include itching, burning, or stinging, any of which may be very severe. There may be mild edema and erythema or scaling and vesiculation, but superimposed infection due to self inflicted trauma is common, resulting in oozing and crusting.

Specific allergens can be identified by patch testing or by response to avoidance.

Elimination of exposure to the offending contactant allergen is necessary for effective treatment, but contact with any potential irritant should be avoided while the reaction continues. Local therapy is similar to that recommended for atopic dermatitis (see Chapter V), consisting of application for 10 minutes every 2-6 hours of cold compresses soaked in aluminum acetate or Burow's solution for the acute, exudative stage, and 1/2% or 1% hydrocortisone cream applied t. i. d. or q. i. d. for milder reactions. Nocturnal sedation with large doses of an antihista-

246

mine may be necessary to prevent scratching. Secondary infection should be treated with an oral antibiotic such as penicillin or erythromycin.

Rarely a very severe reaction may necessitate systemic treatment with adrenal corticosteroids. Their use should be avoided if at all possible because of the numerous possible side effects, including adrenal suppression (see Chapter III). These can be minimized by limiting treatment to the smallest doses and shortest period of time necessary. Even the severest reactions usually respond to treatment with oral corticosteroids within 1 week. Prednisone at a dose of up to 40 mg/day (1-2 mg/Kg body weight) in four divided doses for three days followed by decreasing doses for another 4-7 days is usually sufficient, but daily treatment with prednisone even for this short period also induces adrenal suppression.

ATOPIC DERMATITIS

Atopic dermatitis of the external ear presents as an intensely pruritic eruption consisting of reddish brown papules, xerosis, and fine scales in the concha and outer third of the external auditory canal. Scratching causes excoriations, erythema, and weeping, as the eruption becomes papulovesicular. There may be evidence of atopic dermatitis elsewhere, and fissuring of the skin fold beneath the earlobe is usually due to atopic dermatitis. Allergic rhinitis or asthma may also be present.

Treatment is much the same as for atopic dermatitis in other locations (see Chapter V), including prevention of exposure to offending allergens or irritants, topical hydrocortisone for reactions of mild or moderate severity, and applications of cold aluminun acetate solutions for the acute, exudative stage.

DIFFERENTIAL DIAGNOSIS

The differential diagnosis of allergic otitis externa includes seborrheic dermatitis, psoriasis, infection, and foreign bodies.

Seborrheic dermatitis more frequently causes postauricular fissuring rather than fissuring beneath the earlobe, but it can also be found in the outer third of the external auditory canal. Other areas involved may include the scalp, forehead, eyebrows, eyelid margins, corners of the nose, axillae, umbilicus, and inguinal creases rather than areas typical of atopic dermatitis such as the cheeks, neck, and antecubital and popliteal spaces. Pruritus is absent or mild, and the scales are large and greasy.

Psoriasis can also be found in the concha and outer third of the external auditory canal. The scales are silvery and occur in multiple layers. The typical dull, erythematous plaques are usually found over the elbows, knees, scalp, and sacrum.

Infectious otitis externa with pain, itching, edema, and fever may resemble allergic otitis with superimposed infection, but the usual history of recent swimming may help to identify cause. Drainage of purulent secretions through a perforated tympanic membrane can cause inflammation of the external auditory canal which subsides as the otitis media responds to treatment.

Foreign bodies can also cause inflammation of the external auditory canal, but these are usually easily diagnosed by physical examination.

SECRETORY OTITIS MEDIA

Secretory otitis media or serous otitis media is a chronic or recurrent accumulation of usually sterile fluid behind the tympanic membrane which causes auditory impairment.

The middle ear is normally lined mostly with cuboidal epithelium, but ciliated columnar epithelium interspersed with goblet cells is found near the eustachian tube and throughout its length. Subepithelial mucous glands are also found in the eustachian tube.[1] With secretory otitis media increased gland formation is common in the middle ear, increased numbers of lymphocytes and plasma cells have sometimes been found in the submucosa, and squamous metaplasia can occur.[2]

The fluid itself has been reported to be a transudate, based upon comparisons with serum by protein electrophoresis,[3] but with superimposed infection a mucous exudate with a higher protein concentration is formed.[1] The presence of secretory IgA and other proteins not found in plasma in middle ear secretions obtained from patients with secretory otitis media confirms secretion of proteins by the middle ear mucosa and indicates activity of local immunity.[4]

Middle ear secretions from few children with secretory otitis media have been found to contain IgE by some,[4] while others have reported increased concentrations of IgE in middle ear secretions from most children with secretory otitis media.[5] Some have found eosinophils in middle ear fluid; others have not.[1] The presence of IgE or eosinophils has seemed unrelated to the presence of other evidence of allergy. No IgE forming plasma cells have been identified by immunofluorescent studies of middle ear tissues by some authors while others have apparently identified IgE forming plasma cells.[5]

Ventilation of the middle ear with equalization of pressure with atmospheric pressure is maintained by intermittent opening of the eustachian tube. Contraction of the tensor veli palatini, which occurs often during swallowing, yawning or sneezing, opens the eustachian tube. Obstruction or failure of the tube to open prevents entry of air into the middle ear. As air within the middle ear is absorbed, the reduced pressure may favor transudation, but this is unproved.[1] Measurement of changes in middle ear pressure has demonstrated inefficiency of function of the eustachian tube during the first 7 years, observations which can be related to anatomic characteristics which change in older children to permit more efficient function.[6] Tubal dysfunction due to the recumbent position has also been demonstrated in normal subjects, an observation ascribed to mucosal engorgement due to hydrostatic venous pressure.[7]

Adenoidal hypertrophy is probably seldom responsible for obstruction of the ostia of the eustachian tubes, but may possibly contribute to tubal dysfunction by limiting pressure changes within the eustachian tube.

Both experimental study and clinical observation indicate that fluid can persist indefinitely in the middle ear despite patency of the eustachian tube,[8] although it is probably also possible for fluid to be absorbed by the mucosa of the middle ear, because this has been demonstrated in dogs.[9] There is evidence that fluid can escape through the eustachian tube only if pressure within the middle ear exceeds pressure at the termination of the eustachian tube in the nasopharynx. On the other hand transmission of negative pressure in the nasopharynx to the middle ear may favor subsequent retrograde reflux of fluid from the nasopharynx into the middle ear through the eustachian tube.[10] This might follow sucking a thumb, pacifier, or poorly vented nursing bottle, sniffing, or swallowing with nasal obstruction.

Factors implicated as causes of secretory otitis media include infection and allergy as well as obstruction or dysfunction of the eustachian tube. It is possible that the viscosity or volume of fluid following an episode of acute, suppurative otitis media may exceed the clearance capability of the system.

In some studies most of the subjects with secretory otitis media have been found to have positive family histories for allergy, associated allergic rhinitis, positive skin tests for allergens and favorable responses to allergy treatment.[11,12] Others have reported finding evidence of allergy in only 20-32% of unselected children with secretory otitis media.[13,14] Concentrations of IgE were found to be elevated in the sera and middle ear effusions of 3 of 10 atopic children in one of these studies, but concentrations were higher in the sera, suggesting antibody had reached the middle ear effusion by transudation.[14] Passive transfer testing demonstrated the presence of specific IgE antibody to ragweed and Alternaria in the middle ear secretions of 1 patient whose serum lacked these antibodies, indicating local sensitization. In 6 other children, positive passive transfer tests were found with serum but not with middle ear secretions.

Secretory otitis media or a very similar condition has been produced in guinea pigs previously immunized with bovine serum albumin by injection of this antigen into the middle ear.[15] A condition resembling secretory otitis media has also been produced by insufflation of ragweed pollen into eustachian tubes of monkeys passively sensitized to ragweed by transfusion with serum of a hypersensitive human.[16]

Abnormal tympanograms have been found in as many as 30% of children with allergic respiratory disease, and 5% of the allergic children had type B tympanograms consistent with middle ear effusion, usually unsuspected.[17] Even higher frequencies of abnormal tympanograms have been found in unselected four- and five-year-old kindergarten children than in children of the same age with allergic respiratory disease, however.[18]

Apparently allergy is only one of several important causes of secretory otitis media. Most evidence suggests that it occurs as a complication of the effects of allergic rhinitis upon the nasal mucosa and function of the eustachian tube, but rare primary allergic reactions restricted to the mucosa of the middle ear can also occur.

SYMPTOMATOLOGY

Secretory otitis media usually presents as a loss of auditory acuity which may have been unsuspected until a routine hearing test was done. The loss may occur suddenly following an episode of otitis media or an earache, but usually its onset and progression is insidious. It may fluctuate in severity. The child's response only to loud voices may have been misinterpreted as willful disobedience or disinterest. School achievement often has been poor. Older children may complain of a sensation of fullness in the ears or popping and crackling noises. There may be a history of recurrent episodes of superimposed acute, suppurative otitis media. There is often a history of symptoms of allergic rhinitis (see Chapter IV).

PHYSICAL FINDINGS

The tympanic membrane may appear normal or bulging, but usually is retracted with an abnormally prominent short process of the malleus. It is often dull and may be thickened or wrinkled. The color may be gray, pink, amber, slightly yellow, or deep blue. Occasionally a fluid level or bubbles may be evident behind the tympanic membrane. The handle of

the malleus may appear chalky white, a sign considered pathognomonic of chronic secretory otitis media, or bony landmarks
may be completely obliterated. Limitation of mobility is usually evident to examination with a pneumatic otoscope.

Tuning fork tests disclose that bone conduction is greater
than air conduction. Forks with frequencies of 256, 512, and
1024 can be used; the 256 fork is most sensitive.[1] The Weber
test reveals that the sound is heard better on the side with the
conductive hearing loss when the base of the vibrating fork is
placed on the midline of the skull.

Physical signs of allergic rhinitis are often present (see
Chapter IV).

LABORATORY FINDINGS

Audiometry confirms the presence of a conductive hearing
loss of more than 10 decibels and often 30-50 decibels, usually
relatively constant over all test frequencies.

Tympanometry is the measurement of compliance of the
tympanic membrane during artificially induced changes in air
pressure in the external auditory canal, using an electroacous-
tic impedance bridge or meter. The tympanogram obtained
depends upon the fact that absorption of sound by the tympanic
membrane varies inversely with stiffness of the tympanic membrane. Stiffness and acoustic impedence are least when pressure is equal on both sides of the tympanic membrane. Available
instruments measure the reciprocal of impedance, acoustic admittance. Accordingly it is the ease with which energy flows
that is measured and expressed as acoustic susceptance in mil-
limhos, or as acoustic compliance in cubic centimeters of a
volume of air that has an equivalent compliance. Susceptance
and compliance are essentially equivalent at a frequency of
226 Hz.[19]

Tympanograms are classified as A, B, or C, depending
upon their shape and the pressure at which peak compliance
occurs.[20] Peak compliance of type A tympanograms occurs
at or near pressures of 0 (Fig. 7.1). Type C tympanograms
resemble type A tympanograms, but peak compliance occurs
at or below pressures of -100 mm water. Type B tympanograms are flat and usually indicate the presence of middle
ear effusion, but they can also be due to the presence of im-
pacted cerumen or scarring of the tympanic membranes.[21]
A type C tympanogram indicates an abnormal decrease in
pressure in the middle ear usually due to eustachian tube dysfunction, but type C tympanograms have also sometimes been

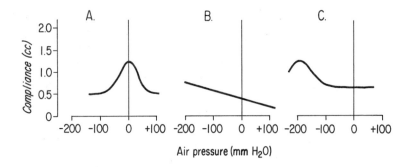

Fig. 7-1. Three common types of tympanograms as obtained by the Teledyne Avionics acoustic impedance meter and plotter.

associated with middle ear effusion. Type A tympanograms are normal but even type A tympanograms may be associated with middle ear effusions if compliance is decreased. Compliance of less than 0.25 cc is probably abnormally decreased when the Teledyne Avionics acoustic impedance meter is used. [22]

Tympanometry has been found to be more sensitive for the detection of middle ear effusion or reduced pressure in the middle ear than either audiometry or pneumatic otoscopy as it is most commonly applied. [21, 23, 24] Tympanometry has been reported to be useful in the evaluation of young infants as well as older children and adults. [25]

Middle ear abnormalities manifested as type B or type C tympanograms often subside spontaneously without treatment within 6 weeks. [22] This must be taken into consideration in assessing the need for therapy and in evaluating responses to therapy.

A lateral roentgenogram of the neck is helpful to establish whether dysfunction of the eustachian tube is due to a nasopharyngeal mass (neoplasm or adenoidal hypertrophy). A roentgenographic method for evaluation of eustachian tube function following injection of contrast material such as Hypaque or Pantopaque through the tympanic membrane has been described. Contrast material is normally cleared from the middle ear within 10 minutes. [26]

Examination of nasal smears for eosinophils is indicated when there is evidence of allergic rhinitis (see Chapter IV).

Allergy skin testing (see Chapter XIII) is most likely to be helpful in identifying specific allergens when the medical history and physical findings suggest allergic rhinitis.

COMPLICATIONS

The commonest complication of secretory otitis media is acute, suppurative otitis media, which usually responds to treatment with antibiotics but may further aggravate the more chronic process. Acute or chronic mastoiditis can also occur.

The commonest serious complication is permanent impairment of auditory acuity due to adhesive otitis media, and this is more likely to occur if treatment is deferred.

If chronic secretory otitis media becomes well established in infancy or early childhood it may cause an extreme delay in the acquisition of speech. Impairment of auditory acuity can have an adverse effect upon social and emotional adjustment as well as acquisition of language skills, and an increased frequency of middle ear abnormalities detected by tympanometry has been reported in children with learning disabilities. [27-29]

A cholesteatoma can occur as a complication of chronic secretory otitis media with or without perforation of the tympanic membrane, but is usually found in association with chronic drainage through a perforated drum.

TREATMENT

When allergy is implicated measures should be instituted to prevent or to minimize exposure to suspected or incriminated allergens (see Chapters IX and XII). When allergens which cannot be avoided, such as pollens and atmospheric molds, are identified, immunotherapy is often beneficial[1, 11, 12] (see Chapter XIV). Pharmacological therapy may also be indicated.

Antihistamines have been shown to block decreases in the patency of canine eustachian tubes induced by histamine, and sympathomimetics with alpha-adrenergic activity can increase patency in eustachian tubes of normal dogs.[30, 31] Nevertheless, there is no conclusive proof that antihistamines or decongestants are effectual in the treatment of secretory otitis media. Direct measurement of pressures in middle ears has demonstrated a definitely beneficial effect of carbinoxamine and pseudoephedrine upon patency of the eustachian tubes of 5 of 13 children.[32] Others have reported no evident, beneficial effect of treatment of children with pseudoephedrine during and after treatment of acute otitis media with several different antibiotics, but the results might have been affected by differences in antibiotic regimens.[33]

Daily use of antihistamines and decongestants is probably most likely to be beneficial if there is evidence of respiratory allergy. If used, topical sympathomimetics should not be continued more than 3 days in succession because of the hazard of rhinitis medicamentosa, and the dose should not be excessive. Details of optimal use of antihistamines and decongestants are found in Chapter IV.

Antibiotics are indicated when infection is present, and aerobic bacteria have been cultured from middle ear effusions in as many as 30% of children with chronic middle ear disease. [34]

Intranasal administration of dexamethasone has been found effective in the treatment of secretory otitis media, [35] but it also causes adrenal suppression at therapeutic doses. [36] Reports of control of symptoms of allergic rhinitis by intranasal beclomethasone dipropionate at doses which do not cause evident adrenal suppression raise the possibility that this may become a useful adjunct in the treatment of secretory otitis media. [37]

Evidence that intranasal treatment with cromolyn sodium is effective in preventing symptoms of allergic rhinitis suggests that this, too, may be found helpful in the treatment of secretory otitis media secondary to allergic rhinitis (see Chapter IV).

Procedures designed to equalize pressure on both sides of the tympanic membrane are of established effectiveness in the treatment of secretory otitis media due to eustachian tube dysfunction. In 1863 Adam Politzer recommended middle ear inflation with a rubber bag while the alae nasi were compressed and the nasopharynx was closed by elevation of the soft palate during swallowing. [38] Subsequent modifications of politzerization have included substitution of compressed air for the rubber bag or bulb and repetition of k-k-k for swallowing water. [39] Simultaneous inspection of the tympanic membrane followed by pneumomassage, utilizing the pneumatic otoscope, and repeated politzerization for more complete removal of fluid has also been recommended. [39] Politzerization should be preceded by meticulous evacuation of mucus from the nose and nasopharynx to minimize introduction of more secretions into the middle ear. Cooperative patients can be taught to do this at home several times each day when there is no perforation of the tympanic membrane, or they can attempt inflation with Valsalva maneuvers, compressing the alae nasi, closing the mouth, and attempting to blow the nose without pouching out the cheeks. [1, 10]

If these methods fail, air pressures can be equalized by myringotomy and fluid can be removed by suction, but recurrence of fluid in the middle ear is frequent after the tympanic membrane heals. When this happens, pressure equalization can be maintained by placing a plastic tube through the tympanic membrane to remain for several weeks or months. [40] Insertion of ventilating tubes is followed by prompt alleviation of conductive hearing loss. Although the tubes are usually extruded spontaneously within a few months, hearing acuity is still good 5-8 years later in all but a very few children. [41] Such long-term follow-up has disclosed normal tympanograms in only 67%, however. Decreased middle ear pressure was the most common abnormality, and effusion had recurred in less than 2%. Adhesive otitis, perforations, and cholesteatoma were found in a few children, but in 25% of the children followed the tympanic membranes were diffusely atrophic, lax, or retracted, possibly increasing the risk of atelectasis and cholesteatoma in the event of a recurrence of acute otitis media. [41]

Resolution of chronic middle ear effusion after treatment with daily prednisone for 1-2 weeks has been found in most of 42 children for whom insertion of ventilating tubes was under consideration. [42]

There is little evidence that adenoidectomy is frequently beneficial. Hypertrophied adenoids may contribute to dysfunction of the eustachian tube by limiting pressure changes but probably only rarely obstruct the ostia. Regrowth of adenoidal tissue often follows adenoidectomy.

Measures which may minimize the likelihood of aspiration of fluid into the middle ear include prohibition of sucking on thumbs, pacifiers, or poorly vented nursing bottles, prevention of sniffing (when possible), [10] and prohibition of self-feeding with liquids in the recumbent position (bottle-propping).

It has been suggested that humidifiers to maintain the relative humidity in the home at 40-50% may help prevent inspissation of nasal secretions and drying of the nose with possible consequent interruption of the integrity of the nasal mucosa. [43] A unit which can be thoroughly cleaned must be chosen, and it should be cleaned regularly to minimize the risk of contamination with molds which could induce hypersensitivity. [44]

INNER EAR

Meniere's disease is an episodic cochleovestibular disorder of undetermined etiology characterized by hearing loss, tinnitus, and vertigo, often associated with nausea and vomiting. There may also be a sensation of intracranial pressure or fullness. Nystagmus may be evident. Most symptoms subside within a few hours. The hearing loss often subsides within a few days but may become permanent after repeated exacerbations. It has been reported only very rarely in children.

The pathogenesis remains obscure. Postmortem examination in subjects who have died of unrelated causes has disclosed distention of the endolymphatic system with distortion of normal relationships, herniations, and rupture of various portions. [45] Rupture of membranes separating the endolymph from the perilymphatic space permitting mixture of the two fluids which differ in ionic composition may account for the observed symptoms.[46]

An allergic etiology in some patients has been suggested by several reports of exacerbations of vertigo or all the symptoms of the syndrome related to exposure to specific allergens, usually foods, and improvement with allergy treatment, including dietary restrictions, environmental control and immunotherapy.[47]

Dietary restriction of sodium and use of diuretics and antihistamines have sometimes been helpful.[48]

REFERENCES

1. Rapp, D. J. , and Fahey, D. : Review of chronic secretory otitis and allergy. J Asthma Res 10:193, 1973.
2. Bernstein, J. M. , and Hayes, E. R. : Middle ear mucosa in health and disease. Arch Otolaryng 94:30, 1971.
3. Tonder, O. , and Gundersen, T. : Nature of the fluid in serous otitis media. Arch Otolaryng 93:473, 1971.
4. Ishikawa, T. , et al.: Secretory otitis media: immunologic studies of middle ear secretions. J All Clin Imm 50:319, 1972.
5. Philips, M. J. , et al.: IgE and secretory otitis media. Lancet ii:1176, 1974.
6. Holborow, C.: Eustachian tubal function. Changes in anatomy and function with age and the relationship of these changes to aural pathology. Arch Otolaryng 92:624, 1970.
7. Rundcrantz, H.: The effects of position change on eustachian tube function. Otolaryng Cl N A 3:103, 1970.
8. Bortnick, E. , et al.: On the egress of fluid from the middle ear. Arch Otolaryng 80:297, 1964.
9. Bortnick, E. , and Proud, G. O.: Experimental absorption of fluids from the middle ear. Arch Otolaryng 81:237, 1965.
10. Lamp, C. B. , Jr.: Chronic secretory otitis media: etiologic factors and pathologic mechanisms. Laryngoscope 83:276, 1973.

11. Whitcomb, N. J.: Allergy therapy in serous otitis media associated with allergic rhinitis. Ann All 23:232, 1965.
12. Dees, S. C., and Lefkowitz, D.: Secretory otitis media in allergic children. Am J Dis Child 124:364, 1972.
13. Davison, F. W.: Middle-ear problems in childhood. JAMA 196:834, 1966.
14. Bernstein, J. M., and Reisman, R.: The role of acute hypersensitivity in secretory otitis media. Trans Am Acad Ophthalmol Otol 78:ORL120, 1974.
15. Hopp, E. S., Elevitch, F. R., Pumphrey, R. E., Irving, T. E., and Hoffman, P. W.: Serous otitis media - An "immune" theory. Laryngoscope 74:1149, 1964.
16. Miglets, A. W., Spiegel, J., and Bernstein, H. A.: Middle ear effusion in experimental hypersensitivity. Ann Otol Rhinol Laryngol 85 (Supp 25, Pt 2):81, 1976.
17. Fernandes, D., Gupta, S., Sly, R. M., and Frazer, M.: Tympanometry in children with allergic respiratory disease. Ann All 40:181, 1978.
18. Zambie, M., Fernandes, D., Sly, R. M., and Frazer, M.: Tympanometry in allergic and in unselected children. J All Clin Immunol 63:200, 1979.
19. Feldman, A. S., and Wilber, L. A.: Acoustic Impedance and Admittance, Baltimore, Williams & Wilkins Co., 1976, p 103.
20. Jerger, J.: Clinical experience with impedance audiometry. Arch Otolaryngol 92:311, 1970.
21. Paradise, J. L., Smith, C. G., and Bluestone, C. D.: Tympanometric detection of middle ear effusions in infants and young children. Ped 58:198, 1976.
22. Sly, R. M., Zambie, M. F., Fernandes, D. A., and Frazer. M.: Tympanometry in kindergarten children. Annals of Allergy 44:1, 1980.
23. McCandless, G. A., and Thomas, G. K.: Impedance audiometry as a screening procedure for middle ear disease. Trans Am Acad Ophthalmol & Otolaryngol 78:ORL98, 1974.
24. Paradise, J. L.: Pediatrician's view of middle ear effusions: More questions than answers. Ann Otol Rhinol Laryngol 85 (Supp 25, Pt 2):20, 1976.
25. Groothuis, J. R., Sell, S. H. W., Wright, P. F., Thompson, J. M., and Altemeier, W. A., III: Otitis media in infancy: Tympanometric findings. Ped 63:435, 1979.
26. Compere, W. E., Jr.: Radiologic evaluation of the eustachian tube. Otolaryngol Cl N A 3:45, 1970.
27. Kaplan, G. J., Fleshman, J. K., Bender, T. R., Baum, C., and Clark, P. S.: Long-term effects of otitis media: a ten year cohort study of Alaskan Eskimo children. Ped 52:577, 1973.

28. Holm, V. A. , and Kunze, L. H. : Effect of chronic otitis media on language and speech development. Ped 43:833, 1969.
29. Masters, L. , and Marsh, G. E. , II: Middle ear pathology as a factor in learning disabilities. J Learning Disabilities 11:104, 1978.
30. Shotts, R. F. , and Jackson, R. T. : Changes in the patency of the dog's eustachian tube induced by histamine and antihistamines. Arch Otolaryngol 96:57, 1972.
31. Davis, L. J. , et al. : Drug-induced patency changes in the eustachian tube. Arch Otolaryng 92:325, 1970.
32. Miller, G. F. : Influence of an oral decongestant on eustachian tube function in children. J All 45:187, 1970.
33. Olson, A. L. , Klein, S. W. , Charney, E. , MacWhinney, J. B. , Jr. , McInerny, T. K. , Miller, R. L. , Nazarian, L. F. , and Cunningham, D. : Prevention and therapy of serous otitis media by oral decongestant: A double-blind study in pediatric practice. Ped 61:679, 1978.
34. Giebink, G. S. , Mills, E. L. , Huff, J. S. , Edelman, C. K. , Weber, M. L. , Juhn, S. K. , nad Quie, P. G. : The microbiology of serous and mucoid otitis media. Ped 63:915, 1979.
35. Lecks, H. I. , et al. : Serous otitis media: Reflections on pathogenesis and treatment. Clin Ped 6:519, 1967.
36. Norman, P. S. , et al. : Adrenal function during the use of dexamethasone aerosols in the treatment of ragweed hay fever. J All 40:57, 1967.
37. Mygind, N. : Local effect of intranasal beclomethasone dipropionate aerosol in hay fever. Brit Med J iv:464, 1973.
38. Ballin, M. J. : Politzer's text-book of the diseases of the ear, 6th ed. , Lea & Febiger, Philadelphia, 1926.
39. Gottschalk, G. H. : Serous otitis: treatment by controlled middle ear inflation. Laryngoscope 72:1379, 1962.
40. Silverstein, H. , et al. : Eustachian tube dysfunction as a cause for chronic secretory otitis in children. (Correction by pressure - equalization). Laryngoscope 76:259, 1966.
41. Tos, M. , and Poulsen, G. : Secretory otitis media. Arch Otolaryngol 102:672, 1976.
42. Schwartz, R. H. , Puglise, J. , and Schwartz, D. M. : Use of a short course of prednisone for treating middle ear effusion. Ann Otol Rhinol Laryngol Suppl (In Press).
43. Sale, C. S. : Control of allergy and humidity in secretory otitis media of children: an analysis of 423 cases. S Med J 63:1042, 1970.
44. Weiss, W. I. , et al. : Hypersensitivity pneumonitis due to contamination of a home humidifier. J All 47:113, 1971.

45. Altmann, F. , and Kornfeld, M. : Histological studies of Meniere's disease. Ann Otol 74:915, 1965.
46. Schuknecht, H. F. : Correlation of pathology with symptoms of Meniere's disease. Otolaryng Cl N A 1:433, 1968.
47. Clemis, J. D. : Cochleovestibular disorders and allergy. Otolaryngol Cl N A 7:757, 1974.
48. Klockhoff, I. , and Lindblom, U. : Glycerol test and diuretics in Meniere's disease. Otolaryngol Cl N A 1:541, 1968.

CHAPTER VIII | ANAPHYLAXIS

During a Mediterranean cruise in 1901 Charles Richet and Paul Portier became interested in seeking to develop an agent which would afford protection (phylaxis) against Physalia toxin. Richet found that injection of an extract of actinaria tentacles into dogs was followed in 2-3 weeks by increased sensitivity. A second injection elicited within a few seconds panting, prostration, diarrhea, and hematemesis. Death often occurred within minutes. The reaction seemed the opposite of the protection which was sought, so Richet coined the term "anaphylaxis".[1]

Type I reactions have been subclassified into generalized or systemic anaphylactic reactions and local anaphylactic reactions such as allergic rhinitis or asthma (see Chapter I). In the United States, however, anaphylaxis is usually used to mean the systemic reaction which is the subject of this chapter.

PATHOGENESIS

Human systemic anaphylaxis is usually mediated by IgE. After antigenic exposure has induced hypersensitivity, reexposure is followed by antigen-antibody interaction and sudden massive release of chemical mediators, probably including histamine and slow reacting substance of anaphylaxis (SRS-A),[2] and formation of kinins. These mediators cause increased capillary permeability, bronchoconstriction, and vasodilation (see Chapter II).

The term "cytotoxic anaphylaxis", (Type II reaction, see Chapter I) has been used to describe the reaction in which complement mediated cellular damage follows reaction of antibody with a component of the cell (acute hemolytic transfusion reactions) or adsorption of a drug-antibody aggregate to the cell (hemolytic and thrombocytopenic reactions induced by Sedormid or quinidine).[2]

Anaphylactoid reactions resemble anaphylactic reactions but do not require prior sensitization and may occur following initial exposure to a substance. Examples include reactions to radiopaque dyes, aspirin, chlortetracycline, polymyxins, thiamine, and most reactions to local anesthetics. [3]

Adverse reactions following intravenous or intramuscular gamma globulin may be anaphylactoid reactions due to histamine release caused by the presence of aggregated IgG in commercial gamma globulin preparations or anaphylactic reactions due to sensitization to IgG aggregates or to IgA. [4]

ETIOLOGY

Anaphylaxis can follow injection, ingestion, inhalation, or contact with a very wide range of substances (Table 8.1), including proteins, carbohydrates, and simple chemicals (haptens). Since therapeutic and diagnostic agents are the commonest causes, anaphylaxis is usually iatrogenic. [5] These agents include antibiotics (especially penicillin), biologicals, and allergy extracts.

Hymenoptera stings are frequent causes of anaphylactic reactions, and foods are sometimes responsible for such reactions. Anaphylaxis has followed sensitization by the products of ethylene oxide gas used for sterilization of plastic tubing used for hemodialysis. [8] It has also been reported to have followed ingestion of chamomile tea, a folk remedy prepared from a plant of the compositae family, which includes ragweed. [9] Anaphylaxis has even been reported to have followed contact with human seminal fluid. [10]

Anaphylaxis has been reported to follow exercise after ingestion of shellfish in a patient whose hypersensitivity to shellfish caused no symptoms without exercise. [11]

Administration of blood transfusions to subjects with or without deficiency of serum IgA has sometimes induced anti-IgA antibodies responsible for anaphylactic reactions following subsequent transfusion. These reactions and those to commercial gamma globulin in patients with IgA deficiency are sometimes mediated by IgG, but are not mediated by IgE antibody.

Fatal or life-threatening reactions have more frequently followed injection of the offending agent than its ingestion or contact with it, but fatal anaphylaxis has also followed oral administration of penicillin. [12]

Data bearing on the question of whether there is an increased susceptibility to anaphylaxis among atopic subjects are contradictory and inconclusive. [13, 14]

CLINICAL MANIFESTATIONS

The early manifestations of anaphylaxis include uneasiness or apprehension, weakness, sweating, sneezing or nasal itching, and generalized pruritus. This may be followed by the ap-

TABLE 8.1 MAJOR CAUSES OF ANAPHYLACTIC AND ANAPHYLACTOID REACTIONS

1. **ANTIBIOTICS**

Penicillin and its derivatives	Polymyxin B
Cephalosporins	Streptomycin
Chloramphenicol	Tetracyclines
Colymycin	Troleandomycin
Kanamycin	Vancomycin
Nitrofurantoin	Amphotericin B

2. **BIOLOGICALS**

Foreign sera (antitoxins, antilymphocyte globulins)	Polypeptide hormones (ACTH, TSH, insulin, parathormone)
Chymopapain	Influenza vaccine
Chymotrypsin	Tetanus toxoid
Penicillinase	Pertussis vaccine
Trypsin	Measles vaccine
Gamma globulin	Typhus vaccine
Asparaginase	

3. **OTHER INJECTABLE MEDICATIONS**

Adrenal corticosteroids	Methylergonovine maleate
Dextran	Protamine
Iron dextran	

4. **LOCAL ANESTHETICS**

Lidocaine	Procaine	Tetracaine

5. **ASPIRIN**

6. **DIAGNOSTIC AGENTS**

Iodinated contrast media	Sulfobromophthalein (BSP)
Sodium dehydrocholate (Decholin)	

7. **HYMENOPTERA STINGS** (Bee, yellow jacket, wasp, hornet, fire ant)

8. **ALLERGY EXTRACTS**

9. **FOODS**

Egg white	banana	Cottonseed	Fish
Milk	mango	Sesame seed	Shellfish
Nuts	orange	Sunflower seed	Beans
			Soybean

10. **INTRAVENOUS NARCOTICS** (Heroin)

pearance of generalized erythema or urticaria and angioedema. Dyspnea and bronchospasm or laryngeal edema may follow quickly. Abdominal cramps may be noted and vomiting or diarrhea (sometimes bloody) may occur. There may be urinary urgency and urinary or fecal incontinence. Vascular collapse may be primary or secondary to respiratory failure, and hypotension is usually present with progression of the reaction. Convulsions and coma may supervene. The pulse may be rapid and weak or unobtainable.

The cutaneous, respiratory, and cardiovascular signs and symptoms may occur individually or in combination and may be mild or so severe that they cause immediate collapse.

Generally there is an inverse relationship between the interval between exposure to the offending agent and the onset of symptoms and the severity of the reaction. Fatal or potentially fatal reactions usually begin within seconds or a few minutes. Less severe reactions may begin several hours later. A fatal reaction to a yellow jacket sting has been reported as long as 96 hours after the sting, however, in a man who had had only nausea for a few minutes immediately after the sting.[15]

Electrocardiographic disturbances recognized during human anaphylaxis include arrhythmias, ST segment elevation or depression, and T wave flattening or inversion.[16] These have usually returned to normal within several days.

DIFFERENTIAL DIAGNOSIS

Anaphylaxis is generally easily diagnosed because of the usually close temporal relationship between signs and symptoms and exposure to the offending agent. Syncope due to fright associated with receiving an injection is the condition most frequently initially confused with anaphylaxis in children. Syncope is usually preceded by pallor but not by cyanosis. The child may begin to perspire and complain of feeling faint or there may be brief loss of consciousness. Mild hypotension is often present but it is associated with bradycardia rather than tachycardia. Progression of a syncopal reaction can be forestalled by placing the child in a recumbent position.

Syncope and urticaria may follow sudden exposure to cold water in a subject with cold urticaria (see Chapter VI). Other forms of urticaria and hereditary angioneurotic edema are usually easily differentiated from anaphylaxis by history and absence of other signs and symptoms of anaphylaxis.

If the patient is seen after unconsciousness has already supervened and no history is available diagnosis is more difficult, but most of the other possibilities to be excluded are rare in the pediatric age group (myocardial infarction, acute adrenal insufficiency, cerebral thrombosis or hemorrhage, insulin-induced hypoglycemia). [5]

TREATMENT

Speed in instituting appropriate therapy is essential to successful management of anaphylaxis. The patient, physician, and necessary equipment and medications must be immediately available. Both patient and physician or someone else qualified to treat anaphylaxis should remain at the physician's office for at least 20 minutes after parenteral administration of penicillin or other antibiotics, biologicals, allergy extracts, or other agents known to be major causes of anaphylaxis (see Table 8.1). The necessary equipment and medications should be immediately available (Table 8.2).

TABLE 8.2   EQUIPMENT AND MEDICATIONS FOR
TREATMENT OF ANAPHYLAXIS[5, 6]

PRIMARY EQUIPMENT AND MEDICATIONS

Tourniquet
Syringes, disposable, 1 ml and 5 ml
Epinephrine solution, aqueous, 1:1000
Diphenhydramine (Benadryl), injectable, 50 mg/ml
Oxygen tank and mask
Normal saline for injection

SUPPORTIVE EQUIPMENT AND MEDICATIONS

Intravenous infusion sets
Intravenous needles
Laryngoscope with interchangeable pediatric and adult blades
Oral airways, infant, child, adult
Endotracheal tubes (Numbers 18, 22, 26, and 30 French)
Needles, No. 12, for temporary airway
Cricothyrotomy tube or tracheostomy set
Suction apparatus
Bag resuscitator for assisted ventilation
Sterile surgical cutdown set
Aminophylline solution, injectable, 25 mg/ml
Hydrocortisone for injection
Glucose, 5% in isotonic saline (two 500 ml bottles)
Metaraminol bitartrate (Aramine), 1% for injection

The choice of therapy will depend upon the nature and severity of the reaction. (Table 8.3). Patients with even the earliest signs of anaphylaxis should be treated immediately. Aqueous epinephrine, 1:1000, is the treatment of choice for anaphylaxis. It should be administered immediately by intramuscular injection into the upper arm (0.01 ml/Kg, maximum dose 0.3 ml for a child or 0.5 ml for an adult) and massaged to hasten absorption from the injection site. Mild reactions can be treated with subcutaneous injection. If necessary the same dose can be repeated at 15-20 minute intervals until 3 doses have been administered by subcutaneous or intramuscular injection. If imperative because of peripheral vascular collapse this dose can be diluted with 10 ml saline and injected intravenously once. Phentolamine (Regitine, 0.1 mg/Kg, maximum adult dose 5 mg) has been recommended for signs and symptoms of overtreatment with epinephrine.[17] If there is evidence of laryngeal obstruction, endotracheal intubation or tracheostomy may become necessary.

TABLE 8.3 TREATMENT OF ANAPHYLAXIS

---

1. Epinephrine, aqueous, 1:1000 (0.01 ml/Kg, maximum dose 0.3 ml in a child or 0.5 ml in an adult) I.M. or S.C. If necessary repeat at 15-20 minute intervals for total of 3 doses.
2. Establish airway.
3. Ventilate if necessary.
4. Tourniquet proximal to site of sting or injection into extremity.
5. Epinephrine, half previous dose, diluted in 2 ml normal saline and infiltrated around site of injection of antigen.
6. Oxygen.

IF RESPONSE TO THESE MEASURES INSUFFICIENT:

7. Glucose, 5%, in isotonic saline.
8. Aminophylline, 7 mg/Kg, I.V., if necessary for bronchospasm.
9. Diphenhydramine (Benadryl), 2 mg/Kg, I.V. or 5 mg/Kg/ 24 hours orally if necessary for urticaria or angioedema.
10. Hydrocortisone, 7 mg/Kg, I.V., initially; then 7 mg/Kg/ 24 hours by infusion.
11. Metaraminol bitartrate (Aramine), 0.4 mg/Kg (0.5-5 mg) added to I.V. fluids if necessary to maintain blood pressure.

If necessary an airway should be established, and ventilation must be started if apnea has occurred.

If the reaction has followed subcutaneous or intramuscular injection of an agent into an extremity a tourniquet should be applied proximal to the injection site to delay venous return. This can be loosened when improvement occurs or temporarily at 3 minute intervals. [18] Half the previously administered dose of aqueous epinephrine can then be diluted with 2 ml normal saline and infiltrated around the site of injection of the offending antigen. [17]

Oxygen should be supplied by mask in moderate or severe reactions involving the respiratory tract. Hypoxemia is known to increase myocardial irritability, and ventricular fibrillation has caused deaths from anaphylaxis. [6]

If response to these measures has been insufficient, intravenous fluids should be started with a rapid infusion of saline or another plasma volume expander to treat hypovolemia.

Aminophylline, 7 mg/Kg, administered intravenously over 10-20 minutes is often effective in relieving any bronchospasm which has not been reversed by epinephrine. [6,17] Additional aminophylline can be administered intravenously at a dose of 4 mg/Kg 6-8 hours later if necessary.

An antihistamine such as diphenhydramine (Benadryl), 2 mg/Kg, can be administered intravenously (or 5 mg/Kg/24 hrs. orally) if necessary for urticaria or angioedema, and continued treatment with antihistamines at 6 hour intervals for 48 hours has been recommended to minimize late recurrence of symptoms. [17]

Adrenal corticosteroids do not have any immediate effect, but their anti-inflammatory activity is helpful a few hours after their administration. Hydrocortisone can be administered intravenously at an initial dose of 7 mg/Kg followed by an infusion of the same dose over the next 24 hours.

Addition of a vasopressor such as metaraminol bitartrate (Aramine) to the intravenous fluids may be necessary to maintain blood pressure. The dosage recommended is 0.4 mg/Kg (0.5-5.0 mg). [6] Close monitoring for cardiac side effects is necessary.

Depending upon the response to these measures, continued close monitoring of blood pressure, central venous pressure, cardiac rhythm, and acid base balance with frequent blood gas determinations may be necessary.

PATHOLOGY

Postmortem examination following fatal anaphylaxis has most frequently disclosed the presence of edema of the larynx and elsewhere in the upper respiratory tract and pulmonary hyperinflation.[3, 15, 18] Eosinophilia has sometimes been found in the spleen, liver, and lungs.[3]

PREVENTION

Prevention is often more effective and always more desirable than treatment of anaphylaxis. No drug or agent which may be responsible for an anaphylactic reaction (see Table 8.1) should be prescribed without a definite indication for its use and an inquiry about previous adverse reactions to it. When a drug is to be administered it should be given by the oral route rather than parenterally if this will provide adequate treatment.

Patients who have had adverse reactions to an agent should wear emblems indicating their hypersensitivity. *

Skin testing or conjunctival testing is not entirely reliable in identifying subjects at risk for anaphylaxis from drugs, and anaphylaxis can follow the test itself, but testing is indicated when there is no suitable substitute for an agent to which the patient has had a previous serious adverse reaction and there is an urgent reason for use of a drug for which testing gives reasonably reliable results (see Chapter X).

Patients with hymenoptera hypersensitivity should observe precautions to minimize the likelihood of reexposure and should receive immunotherapy (see Chapter XI).

*Medic Alert Foundation, P. O. Box 1009, Turlock, California 95380.

REFERENCES

1. Portier, P. , and Richet, C. : De l'action anaphylactique de certains venins. C R Soc Biol 54:170, 1902.
2. Becker, E. L. , and Austen, K. F. : "Anaphylaxis", in Miescher, P. A. , and Muller-Eberhard, H. J. (ed): Textbook of Immunopathology, Vol. 1, Grune & Stratton, New York, 1968, p 76.
3. Lockey, R. F. , and Bukantz, S. C. : Allergic emergencies. Med Cl N A 58:147, 1975.
4. Ellis, E. F. , and Henney, C. S. : Adverse reactions following administration of human gamma globulin. J All 43:45, 1969.
5. Siegel, S. C. , and Heimlich, E. M. : Anaphylaxis. Ped Cl N A 9:29, 1962.
6. American Academy of Pediatrics Committee on Drugs: Anaphylaxis. Ped 51:136, 1973.
7. Mendelson, L. M. , et al. : Anaphylaxis-like reactions to corticosteroid therapy. J All Clin Imm 54:125, 1974.
8. Poothullil, J. , et al. : Anaphylaxis from the product(s) of ethylene oxide gas. Ann Int Med 82:58, 1975.
9. Benner, M. H. , and Lee, H. J. : Anaphylactic reaction to chamomile tea. J All Clin Imm 52:307, 1973.
10. Frankland, A. W. , and Parish, W. E. : Anaphylactic sensitivity to human seminal fluid. Clin Allergy 4:249, 1974.
11. Maulitz, R. M. , Pratt, D. S. , and Schocket, A. L. : Exercise-induced anaphylactic reaction to shellfish. J All Clin Immunol 63:433, 1979.
12. Sparks, R. P. : Fatal anaphylaxis due to oral penicillin. Am J Clin Path 56:407, 1971.
13. Van Arsdel, P. P. , Jr. : The risk of penicillin reactions. Ann Int Med 69:1071, 1968.
14. Stember, R. H. , and Levine, B. B. : Prevalence of allergic diseases, penicillin hypersensitivity and aeroallergen hypersensitivity in various populations. J All Clin Imm 51: 100, 1973.
15. Barnard, J. H. : Allergic and pathologic findings in fifty insect-sting fatalities. J All 40:107, 1967.
16. Criep, L. H. , and Woehler, T. R. : The heart in human anaphylaxis. Ann All 29:399, 1971.
17. Kuehn, L. F. , and Heiner, D. C. : "Anaphylaxis", in Frazier, C. A. (ed): Current Therapy of Allergy, Med Exam Pub Co. , Inc. , Flushing, N. Y. , 1974, p 294.
18. Weiszer, I. : "Allergic emergencies" in Patterson, R. (ed): Allergic Diseases-Diagnosis and Management. J. B. Lippincott Co. , Philadelphia, 1972, p 327.

CHAPTER IX | FOOD ALLERGY

Three millenia before the birth of Christ, the emperor of China, Shen Nung, ascribed a cutaneous eruption to the ingestion of fish, shrimp, chicken, or horsemeat. Hippocrates suspected a relationship between headaches and drinking milk. Subsequently, almost every food has been recognized as an allergen or at least accused of being responsible for allergic symptoms.

ALLERGENIC FOODS

Almost any food can be allergenic, but certain foods are more frequently allergenic than others. Those most frequently implicated include cow's milk, egg, wheat, corn, chocolate, citrus fruit, legumes, nuts, berries, and shellfish. Cooked foods are generally less allergenic than raw foods.

Allergenicity may also be related to the ease with which a particular food is absorbed from the gastrointestinal tract. It has been estimated that 0.02% of egg albumin is absorbed without digestion in normal children, and this may partly account for the importance of egg white as an allergen.[1] Inflammation of the gastrointestinal tract may enhance the rate of absorption of undigested food and thus increase the risk of sensitization or increase the likelihood of the appearance of allergic symptoms in the previously sensitized subject. In children with diarrhea 0.1% of egg albumin has been found to be absorbed unaltered.[1] Ingestion of alcohol is also said to enhance absorption from the gastrointestinal tract, while ingestion of fats or oils may delay absorption.

There is evidence to suggest that binding of antigen by secretory IgA may be important to prevention of passage of foods across the gastrointestinal mucosa with possible subsequent sensitization.[2] The minimal amounts of IgA naturally present in early infancy may contribute to the increased frequency of food allergy in infancy.

Allergy to a particular food is often but not always associated with allergy to other foods in the same biological family (Tables 9.1 and 9.2). Such cross reactivity is more common in some families, such as the citrus family, than others.

269

TABLE 9.1 BIOLOGIC CLASSIFICATION OF PLANT FOODS

Apple Family
Apple
Pear
Quince

Arrowroot Family
Arrowroot

Arum Family
Taro (Poi)

Banana Family
Banana
Plantain

Beech Family
Beechnut
Chestnut

Birch Family
Filbert
Hazelnut
Wintergreen

Brazil Nut Family
Brazil Nut
Paradise Nut

Buckwheat Family
Buckwheat
Rhubarb

Cashew
Cashew
Mango

Citrus
Grapefruit
Kumquat
Lemon
Lime
Orange
Tangelo
Tangerine

Cola Nut
Chocolate
Cola Nut
Karaya

Custard apple
Custard apple
Papaya
Pawpaw

Ebony
Persimmon

Fungus
Mushroom
Truffle
Yeast

Ginger
Cardamom
Ginger
Turmeric

Gooseberry
Currant
Gooseberry

Goosefoot
Beet
Spinach
Swiss chard

Gourd
Cantaloupe
Casaba
Cucumber
Gherkin
Honeydew
Muskmelon
Persian melon
Pumpkin
Squash
Watermelon

Grains
Barley
Corn
Oat
Popcorn
Rice
Rye
Sorghum
Sugar cane
Wheat

Grape
Grape

Heath
Black huckleberry
Blueberry
Cranberry

Honeysuckle
Elderberry

Laurel
Avocado
Bay leaf
Cinnamon
Sassafras

Legumes
Acacia
Beans (Kidney, lima,
   navy, pinto, string)
Black-eyed pea
Carob bean
Chick pea
Lentil
Licorice
Pea
Peanut
Senna
Soybean
Tragacanth

Lily
Asparagus
Chives
Garlic
Leek
Onion
Sarsaparilla
Shallot

Madder
Black guava
Coffee

Mallow
Cottonseed
Marshmallow
Okra

Mint
Basil
Hoarhound
Marjoram
Mint
Oregano
Peppermint
Sage
Spearmint
Thyme

Morning glory
Sweet potato
Yam

Mulberry
Breadfruit
Fig
Hop
Mulberry

Mustard
Broccoli
Brussels sprouts
Cabbage
Cauliflower
Collards
Horseradish
Kale
Kohlrabi
Mustard
Radish
Rutabaga
Turnip
Watercress

Myrtle
Allspice
Clove
Guava
Myrtle
Paprika
Pimento

Nightshade
Bell pepper
Cayenne pepper
Chili
Eggplant
Potato (white)
Tomato

Nutmeg
Nutmeg and mace

Olive
Manna
Olive

Orchid
Vanilla

Palm
Coconut
Date

Parsley
Anise
Caraway seed
Carrot
Celery
Coriander
Cumin
Dill
Fennel
Parsley
Parsnip

Passionflower
Passion fruit

Pedalium
Sesame seeds

Pineapple
Pineapple

Plum
Almond
Apricot
Cherry
Nectarine
Peach
Plum, prune

Pomegranate
Pomegranate

Protea
Macadamia nut

Rose
Blackberry
Boysenberry
Loganberry
Raspberry
Strawberry

Spurge Family
Tapioca

Sunflower
Artichoke
Camomile
Chicory
Dandelion
Endive
Escarole
Lettuce
Sunflower seed

Walnut
Black walnut
Butternut
English walnut
Hickory nut
Pecan

TABLE 9.2   BIOLOGIC CLASSIFICATION OF ANIMAL FOODS

Amphibians	Grouper, white bass, rock fish
Frog	Hake
	Herring, sardine, shad, sprat
Birds	Muskellunge, pickerel, pike
Chicken	Perch
Dove	Pompano
Duck	Porgy, red snapper
Goose	Smelts
Grouse	Sole
Guinea fowl	Sturgeon
Partridge	Swordfish
Pheasant	
Quail	**Mammals**
Squab	Beef
Turkey	Goat
	Horse
Crustaceans	Lamb
Crab	Pork
Crayfish	Rabbit
Lobster	Squirrel
Prawn	Venison
Shrimp	
	Mollusks
Fish	Abalone
Anchovy	Clam
Barracuda, mullet	Cockles
Black bass, crappie, sunfish	Mussels
Bonito, mackerel, tuna	Octopus
Buffalo, carp, chub	Oyster
Bullhead, catfish	Periwinkle
Cod, haddock, pollack, whiting	Scallop
Croaker, drum, redfish	Snail
Eel	Squid
Flounder, halibut	
Grayling, salmon, trout,	**Reptiles**
whitefish	Turtle

COW'S MILK

Milk is one of the commonest allergenic foods, partly because of the frequency with which it is a major item in the diet. Although ingestion of milk as a beverage is less frequent after infancy and childhood, beef and milk products are consumed in large amounts by many adolescents and adults (Table 9.3).

TABLE 9.3   DIETARY SOURCES OF COW'S MILK

1. Milk: whole or skim, buttermilk, cream, condensed milk, evaporated milk, dried milk or powdered milk
2. Other beverages: Chocolate milk, cocomalt, cocoa, malted milk, milkshakes, Ovaltine
3. Bread and pastry containing milk: batters, cake, cookies, pancakes, prepared flours such as Bisquick, rolls, waffles, zwieback, and most bread except Vienna bread and "kosher parve" bread
4. Butter and margarine except that type of Mazola margarine made with soybean oil and Willow Run margarine
5. Candy: caramels, chocolate, filled candy bars, nougat
6. Cereals: Cream of Rice, Instant Cream of Wheat, Special K, Total
7. Cheese
8. Cream sauces made with butter, margarine, milk or cream: gravies, au gratin dishes
9. Cream soups, chowder
10. Ice cream and sherbet, custard, junket, milk pudding
11. Macaroni, spaghetti
12. Meat containing dried skim milk as a binder or butter or margarine: frankfurters, luncheon meats, meatloaf, sausages, wiener schnitzel (unless 100% meat)
13. "Non-dairy" substitutes containing caseinate: Cereal blend, Coffeemate, Coffee-Rich, Cool-Whip, Imo, Preem, Rich'ning, and others
14. Pies with cream fillings or pie-crust containing butter or margarine
15. Yogurt

At least twenty antigens have been found in cow's milk[3] but those which cause most allergic reactions to milk are β-lactoglobulin, α-lactalbumin, casein, bovine gamma globulin, and bovine serum albumin.[4,5] The β-lactoglobulin and α-lactalbumin of cow's milk and those of goat milk are immunologically identical, and the casein of cow and goat milk are almost identical immunologically,[6,7] but children allergic to cow's milk occasionally can tolerate goat milk, possibly because the allergy may be to other components.[7]

There is some evidence that heating reduces somewhat the allergenicity of cow's milk,[8] and spray-dried milk preparations may be less antigenic than fresh whole milk,[3] but both commercial infant formulas subjected to heat during processing and milk reconstitued from powdered milk elicit allergic symptoms in most infants allergic to cow's milk.[4,7] Casein, α -lactalbumin, and β -lactoglobulin have all been found to be antigenically active in heat treated commercial milks and milk formulas.[9]

EGG

Egg is another of the foods most often responsible for allergic reactions, partly due to the frequency with which it occurs in many diets (Table 9.4). Hypersensitivity is usually limited to the egg white, probably because of allergy to the egg albumin. Egg white is often brushed onto breads, rolls, and pretzels to cause a glazed appearance. Egg sensitive children are sometimes allergic also to chicken and other birds.[2]

TABLE 9.4 DIETARY SOURCES OF EGG

1. Eggs: cooked or raw, fritters, souffles
2. Baking powder except Royal and K.C.
3. Beverages: Ovaltine, ovomalt, root beer
4. Candy: chocolate creams, filled candy bars, fondants, marshmallows, nougats
5. Custard
6. Egg noodles
7. Ice cream and sherbet
8. Meats: meatloaf and sausage unless prepared at home without egg
9. Pastries: batters, cake, cookies, doughnuts, French toast, macaroons, meringue, muffins, pancakes, pie crust, pretzels, waffles
10. Prepared flours such as Bisquick and pancake flour
11. Salad dressing and sauces: hollandaise sauce, mayonnaise, tartar sauce

---

CEREALS

Wheat and corn are the cereals most frequently found to be allergens, but any cereal can be allergenic. Both wheat and corn are found in numerous food products (Tables 9.5 and 9.6). Barley and rice are the two grains least frequently implicated.[2]

Sugar cane is also a member of the grain or grass family, and allergy can be induced by brown sugar or molasses although white cane sugar is not antigenic because of its greater purity.[10]

TABLE 9.5   DIETARY SOURCES OF WHEAT

---

1. Bread, cake, cookies, crackers, pretzels
2. Beverages: Malted milk, Ovaltine, Postum, beer, ale
3. Breakfast foods containing wheat, including cream of wheat, farina, grapenuts, Pablum, Pettijohns, puffed wheat, shredded wheat, Wheaties
4. Chili con carne or canned baked beans
5. Flour
6. Macaroni, noodles, ravioli, spaghetti
7. Meats: hamburger, meatloaf, sausage, wiener schnitzel
8. Pastry: batters, bread crumbs, ice cream cones, pancakes, pie, waffles
9. Sauces, chowder, gravies, soups containing flour or noodles

---

TABLE 9.6   DIETARY SOURCES OF CORN

Adhesives (envelopes, stamps, stickers)	Corn fritters
Ale	Corn meal
Aspirin and other tablets	Corn oil
Bacon	Corn soya
Baking mixes & powders	Cornstarch
Batters	Corn sugar
Beer	Corn syrup
Beets, Harvard	Corn Toasties
Bread	Cough syrup
Cake	Cream pies
Candy	Cream puffs
Carbonated beverages*	Dates, confection
Catsup	Dentifrices
Cereals (processed)*	Dextrose
Cheese	Egg nog
Cheerios	Fish, prepared & processed
Chili	Flour, bleached*
Chop suey	French dressing
Chow mein	Fritos
Coffee, instant	Frosting
Colas	Fruit, canned, frozen, or juices
Cookies	Fruit pies
Confectioner's sugar	Frying fats
Corn Flakes	Gelatin capsules
Corn flour	Gelatin dessert

Table 9.5 (cont'd.)

Graham crackers
Gravy
Grits
Gum, chewing
Ham, cured, tenderized
Hominy
Ice cream
Infant formula*
   Mull-Soy, Similac, Sobee
Jam
Jelly
Jello
Karo syrup
Laxatives*
Lemonade
Margarine & shortening*
Mazola margarine
Meat (processed): bacon,
   bologna, ham, sausage,
   wieners
Metrecal cookies & wafers
Milk in paper cartons
Monosodium glutamate
Nabisco
Nescafe
Noodles
Pablum
Paper containers: Boxes,
   cups, plates, milk cartons
Peanut butter
Peas (canned)
Pickles
Pies (cream)
Plastic food wrappers (inner
   surface may be coated with
   cornstarch)

Popcorn
Pork & beans*
Post Toasties
Powdered sugar
Preserves
Pudding*
Ravioli
Rice (coated)
Rice Krispies
Salt (salt cellars in restau-
   rants, A & P "4 Seasons
   salt")
Salad dressings*
Sandwich spreads
Sauces
Sherbet
Soups
Spaghetti*
String beans (canned, frozen)
Sugar, powdered
Syrup
Tablets & lozenges
Tacos
Tamales
Tea, instant
Toothpaste*
Tortillas
Vanillin
Vegetables (canned, creamed,
   frozen)*
Vinegar, distilled
Vitamins
Waffles
Whiskey and gin
Wines, American*
Yeast

---

*Some brands

CHOCOLATE

Chocolate and cola have been called the commonest of all plant allergens, and hypersensitivity to chocolate is probably always associated with hypersensitivity to cola.[10]

LEGUMES

Allergy to legumes is common and may be severe. Peanut is the most frequent offender, but allergy to one legume is often associated with allergy to others. Soybean is an important potential allergen not only because of the frequent use of soybean formulas but also because of the increasingly numerous other dietary sources (Table 9.7).

Subjects with allergy to beans, peas, and peanut may report exacerbations of symptoms following ingestion of honey, an observation ascribed to the importance of alfalfa, clover, and other legumes as souces of honey. [10]

SUNFLOWER SEEDS

Most plants of the sunflower family do not supply frequently allergenic foods, but ragweed is found in this family, and chewing sunflower seeds or eating lettuce sometimes causes exacerbations of symptoms in patients allergic to ragweed. Even systemic anaphylaxis has been reported to follow ingestion of sunflower seeds. [11]

TABLE 9.7   DIETARY SOURCES OF SOYBEAN

---

1. Bread, cake, crackers, pastry, rolls. (Soybean flour containing 1% oil is often added to bakery products to keep them moist)
2. Candy
3. Cereal: Sunlets, Cellu Soy Flakes
4. Ice cream
5. Infant formulas: Isomil, Mull-Soy, NeoMullsoy, Pro-Sobee, Sobee, Soyalac
6. Lecithin (used in candy)
7. Margarine
8. Meats: pork link sausage, luncheon meats
9. Salad dressing
10. Sauces: Heinz Worcestershire Sauce, La Choy Sauce, Lea & Perrins Sauce, Oriental Show-You Sauce
11. Shortening: Crisco, Spry
12. Soups
13. Soybean noodles, macaroni and spaghetti
14. Soybeans roasted, salted, and eaten as peanuts are eaten
15. Vegetables (Fresh soy sprouts, especially in Chinese dishes)

CHEMICALS

Although allergy to chemicals such as ascorbic acid and citric acid may be possible it has rarely if ever been recognized.

Allergy to coal tar and petroleum derivatives approved by the Food and Drug Administration for use in trace amounts as dyes in foods and drugs is well established although the frequency with which such agents cause hypersensitivity is undetermined.[12,13] Tartrazine (FD & C Yellow No. 5) has been incriminated more frequently than any of the other FD & C dyes. It is often found in orange or green foods and drugs as well as those which are yellow. Possible sources and relationships to other food additives and aspirin are discussed in Chapter VI.

PATHOGENESIS

Food allergy is often due to Type I, anaphylactic hypersensitivity. The mechanisms have been discussed in Chapter II. Reports of inhibition of food-induced asthma and urticaria by oral administration of cromolyn suggest that allergic reactions to foods may occur in the gastrointestinal tract, even when respiratory and cutaneous symptoms ensue.[14,15] No more than 1% of an orally administered dose of cromolyn is absorbed, and inhalation of cromolyn may not prevent asthma due to ingested food.[15]

Sensitization usually follows direct ingestion of antigen, but antigens eaten by the mother can apparently be transmitted to an infant by breast milk and there is evidence that intrauterine sensitization to foods in the maternal diet may even occur.[16-18]

The report of evidence of complement activation following challenge with milk in some infants with delayed gastrointestinal or cutaneous symptoms[19] and the association of milk precipitins with milk allergy in others[8] suggest that food allergy may also be mediated by Type III reactions. Other mechanisms may also be involved.

CLINICAL MANIFESTATIONS

The incidence of food allergy in children is unknown. Allergy to cow's milk has been reported in 1-7.5% of unselected infants.[20,21] The frequency of food allergy seems to decrease as infants and children become older.

Clinical manifestations include gastrointestinal symptoms (nausea, vomiting, diarrhea, abdominal pain); urticaria and angioedema; signs and symptoms of the other atopic diseases, allergic rhinitis, asthma, and atopic dermatitis; secretory otitis media; and systemic anaphylaxis (see Chapters III-VIII).

Symptoms may be mild or severe and may occur immediately after ingestion or may be delayed for 48-72 hours. Usually symptoms occur within 1-2 hours after the offending food has been eaten, but allergy to a very frequently eaten food may cause either continuous or recurrent symptoms.[2]

Infants with food allergy are often described as being "hungry all the time". Ingestion of the offending allergen is followed by crying, apparently due to abdominal pain. The infant is then fed again but never seems satisfied.

Diarrhea due to allergy to cow's milk usually begins at 4-6 weeks of age in infants who have received it from birth, but it may occur as early as 2 days of age.[22]

TENSION-FATIGUE SYNDROME

Allergic toxemia or the tension-fatigue syndrome is characterized by lethargy, fatigue, restlessness, irritability, headache, abdominal pain, pallor, arthralgia, and myalgia, often associated with signs and symptoms of allergic rhinitis or asthma. Remissions have followed dietary elimination of foods, especially milk and chocolate, and exacerbations have been reported to follow subsequent challenge with implicated foods.[23] The vagueness of many of these complaints and the fact that most of the evidence that such symptoms can be due to food allergy is anecdotal have raised some questions about the validity of ascribing these symptoms to food allergy, but the presence of food allergy has been confirmed in some of these patients by demonstration of specific IgE antibodies and allergen-induced histamine release.[24] Detection of specific IgG antibodies in an even higher proportion of these patients raises the possibility of mediation by a nonreaginic immune mechanism, but specific IgG antibodies to foods were also found in more than half of the asymptomatic controls. Although food allergy is not the commonest cause of such symptoms, they may apparently be the chief manifestations of allergy in occasional patients.

ENURESIS

Enuresis has occasionally been ascribed to food allergy.[25] Children with enuresis have sometimes responded to dietary restrictions, but this is an uncommon manifestation of allergy and most enuresis is probably not due to allergy.

HEINER'S SYNDROME

A rare syndrome consisting of recurrent vomiting and diarrhea, failure to thrive, and iron deficiency anemia with pulmonary infiltrates and segmental atelectasis has been found to be associated with serum milk precipitins. [8] Iron-containing macrophages have been found in the bronchial secretions. Improvement has followed dietary elimination of cow's milk and subsequent challenge with milk has elicited exacerbations of symptoms. The significance of the serum milk precipitins is uncertain because of subsequent demonstration of milk precipitins in 1-2% of apparently normal subjects[26] and their more frequent occurrence in association with severe mental retardation and several other conditions. [27-29] The occurrence of serum milk precipitins in as many as 75% of subjects with selective IgA deficiency has suggested a protective role of secretory IgA in preventing absorption of food antigens. [30]

ALLERGIC GASTROENTEROPATHY AND EOSINOPHILIC GASTROENTERITIS

These are described as clinical entities characterized by hypoproteinemia and edema due to loss of plasma protein into the gastrointestinal tract. [31, 32] Growth retardation, peripheral eosinophilia, anemia, and manifestations of allergic respiratory and cutaneous diseases have been found. Eosinophilic infiltration of the mucosa of the gastrointestinal tract has been evident, and this eosinophilia has sometimes increased after challenge with food suspected of being allergenic. Improvement has followed dietary elimination of offending foods or treatment with adrenal corticosteroids.

A frequent association of iron deficiency with occult blood loss from the gastrointestinal tract apparently due to ingestion of cow's milk has also been confirmed by others. [33]

NEPHROTIC SYNDROME

Exacerbations of nephrotic syndrome have been ascribed to milk allergy in a few children in whom proteinuria and activation of C3 followed ingestion of milk, and improvement followed its elimination from their diets. [34] Most of these children also had asthma or "eczema."

DIAGNOSIS

The diagnosis of food allergy is established by history, response to dietary elimination followed by challenge, and occasionally allergy skin testing. The diagnosis is most easily made when severe symptoms have immediately followed ingestion of a food eaten only rarely. When symptoms have been delayed or when due to a food eaten daily it is more difficult to identify the offending allergen. Use of a food diary indicating all ingestants within 24-48 hours before the onset of symptoms may be helpful in implicating specific foods.

The occurrence of symptoms may be related to the amount of allergen ingested as well as whether the food was raw or cooked or processed in some other way. Possible allergy to dyes and other food additives complicates the interpretation of the history.

When a specific food has been implicated confirmation of its allergenicity is sought by strict dietary elimination for 3 weeks followed by challenge unless the previous reaction has been severe enough to suggest that challenge might be hazardous. If the history leaves no doubt concerning the identity of the offending allergen challenge may not be necessary.

When no specific allergen can be incriminated but food allergy is suspected, dietary elimination of the common food allergens for 2-3 weeks followed by reintroduction individually at weekly intervals is helpful (Table 9.8). Observation of the response to restoration of the food to the diet is often even more important than the response to its initial elimination. When specific food has been implicated two more 3 week periods of dietary elimination followed by challenge are recommended before concluding that it has been identified as an offending allergen, in order to lessen the possibility of error due to coincidental variations in symptoms.

SKIN TESTING

Although positive skin tests are usually demonstrable to foods which have caused systemic anaphylaxis, allergy skin testing has generally been considered much less reliable for the identification of food allergens than for inhalant allergens. False positive reactions have been ascribed to irritants or histamine in extracts of certain foods, while false negative reactions have been thought to occur possibly because of allergy to a food metabolite. Specific IgE antibodies against products of the digestion of β-lactoglobulin by pepsin or trypsin have been found in the sera of some patients with milk allergy.[36] There is evidence, however, that the results of prick testing with commercial food extracts correlate well with the results of release of histamine from basophils in vitro and with the results of provocative testing by blind administration of the food in opaque capsules.[37]

For the blind challenge opaque, dye-free, size #1 capsules can be filled with dry or powdered food.[38] The food can be masked with some other food for children unable to swallow the capsule. The initial dose may vary from 10 mg to 2 Gm, depending upon the degree of hypersensitivity suspected. Continual observation

TABLE 9.8   MILK, EGG, CEREAL-FREE DIET
(MODIFIED FROM ROWE)[35]

Poi	Apricot
Tapioca	Grapefruit
Breads made from soybean,	Lemon
lima beans, potato starch,	Peach
or tapioca flour	Pears
Soy milk	Pineapple
	Prune
Lamb	
Bacon	Cane or beet sugar
Chicken (no hens)	Maple syrup or cane sugar
Turkey	syrup flavored with maple
	Olive oil
Artichoke	Sesame oil
Asparagus	Soybean oil and Mazola
Beets	margarine made from
Carrots	Soybean oil
Chard	Salt
Lettuce	Gelatin (plain, lemon, lime
Lima beans	or pineapple)
Peas	Baking powder
Spinach	(Cornstarch-free)
Squash	Baking soda
String beans	Cream of tartar
Sweet potato or yam	Lemon extract
Tomato	Vanilla extract
White potato	White vinegar

for 8-12 hours at the physician's office or the hospital is recommended during and after the challenge. If no reaction is observed, successive challenges with two to ten-fold increases in dosage follow on separate days until a reaction occurs or a dose of 8 Gm is reached. If 8 Gm is tolerated, the food can be restored to the diet safely.[38] If a questionable reaction or subjective complaints occur a glucose-placebo is indicated as a control.

Skin testing is at least helpful in indicating possible allergens which may not have been suspected previously, but their clinical significance should then be confirmed by appropriate dietary trials followed by challenge (unless the history suggests that a severe reaction might follow the challenge) if not by observation following double blind administration of the implicated foods.

Radioallergosorbent testing may also be helpful in implicating food allergens. Techniques, interpretation, and limitations of allergy skin testing and RAST are discussed in Chapter XIII.

OTHER TESTS

Limited data have been reported suggesting the direct basophil degranulation test may be useful in identifying food allergens.[39] Other tests which have been employed for the identification of specific food allergens but which are of no proven value include the leukocytotoxic test, leukopenic index, increased heart rate following ingestion, and intracutaneous provocative testing with provoking doses and neutralizing doses.[40,41]

EOSINOPHILIA

Nasal eosinophilia may occur much less often in children with allergic rhinitis due to food allergy than in those with hypersensitivity to inhalants,[42] but eosinophilia has been reported in mucus on the surface of fresh stools or obtained from the rectum by insertion of the finger in infants with gastrointestinal symptoms due to food allergy.[43]

INTESTINAL BIOPSY

Jejunal changes have been reported in infants with milk allergy 12-24 hours following challenge even with doses too small to elicit symptoms. These changes have included shortening and broadening of villi and infiltration with polymorphonuclear leukocytes and mast cells.[44] Immunofluorescent study has disclosed increases in extracellular immunoglobulins, including IgE, and increased numbers of IgE-forming plasma cells. Eosinophilic infiltration of the gastrointestinal mucosa has been found in eosinophilic gastroenteritis.[32]

DIFFERENTIAL DIAGNOSIS

The differential diagnosis depends upon the clinical manifestations. Specific entities to be considered when cutaneous or respiratory symptoms are present are discussed elsewhere (see Chapters III-VI). The differential diagnosis of gastrointestinal symptoms due to food allergy can include most causes of vomiting, abdominal pain, and diarrhea. Many of these are easily differentiated by clinical features. Among conditions which may be mistaken for food allergy are celiac disease, disaccharidase deficiency, and cystic fibrosis.

CELIAC DISEASE

Celiac disease (nontropical sprue, gluten-induced entero-pathy) is a syndrome of unknown pathogenesis due to intolerance to the gliadin fraction of gluten, one of the protein fractions of wheat, rye, barley, and oats. Gliadin precipitins, hemagglu-tinating antibodies, increased concentrations of IgA or IgE, and IgG, IgA, and IgE antibodies against gliadin and milk have been found in the sera of some patients with celiac disease.[45] Ste-atorrhea usually begins within the first two years of life with chronic diarrhea and large, foul-smelling, floating stools. Other symptoms include anorexia, vomiting, irritability, and failure to grow. Abdominal distention is common. Vitamin deficiency may occur.

Decreased intestinal absorption of D-xylose is usually demonstrable, and biopsy of the distal duodenum or proximal jejunum discloses blunting and loss of villi and mononuclear cell infiltration of the lamina propria. Electron microscopy has disclosed a decrease in the size and the number of micro-villi in the brush border.[45]

Improvement occurs within a few weeks after strict dietary elimination of gluten.

DISACCHARIDASE DEFICIENCY

Disaccharidase deficiency may occur as a primary defic-iency of a single enzyme or secondary to injury of the intestinal mucosa in enteritis, celiac disease, giardiasis, and other con-ditions. Deficiency of lactase, the enzyme responsible for hy-drolysis of lactose into glucose and galactose, is the commonest primary disaccharidase deficiency, having been reported in 10% of Caucasian adults and at a much greater frequency in Negroes, Indians, and other ethnic groups.[46] Its frequency increases as children become older. Congenital lactase deficiency is rare and usually associated with other enzyme deficiencies. Symp-toms include chronic, watery diarrhea, abdominal pain and dis-tention, vomiting, and irritability. Steatorrhea may be present.

The incidence of primary sucrase-isomaltase deficiency is unknown. This is sometimes associated with maltase deficiency, and all four of these enzymes as well as others may be reduced when the defect is secondary to another disease.

Diarrhea due to disaccharidase deficiency usually starts after introduction of a lactose or sucrose containing food into the diet. Malabsorption or poor digestion of carbohydrate is indicated by a stool pH of less than 6 and more than 0.5% reduc-ing substance (Clinitest) in the stool ($>0.25\%$ in 15 drops of 1:1 dilution of stool in water tested with Clinitest). These findings may be normal, however, in a breast-fed neonate.[46]

The specific deficiency is indicated by comparison of concentrations of reducing sugars in the blood following oral administration of monosaccharides and disaccharides or analysis of disaccharidase activities in intestinal mucosa obtained by biopsy.

CYSTIC FIBROSIS

Cystic fibrosis is the commonest cause of chronic malabsorption among Caucasian children in the United States. It is characterized by frequent, large, foul-smelling, floating stools and poor weight gain despite an excessive intake of food. Recurrent pneumonia and bronchiectasis are frequently but not invariably present. The diagnosis is established by increased concentrations of chloride in sweat. (See Chapter III for method and interpretation).

TREATMENT

The treatment for food allergy is elimination of the offending food from the diet. Patients can easily avoid certain foods such as chocolate, but they should be informed about related foods which may also cause symptoms. Cola drinks should also be eliminated from the diets of children with allergy to chocolate, for example.

Diets eliminating foods such as milk, wheat, or corn are more difficult to plan. Parents may be supplied with lists of suggested substitutes or suggested menus as well as lists of dietary sources of the offending allergen (see Table 9.3 to 9.7). Recipes for the preparation of breads and pastries without milk, eggs, or wheat facilitate compliance with the diet (Table 9.9), and the parent can be directed to other sources of suggestions for preparation of suitable foods in books on allergy written for parents. [47] Wheat-free, milk-free, and egg-free recipes are also available from the American Dietetic Association (620 N. Michigan Ave., Chicago, Illinois 60611).

A soybean formula is a suitable substitute for cow's milk for most infants with allergy to milk, but allergy to soybean can also occur. When this occurs Pregestimil or Nutramigen is usually tolerated. These are casein hydrolysates with added corn oil, sugar, starch, minerals, and vitamins. It is prudent to offer these formulas at half strength initially, gradually increasing the concentration over 4-8 days to full strength if tolerated. If this precaution is not observed the sudden increase in osmolar load may cause loose stools which might be mistaken for an indication of allergy to the formula. It is possible for allergy to peptides in casein hydrolysates to occur but this is quite rare.

TABLE 9.9	RECIPES FOR USE WITH CEREAL-FREE DIET

SOY-POTATO BREAD: Preheat oven to 350°F. Grease a 4x7x 2 inch, bright tin, aluminum, or aluminum foil loaf pan (not glass) with soy oil and line completely with waxed paper. Sift flours once before measuring and spoon lightly into measuring cups.

Sift together four times:
> 1 cup soy flour
> 1 cup potato starch flour (not potato flour)
> 1/2 tsp. salt
> 2 Tbsp. white or light brown sugar
> 1 tsp. Cellu cereal-free baking powder*

To 1/2 cup this mixture add:
> 5 tsp. Cellu cereal-free baking powder. Sift together four times and set aside.

To remainder of mixture add:
> 2/3 cup cold water. Mix well and beat vigorously 3 minutes by hand or with electric beater at medium speed.
> Add 3 Tbsp. soy oil and beat 3 more minutes.

Add flour and baking powder mixture previously set aside; beat into batter quickly for 1 minute. Batter should be thick and fluffy. Pour into prepared pan and bake at 350°F. for 1 hour 10 minutes. Cool 5 minutes before removing from pan. Do not slice until cold.

Too much liquid or too hot an oven may cause a soggy streak.

SOY-POTATO CAKE

1 cup soy flour	1/2 tsp. salt
3/4 cup potato starch flour	1/4 cup soy oil
3 Tbsp. Cellu cereal-free baking powder*	3 tsp. vanilla or 2 tsp. vanilla & 1 tsp. lemon extract
3/4 cup sugar	1 cup water

Sift soy flour before measuring. Sift together all dry ingredients well, add water, and mix well. Add oil and vanilla and beat 2 minutes. Pour into muffin or cake pan greased with soy oil. Bake at 350°F. 30 minutes. Makes 12 cupcakes or 2 small layers. For cake bake in loaf pan 1 1/2 hours at 300°F.

SOY-POTATO COOKIES: Using recipe for soy-potato cake, decrease water to make stiff dough, and force through cookie

*Chicago Dietetic Supply House, Inc., 1750 W. Van Buren St., Chicago, Ill. 60612

Table 9.9 (cont'd.)

press onto cookie sheet well greased with soy oil. Thinner batter can be dropped from teaspoon onto cookie sheet. Bake at 375-400ºF. 10-15 minutes.
Thicker dough can be rolled and kept in refrigerator for cutting into slices and baking as needed.

SOY COOKIES

1 cup soy flour
2 tsp. Cellu cereal-free baking
  powder
1/4 tsp. salt
1/3 cup sugar

4 Tbsp. soy oil
3-5 Tbsp. water
1/2 tsp. vanilla or lemon
  extract

Mix oil and sugar and add flavoring. Sift soy flour once before measuring and twice more after adding baking powder and salt. Add flour to oil and sugar and sufficient water to make stiff dough. Form into roll and cut into cookies or force through cookie press. Softer dough can be dropped from teaspoon onto cookie sheet well greased with soy oil. Bake at 350ºF. 15 minutes.

Meatbase formula is also a satisfactory substitute for cow's milk, but one which is often refused by infants already accustomed to another formula.

Elemental diets have not been fully evaluated for the treatment of food allergy, but eosinophilic gastroenteritis has been reported to respond.[48]

Following severe, prolonged diarrhea it may become necessary to discontinue all oral feedings for a period during which intravenous maintenance will be necessary. After oral fructose solutions are found to be tolerated, feedings with a protein hydrolysate can be introduced gradually as tolerated.

Highly restrictive diets cannot be imposed for more than short periods of time without careful assessment of their ability to meet the nutritional needs of the child. If milk and cereal are completely eliminated from the diet supplemental B and D vitamins are necessary. Vitamin C must be supplied for the child unable to eat citrus fruit. Although minimal daily requirements for calcium are not well established, and there are other dietary sources of calcium (Table 9.10), infants, young children and adolescents receiving milk-free diets may benefit from a calcium supplement such as Neo-Calglucon syrup.[49] Recommended daily calcium intakes are 300-600 mg for infants and children, 600-1200 mg for adolescents. Vitamins and minerals

TABLE 9.10   "HYPOALLERGENIC" FOOD SOURCES
              OF CALCIUM

FOOD	AMOUNT	WEIGHT (GRAMS)	CALCIUM (MG)
Barley (Gerber)	1 cup	36	231
Broccoli	1 med. stalk		175
Carrot, raw	1 large	100	37
Celery, raw	1 outer stalk or 3 inner stalks	50	20
Collards	1 cup (cooked)		>250
Dates, domestic, natural	10 medium	100	59
Dates, pitted, cut	1 cup	178	105
Kale	1 cup (cooked)		125
Lamb, cooked	2 chops	114	9
Maple syrup	1Tbsp	20	33
Mustard greens	1 cup (cooked)		175
Olives, green	2 medium	10	9
Pineapple, raw, diced	3/4 cup	100	17
Pineapple, raw, sliced	1 slice	84	14
Prunes, dehydrated	8 large	100	90
Rhubarb	1 cup (cooked)		225
Rice cereal (Gerber)	3/4 cup	27	179
Spinach	1/2 cup	100	158
Turkey, roasted, lean	1 slice	30	9
Turnip greens	1 cup (cooked)		>250

are already added to most milk substitutes available for infants, so further supplementation is unnecessary if the substitute formula is accepted in large enough amounts.

PHARMACOLOGICAL THERAPY

Drug therapy for systemic anaphylaxis and cutaneous and respiratory manifestations of food allergy is discussed elsewhere (see Chapters III-VIII). Most forms of drug therapy are not beneficial for gastrointestinal manifestations of food allergy, but oral administration of a solution of cromolyn sodium at a dose of 50 mg. q.i.d. has been reported to have prevented symptoms in four infants with cow's milk allergy.[50] Diarrhea due to systemic mastocytosis has been controlled with 40 mg. q. i. d. [51] Even allergic respiratory and cutaneous manifestations are reported to have responded to orally administered cromolyn. [14, 15]

IMMUNOTHERAPY

Immunotherapy and oral hyposensitization are not of proven effectiveness in the treatment of food allergy.

PREVENTION

There is evidence that avoidance of cow's milk, beef, veal, egg, and wheat during the first 9 months of life may reduce the likelihood of the development of food allergy during this period when antigens are most readily absorbed from the gastrointestinal tract (see Chapter V). [52] It is probably wise also to withhold citrus fruit and chocolate or cola drinks during the first 9-12 months. Breast feeding should be encouraged, but the mother should be advised to limit her own intake of these highly allergenic foods until her infant has been weaned. Cow's milk hypersensitivity found in nursing infants of mothers consuming large amounts of milk is probably due to passage of cow's milk protein into the breast milk. [53, 54] Infants nursed in early infancy have been reported to have lower total serum IgE concentrations at 2 years of age than control infants. [55] When breast feeding is impossible, a casein hydrolysate or soybean formula is safer to use than cow's milk. Whenever foods are introduced into the infant's diet, they should be offered individually with intervals of at least 1 week between new foods to facilitate prompt identification of any food which is not tolerated.

Most of these precautions may be unnecessary for most infants, but it may be prudent to recommend them at least when there is an immediate family history of atopic diseases or food allergy.

It is also wise to restrict ingestion of highly allergenic foods during episodes of acute gastroenteritis, when absorption of undigested food is enhanced and to discourage overindulgence in any particular food even when the child is well.

PROGNOSIS

The prognosis is somewhat dependent upon the specific manifestations of the allergy, possibly the number and identity of food allergens, and probably early diagnosis and treatment. Cow's milk allergy is reported usually to subside within 1-2 years, but may occasionally persist throughout the subject's life.

REFERENCES

1. Gruskay, F. L. , and Cooke, R. E. : The gastrointestinal absorption of unaltered protein in normal infants and in infants recovering from diarrhea. Ped 16:763, 1955.
2. Tomasi, T. B. , and Katz, L. : Human antibodies against bovine immunoglobulin M in IgA deficient sera. Clin Exp Immunol 9:3, 1971.
3. Hanson, L. A. , and Mansson, I. : Immune electrophoretic studies of bovine milk and milk products. Acta Paed 50: 484, 1961.
4. Goldman, A. S. , et al.: Milk allergy: I. Oral challenge with milk and isolated milk proteins in allergic children. Ped 32:425, 1963.
5. Lebenthal, E.: Cow's milk protein allergy. Ped Cl N A 22:827, 1975.
6. Crawford, L. V. , and Grogan, F. T.: Allergenicity of cow's milk protein. J Ped 59:347, 1961.
7. Freier, S. , et al.: Intolerance to milk protein. J Ped 75: 623, 1969.
8. Heiner, D. C. , et al.: Multiple precipitins to cow's milk in chronic respiratory disease. Am J Dis Child 103:634, 1962.
9. Saperstein, S. , and Anderson, D. W. : Antigenicity of milk proteins of prepared formulas measured by precipitin ring tests and passive cutaneous anaphylaxis in the guinea pig. J Ped 61:196, 1962.
10. Speer, F. : "Intolerance to foods", in Speer, F. , and Dockhorn, R. J. , (ed): Allergy and Immunology in Children, Chas. C. Thomas, Springfield, 1973, p 273.
11. Noyes, J. H. , Boyd, G. K. , and Settipane, G. A.: Anaphylaxis to sunflower seed. J All Clin Immunol 63:242, 1979.
12. Lockey, S. D. : Allergic reactions due to FD & C Yellow No. 5, tartrazine. Ann All 17:718, 1959.
13. Michaelsson, G. , and Juhlin, L. : Urticaria induced by preservatives and dye additives in food and drugs. Brit J Derm 88:525, 1973.
14. Dannaeus, A. , Foucard, T. , and Johansson, S. G. O. : The effect of orally administered sodium cromoglycate on symptoms of food allergy. Clin All 7:109, 1977.
15. Dahl, R. : Disodium cromoglycate and food allergy. Acta Allergol 33:120, 1978.
16. Ratner, B. : A possible causal factor of food allergy in certain infants. Am J Dis Child 36:277, 1928.
17. Matsumura, T. , et al.: Congenital sensitization to food in humans. Jap J All 16:858, 1967.
18. Matsumura, T. , et al: Egg sensitivity and eczematous manifestations in breast-fed newborns with particular reference to intrauterine sensitization. Ann All 35:221, 1975.

19. Matthews, T. S., and Soothill, J. F.: Complement activation after milk feeding in children with cow's milk allergy. Lancet ii:893, 1970.
20. Bachman, K. D., and Dees, S. C.: Milk allergy. I. Observations on incidence and symptoms in "well" babies. Ped 20:393, 1957.
21. Gerrard, J. W., et al.: Cow's milk allergy: Prevalence and manifestations in an unselected series of newborns. Acta Paed Scand Supp 234, 1973.
22. Gryboski, J. D.: Gastrointestinal milk allergy in infants. Ped 40:354, 1967.
23. Speer F.: The allergic tension-fatigue syndrome in children. Int Arch All 12:207, 1958.
24. Galant, S. P., et al.: An immunological approach to the diagnosis of food sensitivity. Clin All 3:363, 1973.
25. Esperanca, M., and Gerrard, J. W.: Nocturnal enuresis: Comparison of the effect of Imipramine and dietary restriction on bladder capacity. Canad Med Assn J 101:721, 1969.
26. Buckley, R. H., and Dees, S. C.: Nutritional and antigenic effects of two bovine milk preparations in infants. J Ped 69:238, 1966.
27. Nelson, T. L.: Spontaneously occurring milk antibodies in mongoloids. Am J Dis Child 108:494, 1964.
28. Handelman, N. I., and Nelson, T. L.: Association of milk precipitins with esophageal lesions causing aspiration. Ped 34:699, 1964.
29. McCrea, M. G., et al.: Milk precipitins. JAMA 203:557, 1968.
30. Buckley, R. H., and Dees, S. C.: Correlation of milk precipitins with IgA deficiency. NEJM 281:465, 1969.
31. Waldmann, T. A., Wochner, R. D., Laster, L., and Gordon, R. S., Jr.: Allergic gastroenteropathy. New Eng J Med 276:761, 1967.
32. Klein, N. C., Hargrove, R. L., Sleisenger, M. H., and Jeffries, G. H.: Eosinophilic gastroenteritis. Med 49:299, 1970.
33. Woodruff, C. W., et al.: The role of fresh cow's milk in iron deficiency. II. Comparison of fresh cow's milk with prepared formula. Am J Dis Child 124:26, 1972.
34. Sandberg, D. H., McIntosh, R. M., Bernstein, C. W., Carr, R., and Strauss, J.: Severe steroid-responsive nephrosis associated with hypersensitivity. Lancet 1:388, 1977.
35. Rowe, A. H., and Rowe, A., Jr.: Food Allergy, Chas. C. Thomas, Springfield, 1972.
36. Haddad, Z. H., Verma, S., and Kalra, V.: IgE antibodies to peptic and peptic-tryptic digests of beta-lactoglobulin: Significance in food hypersensitivity. J All Clin Immunol 63:198, 1979.

37. Lee, W. Y., Ramigio, L. K., and May, C. D.: Studies of hypersensitivity reactions to foods in infants and children. J All Clin Immunol 62:327, 1978.

38. May, C. D., and Block, S. A.: A modern clinical approach to food hypersensitivity. Allergy 33:166, 1978.

39. Soifer, M. M., and Hirsch, S. R.: The direct basophil degranulation test and the intracutaneous test: A comparison using food extracts. J All Clin Imm 56:127, 1975.

40. Bronsky, E. A., et al.: Evaluation of the provocative food skin test technique. J All 47:104, 1971.

41. Lieberman, P., et al.: Controlled study of the cytotoxic food test. J All Clin Imm 53:89, 1974.

42. Murray, A. B.: Nasal secretion eosinophilia in children with allergic rhinitis. Ann All 28:142, 1970.

43. Rosenblum, A. H., and Rosenblum, P.: Gastrointestinal allergy in infancy. Significance of eosinophiles in the stools. Ped 9:311, 1952.

44. Shiner, M., et al.: Intestinal biopsy in the diagnosis of cow's milk protein intolerance without acute symptoms. Lancet ii:1060, 1975.

45. Goldstein, G. B., and Heiner, D. C.: Clinical and immunological perspectives in food sensitivity. J All 46:270, 1970.

46. Poley, J. R.: Chronic diarrhea in infants and children. So Med J 66:1035, 1973.

47. Frazier, C. A.: Parent's Guide to Allergy in Children. Doubleday & Co., Garden City, New York, 1973.

48. Nelson, T. L., Klein, G. L., and Galant, S. P.: Severe eosinophilic gastroenteritis successfully treated with an elemental diet (Vivonex). J All Clin Immunol 63:198, 1979.

49. Hadley, R. A.: Calcium and hypo-allergenic diets. Ann All 30:36, 1972.

50. Freier, S., and Berger, H.: Disodium cromoglycate in gastrointestinal protein intolerance. Lancet 1:913, 1973.

51. Dolovich, J., et al.: Systemic mastocytosis: control of lifelong diarrhea by ingested disodium cromoglycate. C M A Journal 111:684, 1974.

52. Glaser, J., and Johnstone, D. E.: Prophylaxis of allergic disease in the newborn. JAMA 153:620, 1953.

53. Kaplan, M. S., and Solli, N. J.: IgE to cow's milk protein in breast-fed atopics. Ann All 39:75, 1977.

54. Frick, O. L., German, D. F., and Mills, J.: Development of allergy in children. I. Association with virus infections. J All Clin Immunol 63:228, 1979.

55. Ziering, R. W., O'Connor, R., Mellon, M., Cook, D., Tomaszewski, M., Street, D. H., and Hamburger, R. N.: University of California in San Diego Prophylaxis of allergy in infancy study: an interim report. J All Clin Immunol 63:199, 1979.

CHAPTER X | DRUG ALLERGY

Adverse reactions to drugs are estimated to have been responsible for 5% of hospitalizations and to occur in 10-15% of hospitalized patients.[1,2] Although most of these reactions have occurred in adults and not more than 7% have been fatal or life-threatening, the possibility of a subseuqnet adverse reaction exists whenever a prescription is written or a drug administered.

CLASSIFICATION OF ADVERSE REACTIONS

A drug can be defined as any agent administered for the purpose of diagnosis, treatment, or prevention of disease, while an adverse drug reaction is an unintended or undesired consequence of drug therapy.[3] Adverse reactions include those due to overdosage or toxicity, side effects, secondary effects, drug interactions, teratogenicity, intolerance, idiosyncrasy, and allergy or hypersensitivity.

OVERDOSAGE

Toxic effects of a drug are directly related to the total amount of the drug in the body and often differ only in degree from the desired pharmacologic effect. Toxicity may be due to accidental or deliberate administration of an excessive dose or a decreased rate of metabolism or excretion of the drug.

SIDE EFFECTS

Side effects are undesirable pharmacologic actions of a drug which often occur when it is administered at the usual dosage, such as the drowsiness caused by antihistamines.

SECONDARY EFFECTS

Secondary effects are indirect effects which are undesirable but may not occur in all patients, such as overgrowth of drug-resistant staphylococci in the gastrointestinal tract due to alteration of the intestinal flora by the action of broad spectrum antibiotics.

DRUG INTERACTIONS

A drug interaction occurs whenever the action of a drug is modified by another drug or some other exogenous chemical. The effect may be beneficial or adverse. Effects may be additive, synergistic, or antagonistic and may affect absorption, metabolism, or excretion of one or both drugs.

TERATOGENICITY

Administration of certain drugs early in pregnancy can cause developmental defects in the fetus.

INTOLERANCE

Intolerance consists of occurrence of a characteristic pharmacologic effect of a drug following an unusually small dose, such as the tinnitus which is noticed by some subjects even after small doses of aspirin.

IDIOSYNCRASY

Drug idiosyncrasy is a qualitatively abnormal response which is not mediated by an immunologic mechanism but may be due to a genetically determined enzyme deficiency or metabolic defect. One example is hemolytic anemia due to deficiency of glucose-6-phosphate dehydrogenase in erythrocytes.

HYPERSENSITIVITY

Allergic reactions are also qualitatively abnormal responses which are unrelated to the pharmacologic action of the drug, but these are mediated by immunologic mechanisms.

MECHANISMS OF DRUG ALLERGY

Most allergic drug reactions follow stimulation of antibody production by a combination of the drug or more often one of its metabolites with an endogenous protein or another macromolecule. This need for conjugation with a metabolite probably accounts for the relatively low frequency of drug allergy, the extreme variation in frequency of sensitization among different drugs, and the occurrence of hypersensitivity reactions limited to single organs or tissues. Metabolism of a drug in a certain organ might result in accumulation of the antigenic conjugate in that organ, and conjugation with an organ-specific protein might induce formation of antibody with specificity for that protein as well as the haptenic group, resulting in autoimmunity.[4]

Although the hapten-protein conjugate is usually necessary for immunogenicity, the antibody formed is usually directed primarily against the drug, although there may also be some reactivity against the protein carrier.

Only bivalent or multivalent antigens which can form bridges between antibody molecules can elicit allergic reactions. Such bridging is necessary for soluble antibody molecules to react with complement to release cytoactive peptides or to activate mediator release from mast cells or lymphocyte transformation. Univalent haptens not only fail to elicit allergic reactions but inhibit such reactions by competition with multivalent antigens for antibody.[4]

Allergic drug reactions may be due to Type I hypersensitivity (systemic anaphylaxis), Type II hypersensitivity (penicillin-induced hemolytic anemia), Type III hypersensitivity (serum sickness), or Type IV hypersensitivity (contact dermatitis). These types of reactions are discussed in Chapter I.

CLINICAL MANIFESTATIONS

ANAPHYLAXIS

The clinical features, differential diagnosis, and treatment of systemic anaphylaxis are discussed in Chapter VIII.

Penicillin is the commonest cause of systemic anaphylaxis, estimated at one time to have accounted for as many as 300 fatalities each year in the United States.[5] Less frequent causes of systemic anaphylaxis include insect stings, allergen extracts, foreign antisera, organic mercurials, heroin and other opiates, iodinated radiographic contrast material, local anesthetics, streptomycin, sulfobromophthalein (BSP), dehydrocholate sodium (Decholin), fluorescein, Congo red, dextran, aspirin, heparin, vitamin B_{12}, demethylchlortetracycline and other tetracyclines, cephalosporins, enzymes, hormones, and vaccines.[3,4]

SERUM SICKNESS

When antigens are still present in the circulation when antibody is produced, circulating antigen-antibody complexes may form and may cause tissue injury and symptoms of serum sickness (see Chapter I). The antibody is probably usually of the IgG class, but IgM and IgE antibodies have also been implicated.[4] Following initial exposure to the drug, symptoms may occur after a latent period of at least 6 days (usually 7-12 days) and usually persist for approximately 7 days. Long acting penicillin or sulfonamides may cause symptoms beginning as long as 3 weeks after the last dose of drug and persisting for as long as 3-4 weeks.[4]

Serum sickness is characterized by fever, cutaneous eruptions, lymphadenopathy, and arthritis. Pruritus may be the initial symptom, and erythema and swelling may be evident at the injection site. Urticaria and angioedema are the commonest cutaneous manifestations, but morbilliform, scarlatiniform or purpuric eruptions or erythema multiforme may occur. Cutaneous eruptions are estimated to occur in 90% of patients with serum sickness.[3]

Joint symptoms, usually arthralgias of the knees, ankles, or wrists, occur in approximately 50% of patients.

Tenderness and enlargement of lymph nodes draining the site of injection of an offending drug are often present, but generalized lymphadenopathy and splenomegaly may occur.

Less common manifestations include peripheral neuropathy, nephritis, and vasculitis involving the myocardium, kidneys, liver, pancreas, adrenals, muscle, and skin.

In the subject already sensitized by prior exposure to the drug severe clinical manifestations may occur within a few days after reexposure (usually 2-4 days).

Laboratory findings may include mild leukocytosis, mild eosinophilia, and slight elevations in the sedimentation rate. The smear of the peripheral blood may disclose the presence of atypical lymphocytes and plasmacytes.[3] Serum complement is sometimes reduced in concentration.

Serum sickness has followed administration of foreign sera, penicillin, sulfonamides, thiouracils, diphenylhydantoin, aminosalicylic acid, and streptomycin.

CUTANEOUS ERUPTIONS

Cutaneous eruptions are the commonest manifestations of drug allergy. These include contact dermatitis, urticaria or angioedema, exfoliative dermatitis, erythema multiforme, and maculopapular, morbilliform, or erythematous eruptions. Pruritus may occur without any evident eruption. Other manifestations include erythema nodosum, fixed drug eruptions, photosensitivity, Stevens-Johnson syndrome, toxic epidermal necrolysis, and allergic vasculitis.

Contact dermatitis can follow topical application of drugs to the skin or mucous membranes following previous sensitization. It usually presents as an erythematous, papular, vesicular eruption with edema and sometimes bullae, restricted to the area of contact. The diagnosis may be obscured by the fact that the drug has often been applied as treatment for another dermatitis, but contact dermatitis should be suspected from aggravation of the previous eruption. Agents commonly implicated include local anesthetics, antihistamines, penicillin, sulfonamides, streptomycin, neomycin, mercurials, and parabens, which are used as preservatives in many topical medications. It is prudent to avoid topical use of antibiotics, anesthetics, and antihistamines because of the frequency with which topical use has caused sensitization.

Urticaria and angioedema can occur alone or as symptoms of serum sickness. Their clinical manifestations and treatment are discussed in Chapter VI. Almost any drug can cause urticaria, but those most commonly incriminated include penicillin, salicylates, sulfonamides, organ extracts, foreign sera, and allergen extracts.

Exfoliative dermatitis is a generalized, erythematous, scaly eruption causing loss of the superficial layers of skin and often associated with fever and malaise. It may follow other drug-induced cutaneous eruptions and is often fatal. This dermatitis may persist for months after withdrawal of the offending drug. Commonly implicated drugs include penicillin, sulfonamides, barbiturates, phenothiazines, and hydantoins.

Erythema nodosum usually presents as bilaterally symmetrical, warm, tender, erythematous nodules over the anterior aspects of the legs. The lesions may resemble bruises and may persist for a few days or several weeks. Fever, malaise, arthralgia, and myalgia may be present. Iodides, and bromides are the drugs most often implicated, but others which have been suspected include penicillin, sulfonamides, antipyrine, and salicylates.[3]

Fixed drug eruptions are round or oval areas of edema followed by erythema and then a reddish-purple, elevated lesion or scaly, urticarial, vesicobullous, hemorrhagic, or nodular lesions which recur at the same sites with each reexposure to the same drug. Lesions may be single or multiple and are sometimes mildly pruritic. They usually subside within 3 weeks after discontinuation of the drug, but may leave residual hyperpigmentation. Common causes include phenolphthalein, barbiturates, sulfonamides, tetracyclines, antipyretics, and quinine.[3]

Photosensitivity, due to interaction between a drug and light energy, may be due to phototoxic reactions or photoallergic reactions. Phototoxic reactions are not immunologic and may follow initial simultaneous exposure to light and drug in adequate concentrations. Erythema occurs, sometimes with vesiculation, and residual hyperpigmentation may remain. Lesions are limited to areas exposed to light. Drugs most often responsible have been topical coal tar preparations and oral demethylchlortetracycline (Declomycin).

Photoallergic reactions are immunologic reactions, requiring prior sensitization. The lesions resemble those of contact dermatitis and may recur over days or months following each exposure to light even without further drug administration. The drugs most often implicated include phenothiazines, sulfonamides, and griseofulvin. Bithional and halogenated salicylamides, which are bacteriostatic agents often used in soaps, antiseptics, and topical medications, also cause photoallergic reactions.

Stevens-Johnson syndrome, erythema multiforme exudativum, is characterized by erythematous, papular lesions which enlarge and become vesicular or bullous. The eruption involves not only most of the skin but also the mucous membranes, of the conjunctivae, nose, mouth, and genitalia. Respiratory tract involvement may cause bronchitis or pneumonia. Fever and malaise or severe prostration are common. Corneal ulceration may be followed by scarring and blindness. The process may continue for 4-6 weeks or even longer, and the mortality may be as high as 10%. When drug allergy has been suspected, the drugs most often implicated have been long acting sulfonamides and barbiturates. A relationship to infection with Myco- plasma pneumoniae, herpes simplex, and other viruses has also been suspected.

Henoch-Schonlein purpura, anaphylactoid purpura, is another condition of unknown etiology possibly due to drug allergy. The cutaneous lesions may initially be pruritic, maculopapular, or urticarial, but then become purpuric. The diagnosis is usually evident from the typical distribution over the buttocks and lower extremities. Arthralgia and abdominal pain indicate involvement of the small blood vessels of joints and the gastrointestinal tract, and renal involvement is also common. Fever, leukocytosis, and hematuria are often present. Salicylates are the most commonly implicated drugs. Food allergy and antecedent respiratory infections have also been suspect.

Toxic epidermal necrolysis, Lyell's syndrome, begins as generalized erythema that is followed by desquamation. Healing without scarring usually occurs within 2 weeks, but the mortality rate may be as high as 25%. Death is usually due to sepsis or electrolyte imbalance. Infection with phage group 2 staphylococci has been associated with toxic epidermal necrolysis in infants, but drug allergy has been implicated in older children and adults. Suspected drugs include penicillin, sulfonamides, barbiturates, isoniazid, and hydantoins. [3]

PULMONARY MANIFESTATIONS

Asthma may occur as a manifestation of systemic anaphylaxis or following inhalation of penicillin or other drugs.

Loeffler's syndrome is characterized by widespread, transient, often migratory pulmonary infiltrates and peripheral eosinophilia, usually due to invasion by roundworm larvae, but sometimes due to drug allergy. The process may continue for several weeks after discontinuation of use of the offending drug. Loeffler's syndrome is reported to have followed administration of para-aminosalicylic acid, penicillin, sulfonamides, and mephenesin.[3]

Pulmonary reactions to nitrofurantoin, methotrexate, and bleomycin have been largely limited to adults. These are of unknown etiology, but hypersensitivity has been suspected. Nitrofurantoin reactions may occur within hours or days after exposure with findings including chills and fever, dyspnea, pleural effusion, and pulmonary infiltrates due to interstitial fibrosis, often associated with peripheral eosinophilia. A chronic form of nitrofurantoin lung is not usually associated with eosinophilia, but fever, dyspnea, and roentgenographic evidence of interstitial fibrosis are found. Interstitial pulmonary infiltrates are also found in patients with pulmonary reactions to either methotrexate or bleomycin.

HEMOLYTIC ANEMIA

Penicillin-induced hemolytic anemia is seen in patients receiving treatment with large doses of penicillin especially if renal function is poor. It is associated with a positive Coombs reaction. Improvement is rapid after therapy has been stopped.

Other agents that cause immune hemolytic anemias include quinine, quinidine, dipyrone, aminosalicylic acid, mephenytoin, stibophen, cephalothin, and phenacetin.

THROMBOCYTOPENIA

Immunologically mediated thrombocytopenia may be associated with fever and arthralgia as well as petechiae and hemorrhage. The commonest causes are quinine, quinidine, meprobamate, chlorothiazide, thiouracils, chloramphenicol, and sulfonamides.[4]

GRANULOCYTOPENIA

Immunologically mediated granulocytopenia can be caused by aminopyrine, phenylbutazone, phenothiazines, thiouracils, sulfonamides, chloramphenicol, and anticonvulsants.[3,4]

FEVER

Fever may occur as the only manifestation of drug allergy. If there has been no previous exposure to the drug, fever usually begins 7-10 days after treatment has started and persists until within 2-3 days after it has been discontinued. There may be an associated leukocytosis, sometimes as high as 30, 000 per cubic millimeter and often consisting predominantly of neutrophils. Fever may occur within a few hours after administration of the drug if previous sensitization has occurred.

Drug fever may precede other manifestations of drug allergy such as anaphylaxis or exfoliative dermatitis, and arteritis and focal necrosis have been found in the myocardium, liver, lungs, and spleen when patients have died with drug fever. [6]

Drugs most commonly implicated include sulfonamides, para-aminosalicylic acid, iodides, thiouracils, quinidine, procainamide, mercurial diuretics, streptomycin, isoniazid, anticonvulsants, barbiturates, salicylates, penicillin, and other antibiotics. [3,4,6] Digitalis, chloramphenical, and tetracyclines have rarely, if ever, caused fever. [6]

HEPATITIS

Hepatitis due to administration of aminosalicylates, sulfonamides, phenothiazines, and other drugs is suspected of being due to drug allergy. [7]

PNEUMONITIS

Nitrofurantoin-induced pneumonitis is characterized by fever, coughing, diffuse pulmonary infiltration, pleural effussion, hilar adenopathy, and sometimes asthma. This reaction is probably due to allergy.

NEPHRITIS

Interstitial nephritis occurs rarely in patients treated with large doses of methicillin or penicillin. There may be associated cutaneous eruptions, fever, or eosinophilia beginning 3-10 days after treatment with the drug has started. The reaction may be fatal if the drug is not discontinued. It has been ascribed to a drug-induced autoimmune reaction. [7]

Other drugs implicated as possibly responsible for interstitial nephritis include sulfonamides, furosemide, or thiazides.

DRUG-INDUCED
LUPUS ERYTHEMATOSUS

A syndrome resembling systemic lupus erythematosus has followed administration of hydralazine or procainamide or less frequently isoniazid, oral contraceptives, griseofulvin, tetracycline, thiouracil, diphenylhydantoin, and other anticonvulsants, and chlorpromazine.[8] Cutaneous, central nervous system, and renal involvement do not usually occur in contrast to their more frequent occurrence in systemic lupus erythematosus.

PENICILLIN

Penicillin and its derivatives are the commonest causes of drug allergy and of systemic anaphylaxis. The frequency of penicillin allergy is unknown, but estimates have ranged from 0.7-10%. Systemic anaphylaxis has been reported in 15-40 patients per 100,000 treated with penicillin; fatal anaphylaxis in 1.5-2/100,000.[5] Other clinical manifestations include urticaria, other cutaneous eruptions, fever, serum sickness, and more rarely hemolytic anemia,[9] nephritis,[10] granulocytopenia, thrombocytopenia, or neuritis.

CLASSIFICATION OF REACTIONS

The common allergic reactions to penicillin have been classified as immediate, accelerated, or late reactions.[11] Immediate reactions begin within 30 minutes, and these are the most dangerous, including urticaria and systemic anaphylaxis.

Accelerated allergic reactions are those that begin 2-72 hours after penicillin therapy has started. Accelerated reactions usually are manifested as pruritus or urticaria, wheezing or laryngeal edema, or local inflammatory reactions. These are usually less serious reactions, but death from asphyxia can follow laryngeal edema.

Late reactions are the commonest allergic reactions to penicillin, accounting for 80-90% of reactions. These usually begin more than 72 hours and sometimes weeks after initiation of penicillin therapy and are manifested as morbilliform, urticarial, or erythematous eruptions, serum sickness, or local inflammatory reactions.

Immediate and accelerated reactions are mediated by skin sensitizing antibodies, but these antibodies are not all directed against the same antigenic determinants.

ANTIGENIC DETERMINANTS

Approximately 95% of penicillin is degraded in vitro to ben-
zylpenicillenic acid, which combines with proteins to form ben-
zylpenicilloyl (BPO) haptenic groups. This conjugate is therefore
known as the major antigenic determinant. Benzylpenicillin can
also react directly with proteins to form this conjugate. Reaction of benzylpenicillin with a synthetic polypeptide, polylysine,
results in the formation of a derivative that is not immunogenic but can react with skin sensitizing antibody with specificity
for the BPO group.

Other penicillin degradation products can also react with
proteins to form small amounts of hapten-protein conjugates,
the minor determinants. It is these minor determinants that
are usually responsible for immediate and accelerated allergic
reactions to penicillin. A minor determinant mixture (MDM)
containing benzylpenicillin, benzylpenicilloate, benzylpenilloate,
and α -benzylpenicilloylamine has been recommended for skin
testing to detect hypersensitivity to minor determinants.[12]
Others have used a sterile solution of benzylpenicillin diluted
with alkaline buffered saline and stored at room temperature
for 2-4 weeks for detection of hypersensitivity to minor determinants.[13] A major determinant concentration of $1x10^{-6}$ and
minor determinant concentrations of $1x10^{-2}$ (for each ingred-
ient) have been recommended for skin testing.[14]

Skin sensitizing antibodies with specificity for minor determinants are responsible for most immediate reactions; those
with specificity for the major determinant, late reactions. Accelerated reactions may be mediated by either.[13, 14]

BPO specific antibodies of the IgG class are also found in
almost all patients with BPO specific reaginic antibodies. These
apparently at least include blocking antibodies; accelerated urticarial reactions may subside when specific IgG antibody titers
increase.[14] High titers of IgG antibodies have also been associated with penicillin-induced hemolytic anemia.

BPO specific IgM antibodies are found in almost everyone
treated with penicillin. High titers have been associated with
late maculopapular or erythematous eruptions.

It has also been suggested that protein or polypeptide im-
purities present in penicillin in trace amounts may be immunogenic and may cause allergic reactions,[15] but the significance
of this possibility has not yet been determined.

SKIN TESTING

Skin testing can be done with sterile solutions of benzylpenicillin, and use of a solution prepared 2-4 weeks before testing
may be more likely to contain benzylpenicilloate.[3] Serial ten-

fold dilutions containing 1, 10, 100, 1,000, and 10,000 units/ ml. are prepared. An even more dilute solution is indicated if severe penicillin hypersensitivity is suspected. All testing is done on the upper extremities with medications and equipment for the treatment of anaphylaxis immediately available. If the initial prick or scratch test with the most dilute solution (1 unit /ml.) is negative when compared with the diluent control, an intradermal test with the same dilution is done. If this is negative when compared with the intradermal control at 15 minutes, intradermal testing is continued at 15-30 minute intervals with successive ten-fold increases in the concentration of the test solution until a positive reaction occurs or until the highest concentration has been reached.

Penicilloyl polylysine (PPL) is available commercially for testing for hypersensitivity to the major determinant.

A negative skin test with both PPL and MDM indicates that an immediate reaction following treatment with penicillin is very unlikely but not impossible, and the likelihood of an accelerated reaction or late urticarial reaction is also reduced. A positive reaction to MDM indicates that an immediate, anaphylactic reaction is likely if penicillin is administered. A positive reaction to PPL indicates an increased risk of an accelerated or late urticarial reaction if penicillin is administered. Skin testing has not generally been helpful in identifying patients at risk for allergic reactions such as hemolytic anemia, serum sickness, or exanthematous eruptions that are not mediated by reaginic antibody.

Skin testing may induce penicillin hypersensitivity and may cause systemic anaphylaxis. It is helpful only in assessing the likelihood of hypersensitivity at the time it is done and the results are irrelevant to the safety of administration of penicillin at some indefinite future time. Since desensitization may have occurred during the testing procedure, if the skin tests have been negative, treatment with penicillin should be started at once. Continued observation is necessary because of the possibility of systemic anaphylaxis despite negative skin test results. Skin testing is probably indicated in someone with suspected penicillin hypersensitivity only when there is need for treatment of a serious or life-threatening illness with penicillin and no other drug can be reasonably substituted.

OTHER TESTS

Direct skin testing has been found generally to be more sensitive for the detection of penicillin hypersensitivity than passive transfer testing. Occasional exceptions have been observed when sensitization has occurred only very recently.

Direct skin testing may then be negative, while passive transfer testing demonstrates the presence of circulating antibody. [16]

Because of the potential hazards of skin testing other methods
of detecting penicillin hypersensitivity have been sought. Results of the radioallergosorbent test[17] and histamine release
from leukocytes in vitro[18] have been found to correlate well
with the results of skin testing, but a major disadvantage to
their use is the delay before the results are known. When evaluation for penicillin hypersensitivity is necessary, results are
usually needed immediately.

Other methods of testing that have been recommended include rat mast cell degranulation, production of migration inhibitory factor by lymphocytes, the lymphocyte transformation
test and the skin window technique.

Delayed hypersensitivity demonstrated by skin testing with
penicillin has been associated sometimes with reactions to penicillin consisting of late, nonurticarial cutaneous eruptions. [19]

AMPICILLIN

Ampicillin is associated more frequently with cutaneous
eruptions (7.7%) than is penicillin (2.7%). [20] Most of these are
erythematous, maculopapular eruptions, which may be dose
related[21] and are especially frequent in patients with infectious
mononucleosis. These maculopapular eruptions usually begin
during the second and third weeks after initial exposure and are
apparently rarely due to reagin-mediated allergic reactions,
while urticarial eruptions due to ampicillin are often manifestations of allergy to the drug. [22]

Interstitial nephritis and many of the other types of allergic
reaction that have followed treatment with penicillin have also
been associated with treatment with ampicillin. [23]

CROSS REACTIVITY

Patients who are allergic to penicillin are often also allergic to ampicillin and other semisynthetic derivatives of penicillin. The results of skin testing with major and minor determinant
reagents for penicillin, ampicillin, and methicillin have indicated, however, that often allergy to penicillin may not be
associated with allergy to either of the other two drugs, and allergy to either ampicillin or methicillin may occur without allergy to penicillin. [24]

Many if not most patients with penicillin allergy have also
been found to be allergic to cephalosporins, possibly because
both drugs have β-lactam rings.[25]

If either a semisynthetic penicillin or a cephalosporin must be administered to a patient with a history of penicillin allergy, preliminary skin testing should be done with several serial dilutions of the drug as recommended for penicillin testing. Suitable concentrations of cephalothin for skin testing are 0.25, 2.5, and 25 mg./ml.[3]

DESENSITIZATION

Although allergy to penicillin is an indication for substitution of another equally effective antibiotic that does not cross react with penicillin, occasionally there may be no suitable alternative to treatment of a life-threatening infection with penicillin. Desensitization is the procedure whereby administration of gradually increasing doses of penicillin may enable the patient to receive therapeutic doses without developing a serious allergic reaction. Urticaria may occur during treatment of such patients and fatal anaphylaxis has occurred during attempted desensitization.[26] Antihistamines, sympathomimetics, and adrenal corticosteroids have sometimes been administered simultaneously, but there is no evidence that they prevent anaphylaxis.[3] Tolerance of penicillin may be due either to loss of skin sensitizing antibody through competition for antigen (desensitization) or stimulation of production of IgG blocking antibody.[26]

If desensitization is attempted it should follow immediately the previously described procedure for skin testing with solutions of penicillin of increasing concentration (Table 10.1). With the last intradermal test (0.02ml/10,000u/ml.) 200 units of penicillin will have been administered, but a smaller dose will have been administered if a positive reaction has occurred at a lower concentration. Because of the reduced rate of absorption from the intradermal site, it may be best to continue desensitization with a somewhat smaller dose when subcutaneous administration is started. Larger doses than this have sometimes been given intradermally during desensitization.[26]

Successively increasing doses are administered at 15 minute intervals (see Table 10.1) if tolerated. If the final subcutaneous dose is delivered without any serious reaction, continuous intravenous therapy can then be started immediately.[27] Medications, equipment, and personnel must be immediately available for the treatment of anaphylaxis, and any reactions that occur must be treated immediately (see Chapter VIII).

ASPIRIN

Aspirin probably is second only to penicillin as a cause of adverse reactions. Urticaria and angioedema are the most commonly recognized reactions resembling allergic reactions,

TABLE 10.1   PENICILLIN DESENSITIZATION

SOLUTION INJECTED AT 15 MINUTE INTERVALS

ROUTE	CONCENTRATION (UNITS/ML)	VOLUME (ML)	DOSE (UNITS)
Scratch or Prick (Test)	1	0.02	0.02
Intradermal (Test)	1	0.02	0.02
Intradermal (Test)	10	0.02	0.2
Intradermal (Test)	100	0.02	2
Intradermal (Test)	1000	0.02	20
Intradermal (Test)	10,000	0.02	200
Subcutaneous	100	0.05	5
Subcutaneous	100	0.1	10
Subcutaneous	100	0.2	20
Subcutaneous	100	0.4	40
Subcutaneous	100	0.8	80
Subcutaneous	1000	0.15	150
Subcutaneous	1000	0.3	300
Subcutaneous	1000	0.6	600
Subcutaneous	1000	1.0	1000
Subcutaneous	10,000	0.2	2000
Subcutaneous	10,000	0.4	4000
Subcutaneous	10,000	0.8	8000
Subcutaneous	100,000	0.15	15,000
Subcutaneous	100,000	0.3	30,000
Subcutaneous	100,000	0.6	60,000
Subcutaneous	100,000	1.0	100,000
Subcutaneous	1,000,000	0.2	200,000
Subcutaneous	1,000,000	0.4	400,000
Subcutaneous	1,000,000	0.8	800,000

but vasomotor rhinitis and asthma can also occur. Other adverse reactions include systemic anaphylaxis, nephrotoxicity following salicylate abuse, abnormal hemostasis, toxic effects on the gastrointestinal tract, hepatitis, and pancytopenia.[28]

The frequent association of asthma, nasal polyposis, and aspirin-induced wheezing may sometimes be transmitted as an autosomal recessive trait.[29] Although this triad usually has begun in adults, asthmatic children with the sudden onset of asthma in late childhood who are girls, have no personal or family history of atopy and have nasal polyposis are those children with the highest risk of having aspirin intolerance.[30]

The incidence of aspirin intolerance among asthmatics has generally been estimated at 2-4%, [3], [31] but measurement of pulmonary function before and after aspirin challenge in adult asthmatic patients with steroid dependent asthma, nasal polyps, or sinusitis but no history of aspirin intolerance has identified aspirin intolerance in 20%. [32] Aspirin intolerance has been reported in as many as 28% of children with severe asthma. [33] Its frequency among subjects without atopic disease has been estimated at 0.9%. [31]

The mechanism through which aspirin intolerance is mediated is unknown, but it is apparently not usually immunologic. [28], [34] Skin testing is usually negative, although skin testing with aspiryl-polylysine has occasionally elicited positive reactions in patients who have had urticaria or angioedema following aspirin administration. [35] Serum IgE concentrations in patients with aspirin-induced asthma have been normal, and attempts to transfer aspirin intolerance to monkeys with plasma transfusions have been unsuccessful. [34]

Mediation by a pharmacologic mechanism is suggested by the observation that reactions are also provoked in these patients by several chemicals whose structures do not resemble that of aspirin. These include indomethacin, antipyrine, tartrazine (a yellow dye added to foods and drugs), and benzoic acid derivatives, which are also found in many foods. A relationship to aspirin's inhibition of prostaglandin synthesis has been suspected, but tartrazine does not inhibit prostaglandin synthesis. [36]

Complete avoidance of these is difficult (see Table 6.3, 6.4) but necessary for the patient with intolerance, and avoidance of aspirin is generally wise for any patient with asthma or chronic urticaria. Acetaminophen is usually a suitable substitute analgesic and antipyretic, but obstructive changes in pulmonary function are reported to have followed administration of acetaminophen to some patients with aspirin sensitivity. [37]

Skin testing with aspirin is contraindicated because of the possibility of anaphylactic reactions. [3]

RADIOGRAPHIC CONTRAST MEDIA

Adverse reactions to iodinated contrast media include flushing, nausea, vomiting, generalized pruritus, urticaria, angioedema, rhinorrhea, sneezing, wheezing, hypotension, convulsions, cardiac arrest. Their incidence has been estimated at 5-8% of patients receiving intravascular contrast media with moderate or severe reactions occurring in 0.9-1.7%. [38-40] A fatal reaction may occur once in 50,000 studies. [41] The frequency of generalized reactions in patients with histories of a previous generalized reaction has been found to be as high as 30-35%. [39,41]

Despite the similarity of many of these reactions to allergic reactions, there is no evidence that they are mediated by immunologic mechanisms. Skin testing is not helpful in identifying patients at risk and a serious reaction may follow initial exposure to contrast material. Injection of iodinated contrast media has often been found to elicit a nonsequential activation of the complement system with decreases in total hemolytic complement activity, but no relationship to clinical reactions has been established. [42] It is most likely that these anaphylactoid reactions are due to nonspecific release of histamine from mast cells and basophils.

No reliable method of identifying patients at risk for anaphylactoid reactions to contrast media is available, although the risk is increased in those with histories of previous reactions to contrast material. Neither atopy nor a history of adverse reactions to iodides (see Chapter III) is a contraindication. Preliminary intravenous injection of 1 ml of contrast material to observe the patient's response cannot be recommended because such test doses have been followed by fatal reactions themselves, and fatal reactions have followed administration of the full dose when the pretest has been negative. [41]

Unfortunately there is no non-crossreacting substitute for iodinated radiographic contrast materials, and studies with such agents are often essential in directing appropriate management of patients. There is evidence that it may be possible to minimize risks in patients who have previously had anaphylactoid reaction s to contrast materials by pretreatment with adrenal corticosteroids or diphenhydramine. [40,44] When a previous reaction has been severe pretreatment may be combined with cautious, graded, intravenous administration of the contrast material at 10 minute intervals: 0.1 ml/1:100, 0.1 ml/1:10, 1 ml (undiluted), 5 ml, 20 ml. [44] Some have recommended pretreatment of adults at risk with prednisone, 50 mg q6hx3, starting 18 hours before the study, and diphenhydramine, 50 mg. I. M., 1 hour before the study. [45] Equivalent doses for children would probably be approximately 1 mg/Kg.

LOCAL ANESTHETICS

Adverse reactions to local anesthetics are usually due to toxicity, which may follow overdosage, rapid absorption, or inadvertent intravascular injection.

The symptoms include excitation, nervousness, euphoria, slurring of speech, dizziness, nausea, vomiting, disorientation, convulsions, coma, and respiratory and cardiac failure. Myocardial depression and peripheral vasodilation may cause shock. Toxic reactions are occasionally fatal.[3]

Toxic effects can be minimized by addition of epinephrine to the agent to be used to cause local vasoconstriction, slowing systemic absorption, but the epinephrine can also cause toxic effects: nervousness, tremor, tachycardia, and hypertension.

Contact dermatitis is the commonest allergic reaction to local anesthetics. The use of these agents in topical preparations is to be decried. Other manifestations of allergic reactions include urticaria, angioedema, conjunctivitis, rhinitis, bronchospasm, and systemic anaphylaxis, but these reactions are extremely rare. Delayed hypersensitivity may cause delayed swelling at the injection site, but such reactions are usually due to the trauma of the procedure.[3]

Cross reactivity is frequently seen among local anesthetics with p-aminophenyl groups (Table 10.2). Lidocaine and other agents chemically unrelated to procaine are usually well tolerated by patients with hypersensitivity to procaine.

TABLE 10.2   CHEMICAL RELATIONSHIPS
OF LOCAL ANESTHETICS

Frequent Cross-reactivity (contain p-aminophenyl group):

Procaine (Novocaine)	Monocaine
Benzocaine	Butyn
Pontocaine (Tetracaine)	Borocaine
Tantocaine	Butesin
Larocaine	Chloroprocaine

No Cross-reactivity with Procaine Group:

Xylocaine (Lidocaine)	Stovaine
Carbocaine (Mepivicaine)	Diothane
Dibucaine (Nupercaine)	Apothesine
Holocaine	Cocaine
Metycaine	Intracaine
Alypine	Prilocaine
Bupivacaine	

Skin testing has sometimes been reported helpful in identifying local anesthetics that can be tolerated by patients who have had allergic reactions,[46] but results have been variable and it is usually possible to substitute a chemically unrelated agent.

VACCINES

TETANUS TOXOID

Adverse reactions to administration of tetanus toxoid include urticaria, angioedema, and large local reactions that may be associated with fever and malaise as well as peripheral neuropathy rarely.[3] Reactions due to Type I hypersensitivity are associated often with positive skin tests and may necessitate an attempt at desensitization if the patient is not already immune. Successive intradermal test doses with 0.1 ml of 1:1,000; 1:100, and 1:10 dilutions of tetanus toxoid have been recommended to determine the strongest concentration that fails to elicit a reaction.[47] Subsequent doses, starting with this dilution, are administered once or twice each week with gradual increases in dosage as tolerated until 0.1 ml of the undiluted toxoid has been reached. This dose is then repeated monthly until adequate immunization has been achieved as determined by assay of the antitoxin titer.[3]

If the usual initial series of tetanus toxoid immunizations has been completed in infancy and early childhood, further routine boosters are recommended only at 10 year intervals after 6 years of age. Avoidance of unnecessary hyperimmunization is expected to lessen the frequency of allergic reactions.

CHICK EMBRYO VACCINES

Vaccines prepared from viruses grown in embryonated chicken eggs or tissue cultures of chick embryo cells may contain very small amounts of egg protein. Administration of such vaccines is not contraindicated unless there is a history of allergic symptoms following ingestion of egg. A positive skin test to egg is not a contraindication, but skin testing with the vaccine before administration of the full dose might be prudent in such children. Administration of rubeola vaccine prepared in tissue cultures of chick embryo cells has been tolerated by children allergic to egg.[48]

DIAGNOSIS

The diagnosis of drug allergy is usually made by history. This causes frequent overdiagnosis of penicillin allergy, especially when the only manifestation has been a cutaneous eruption. Only 7-10% of children with histories of penicillin allergy have been found to have immunological evidence of hypersensitivity.[13,49] On the other hand, as many as 4-8% of adult patients without histories of penicillin allergy have been found to have positive immediate skin tests.[50,51]

Allergy skin testing for Type I hypersensitivity is reliable for high molecular weight compounds but unreliable for most low molecular weight compounds that act as haptens. Skin testing is helpful for detecting penicillin hypersensitivity, however, although not without risk. Skin testing elicits false positive reactions from nonspecific irritation or nonimmunologic release of histamine with some drugs.

Skin testing for Type IV hypersensitivity is rarely helpful, but may correlate with delayed hypersensitivity to procaine.

Patch testing or photopatch testing is very useful in the diagnosis of contact dermatitis or photosensitivity.

The radioallergosorbent test, release of histamine from leukocytes, basophil degranulation test, and other in vitro methods of identifying drug allergens are still largely experimental. The radioallergosorbent test seems to be the most promising of these.

PREVENTION

No drug should be prescribed without a definite indication and without inquiry concerning previous adverse reactions to it or to related drugs. When there is a history of a previous adverse reaction, an equally effective, non-crossreacting drug should be substituted if at all possible. If this is impossible, appropriate tests should be done to assess the subject's risk of having an allergic reaction, depending upon the history and if the drug is one for which testing is possible.

It is not known whether there is an increased frequency of allergy to most drugs among atopic patients although aspirin should be avoided by asthmatics. Drug allergy has been reported in 17% of patients with atopic respiratory disease; penicillin allergy, in 10-11%.[52] Skin testing, however, has failed to demonstrate any increase in the frequency of penicillin hypersensitivity in patients with asthma or ragweed hay fever.[53] Systemic anaphylaxis is thought to occur more frequently among atopic subjects, on the other hand.[3,7] It may be prudent to avoid administration of penicillin by intramuscular injection to this population.

Administration of a drug by the oral route is least likely to cause sensitization or to provoke systemic anaphylaxis, but fatal anaphylaxis has been caused by oral penicillin.[54]

Patients should be observed for 20 minutes after injection of penicillin or another drug, and medications, equipment, and personnel should be immediately available for treatment of systemic anaphylaxis (see Chapter VIII).

Patients who have had adverse reactions to drugs should wear emblems indicating their hypersensitivity. *

PROGNOSIS

The natural history of drug allergy is unknown. Immunologic evidence of penicillin hypersensitivity is rarely found more than 2 years after the adverse reaction in children[49] despite possible frequent reexposure to penicillin through ingestion of milk.[55] The frequency of positive skin tests for penicillin in adults is reported to decline from 90% within 3 months after the reaction to 25% at 5-10 years.[56] If skin testing is not done or not possible it cannot be concluded that allergy is no longer present even after several years because marked sensitivity is known occasionally to have persisted for several years without recognized reexposure to the drug.[7]

*Medic Alert Foundation, P. O. Box 1009, Turlock, California 95380.

REFERENCES

1. Seidl, L. G. , et al.: Studies on the epidemiology of adverse drug reactions. Bull Johns Hopkins Hosp 119:299, 1966.
2. Hurwitz, N. , and Wade, O. L.: Intensive hospital monitoring of adverse reactions to drugs. Brit Med J 1:531, 1969.
3. DeSwarte, R. D.: "Drug allergy", in Patterson, R. (ed): Allergic Diseases, J. B. Lippincott Co., Philadelphia, 1972.
4. Parker, C. W.: Drug allergy. NEJM 292:511, 1975.
5. Idsoe, O. , et al.: Nature and extent of penicillin side reactions, with particular reference to fatalities from anaphylactic shock. Bull WHO 38:159, 1968.
6. Cluff, L. E. , and Johnson, J. E. , III: "Drug fever", in Kallos, P. , and Waksman, B. H. (ed): Progress in Allergy 8:149, S. Karger, Basel, 1964.
7. Parker, C. W.: Drug allergy. NEJM 292:732, 1975.

8. Harpey, J. P.: Lupus-like syndromes induced by drugs. Ann All 33:256, 1974.
9. Petz, L. D., and Fudenberg, H. H.: Coombs-positive hemolytic anemia caused by penicillin administration. NE JM 274:171, 1966.
10. Gilbert, D. N., et al.: Interstitial nephritis due to methicillin, penicillin, and ampicillin. Ann All 28:378, 1970.
11. Levine, B. B., et al.: Prediction of penicillin allergy by immunological tests. Ann N Y Acad Sci 145:298, 1967.
12. Levine, B. B., and Redmond, A. P.: Minor haptenic determinant-specific reagins of penicillin hypersensitivity in man. Int Arch All Appl Imm 35:445, 1969.
13. Bierman, C. W., et al.: Penicillin allergy in children: The role of immunological tests in its diagnosis. J All 43: 267, 1969.
14. Levine, B. B., and Zolov, D. M.: Prediction of penicillin allergy by immunological tests. J All 43:231, 1969.
15. Stewart, G. T.: Allergenic residues in penicillins. Lancet 1:1177, 1967.
16. Redmond, A. P., and Levine, B. B.: The relationship between direct immediate skin tests and passive transfer tests in man. J All 39:51, 1967.
17. Wide, L., and Juhlin, L.: Detection of penicillin allergy of the immediate type by radioimmunoassay of reagins (IgE) to penicilloyl conjugates. Clin All 1:171, 1971.
18. Perelmutter, L., and Eisen, A. H.: Studies on histamine release from leukocytes of penicillin-sensitive individuals. Int Arch All 38:104, 1970.
19. Fellner, M. J., et al.: Delayed hypersensitivity to penicillin. Clinical significance and hyposensitization after therapy. JAMA 210:2061, 1969.
20. Shapiro, S., et al.: Drug rash with ampicillin and other penicillins. Lancet 2:969, 1969.
21. Bass, J. W., et al.: Adverse effects of orally administered ampicillin. J Ped 83:106, 1973.
22. Bierman, C. W., et al.: Reactions associated with ampicillin therapy. JAMA 220:1098, 1972.
23. Woodroffe, A. J., et al.: Acute interstitial nephritis following ampicillin hypersensitivity. Med J Austr 1:65, 1975.
24. Van Dellen, R. G., et al.: Differing patterns of wheal and flare skin reactivity in patients allergic to penicillins. J All 47:230, 1971.
25. Assem, E. S. K., and Vickers, M. R.: Tests for penicillin allergy in man. II. The immunological cross-reaction between penicillins and cephalosporins. Immunol 27:255, 1974.

26. Fellner, M. J. , et al.: Mechanisms of clinical desensitization in urticarial hypersensitivity to penicillin. J All 45: 55, 1970.
27. Stewart, G. T. , and McGovern, J. P.: Penicillin Allergy. Chas. C. Thomas, Springfield, 1970.
28. von Maur, K. , et al.: Aspirin intolerance in a family. J All Clin Imm 54:380, 1974.
29. Lockey, R. F. , et al.: Familial occurrence of asthma, nasal polyps, and aspirin intolerance. Ann Int Med 78:57, 1973.
30. Falliers, C. J.: Aspirin and subtypes of asthma: Risk factor analysis. J All Clin Imm 52:141, 1973.
31. Settipane, G. A. , et al.: Aspirin intolerance. II. A prospective study in an atopic and normal population. J All Clin Imm 53:200, 1974.
32. McDonald, J. R. , et al.: Aspirin intolerance in asthma. J All Clin Imm 50:198, 1972.
33. Rachelefsky, G. S. , et al.: Aspirin intolerance in chronic childhood asthma: detected by oral challenge. Ped 56:443, 1975.
34. Vatanasuk, M. , et al.: Serum IgE and passive transfer in aspirin intolerance. J All 47:109, 1971.
35. De Weck, A. L.: Immunological effects of aspirin anhydride, a contaminant of commercial acetylsalicylic acid preparations. Int Arch All 41:393, 1971.
36. Gerber, J. G. , Payne, N. A. , Oelz, O. , Nies, A. S. , and Oates, J. A.: Tartrazine and the prostaglandin system. J All Clin Immunol 63:289, 1979.
37. Delaney, J. C.: The diagnosis of aspirin idiosyncrasy by analgesic challenge. Clin All 6:177, 1976.
38. Ochsner, S. F. , and Calonje, M. A.: Reactions to intravenous iodides in urography. So Med J 64:907, 1971.
39. Witter, D. M. , et al.: Acute reactions to urographic contrast medium. Am J Roentgenol Rad Ther 119:832, 1973.
40. Zweiman, B. , and Hildreth, E. A.: An approach to the performance of contrast studies in contrast material-reactive persons. Ann Int Med 83:159, 1975.
41. Fischer, H. W. , and Doust, V. L.: An evaluation of pretesting in the problem of serious and fatal reactions to excretory urography. Rad 103:497, 1972.
42. Arroyave, C. M. , Schatz, M. , and Simon, R. A.: Activation of the complement system by radiographic contrast media. Studies in vivo and in vitro. J All Clin Immunol 63:276, 1979.
43. Lasser, E. C. , et al.: Histamine release by contrast media. Rad 100:683, 1971.

44. Schatz, M., et al.: The administration of radiographic contrast media to patients with a history of a previous reaction. J All Clin Imm 55:358, 1975.

45. Patterson, R., and Schatz, M.: Administration of radiographic contrast medium. J All Clin Imm 56:328, 1975.

46. Aldrete, J. A., and Johnson, D. A.: Evaluation of intracutaneous testing for investigation of allergy to local anesthetic agents. Anesth & Analg 49:173, 1970.

47. Tuft, L.: Allergic reactions following immunization procedures. Arch Environ Health 13:91, 1966.

48. Kamin, P. D., et al.: Use of live, attenuated measles virus vaccine in children allergic to egg protein. JAMA 193, 1125, 1965.

49. Rosh, M. S., and Shinefield, H. R.: Penicillin antibodies in children. Ped 42:342, 1968.

50. Adkinson, N. F., et al.: Routine use of penicillin skin testing on an inpatient service. NEJM 285:22, 1971.

51. Stember, R. H., and Levine, B. B.: Frequency of skin reactivity to penicillin haptens in patients without histories of penicillin allergy. J All Clin Imm 49:96, 1972.

52. Miller, F. F.: History of drug sensitivity in atopic persons. J All 40:46, 1967.

53. Stember, R. H., and Levine, B. B.: Prevalence of allergic diseases, penicillin hypersensitivity, and aeroallergen hypersensitivity in various populations. J All Clin Imm 51: 100, 1973.

54. Sparks, R. P.: Fatal anaphylaxis due to oral penicillin. Am J Clin Path 56:407, 1971.

55. Wicher, K., et al.: Allergic reaction to penicillin present in milk. JAMA 208:143, 1969.

56. Budd, M. A., et al.: Evaluation of intradermal skin tests in penicillin hypersensitivity. JAMA 190:203, 1964.

The first recorded death from an insect sting occurred in
2641 BC, when King Menes of Egypt was stung by a hornet during a visit to Britain.[1] Presumably even earlier deaths of less
prestigous subjects have remained unrecorded. Fatal reactions
continue to follow insect stings, almost always due to anaphylactic reactions following the stings of insects of the order Hymenoptera.[2] At least 30 deaths from Hymenoptera are reported
each year in the United States,[3,4] and it is likely that many
more deaths from this cause are incorrectly ascribed to cardiovascular disease.

There may be some increase in the frequency of insect
sting hypersensitivity among atopic subjects,[5] and fatal reactions may be more frequent among such subjects,[3] but most insect sting allergy apparently occurs in patients with no history
of hay fever, asthma, or other atopic diseases.[6,7]

HYMENOPTERA

The number of different species of Hymenoptera has been
estimated at more than 100,000. The four families responsible
for most insect sting hypersensitivity are the Apidae (honeybees), Bombidae (bumblebees), Vespidae (wasps, hornets, yellow jackets), and Formicidae (ants) (Figure 11.1). Identification
of the insect responsible for a sting is often impossible or
erroneous. At best it has usually been glimpsed only fleetingly.
If the insect has been killed, however, it may be submitted for
identification. Only the honeybee leaves its stinger in the victim, but it may be brushed off before its presence is recognized.
The type of insect may also be suspected from the circumstances
and surroundings in which the attack occurred. Bees usually
sting only in self defense, while yellow jackets are more ag-
gressive. Bees, wasps, yellow jackets, and hornets all feed
on nectar, but wasps feed mostly upon other insects. Wasps,
yellow jackets, and hornets also eat overripe fruit. Honeybees,
hornets, and wasps usually nest in trees or shrubs, while yel-

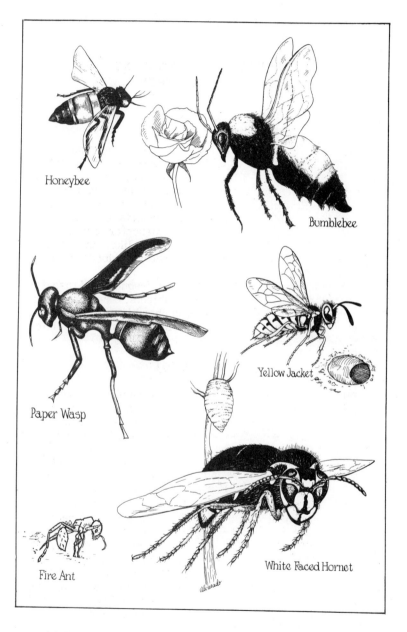

Honeybee

Bumblebee

Paper Wasp

Yellow Jacket

Fire Ant

White Faced Hornet

Fig. 11-1. Hymenoptera which most frequently cause anaphylactic reactions.

low jackets usually build their nests underground. Paper wasps often nest under the eaves of buildings or in attics. The white faced hornet can be recognized from the distinctive, large, football-shaped nest hanging from the branch of a tree. Fire ants build mounds of varying height, depending upon the consistency of the soil, and their sting is followed by the appearance of a pustule.

Honeybees, yellow jackets, and wasps have most often been identified as responsible for allergic reactions when some identification has been possible. [9]

It has been estimated that approximately 0.05 ml of venom is usually injected during an insect sting. [10] The content of bee, wasp, yellow jacket, and hornet venom varies with the insect. The major allergen of honeybee venom is reported to be phospholipase A, but hyaluronidase is also allergenic, and honeybee venom also contains melittin and smaller amounts of apamin, an acid phosphatase, and several poorly defined, higher molecular weight molecules. [11] The major allergen of vespid venoms is a protein known as antigen 5, but vespid venoms contain a phospholipase and a hyaluronidase which are also allergenic. [12] Vespid venoms also contain histamine, serotonin, kinins, and acetylcholine. Cross-reactivity between the various vespid venoms has been found, but there is no cross-reactivity between the allergenic components of vespid venoms and those of honeybee venom. [13]

It is evident from the variety of pharmacologically active agents found in hymenoptera venom that some local reaction is to be expected even without hypersensitivity, and multiple stings can elicit an anaphylactoid reaction.

CLINICAL MANIFESTATIONS

The normal reaction to a bee, wasp, hornet, or yellow jacket includes pain subsiding within a few minutes and followed by local erythema and a pruritic wheal, which subsides within a few hours. [8] Multiple stings can cause systemic symptoms of toxicity, including vomiting, diarrhea, syncope, edema, headache, fever, and convulsions. It has been estimated that 500 stings usually deliver a lethal dose of venom, [7] but survival has followed thousands of honeybee or fire ant stings. [10,14]

Local reactions consist of edema which may be limited to a small area or may involve an entire extremity and may persist for as long as several days. Wasp, yellow jacket, and hornet stings often transmit bacteria which occasionally cause a cellulitis evident a few hours or days after the stings. [8]

Signs and symptoms of systemic anaphylaxis (see Chapter VIII) may appear within seconds or minutes, and fatal anaphylaxis usually causes death within 6 hours although death may occur within a few minutes.

"Delayed reactions" in which there are no signs or symptoms within the first hour are estimated to comprise less than 3% of allergic reactions. [6] Such reactions may occur several days after the sting. These have been reported to include such diverse entities as thrombocytopenic purpura, bloody diarrhea, fatal necrotizing angiitis, nephrotic syndrome, hemorrhagic brain infarcts, peripheral neuropathies, and polyneuritis with transverse myelitis. [15] One adult who has been reported experienced nausea for a few minutes after a yellow jacket sting but 96 hours later suddenly became delirious and died. [3] Serum sickness may occur 10-14 days after the sting with fever, lymphadenopathy, headache, malaise, polyarthritis and urticaria.

FIRE ANT

A fire ant sting is normally followed by the appearance of a wheal within a few minutes, but this is followed within 24 hours by the development of a sterile pustule 2-3 mm in diameter. The pustule may persist 3-8 days, and a pink macule may be evident for several weeks. This necrotic local reaction distinguishes the venom of fire ants from that of other ants. Excessive local swelling, generalized urticaria, and systemic anaphylaxis sometimes with fatalities have been reported to have followed fire ant stings. [16] Severe allergic reactions have followed fire ant stings much more frequently than the stings of other ants.

TESTING

Substantial numbers of subjects without histories of hypersensitivity to stinging insect venom have been reported to show positive reactions to allergy skin testing with whole body extract, mostly at concentrations of 1:1000 or 1:100, and positive intradermal skin tests to venom at concentrations of $0.1 \mu g/ml$ or greater have been found in some subjects without histories of hypersensitivity to Hymenoptera venom. [17,18] More than half of patients experiencing life-threatening systemic anaphylaxis have reported having had no previous systemic reaction to Hymenoptera stings, however. [6] On the other hand, as many as 40% of patients with histories of systemic reactions and positive skin tests may experience no reaction after the next Hymenoptera sting. [19] Specific IgE antibody concentrations in serum have been found to decrease spontaneously to insignificant levels within a few weeks after systemic reactions in some patients, although anamnestic responses with sudden increases in specific IgE can occur in some of these if they are restung. [20]

Five individual Hymenoptera venoms are commercially available for diagnosis and treatment. * The freeze-dried preparations are reconstituted with diluent containing 0.03% normal human serum albumin as a stabilizer to prevent adsorption to glass, and thus to maintain antigenic potency. One manufacturer recommends storage of venom extracts reconstituted at concentrations of 1.0-100 μg/ml for not more than one month; 0.1 μg/ml, 14 days; and less than 0.1 μg /ml for only 24 hours, but other highly diluted allergen extracts stabilized with 0.03% human serum albumin have been reported to retain their potency for 6 months or more. [21]

Testing is started with scratch or prick tests with venoms at concentrations of 0.01 μg /ml. If these are negative as compared with the diluent control, intradermal testing is started with concentrations of 0.001 μg /ml. If these are negative as compared with the intradermal diluent control, this is followed by additional intradermal testing with successive ten-fold increases in concentration until a positive reaction is obtained or until the concentration of 1 μg /ml has been reached. If the initial scratch or prick test is positive intradermal testing is started at a concentration of 0.0001 μg /ml if necessary for confirmation. Use of a positive histamine control is also recommended. See Chapter XIII for further details of testing technique.

Because a refractory period may follow allergic reactions to Hymenoptera stings it may be best to defer skin testing for 2-4 weeks to minimize the possibility of false negative reactions. [22] On the other hand, if testing is deferred for more than a few months decreased reactivity may have occurred. [23]

Facilities for treatment of anaphylaxis must be immediately available while testing is being done, and testing for Hymenoptera hypersensitivity should be done on an extremity to permit application of a tourniquet if a serious reaction occurs.

Human leukocyte histamine release has been reported to correlate well with results of skin testing to Hymenoptera venom, and the correlation with histories is better than when whole body extract is used. [24,25] The cells of as many as 15% of patients with allergy to Hymenoptera venom do not release histamine even after challenge with anti-IgE, however. [26]

Use of the RAST has been limited by as many as 20% false-positive and 20% false-negative tests as compared with allergy skin testing. [27]

*Hollister Stier Laboratories, Spokane, Washington 99220; Pharmacia Diagnostics, Piscataway, New Jersey 08854

TREATMENT

Treatment of the acute anaphylactic reaction is the same as that for anaphylaxis due to other causes (see Chapter VIII). If the stinger of a honeybee has been left in the skin it should be flicked away carefully with a blade or fingernail to prevent injection of more venom by application of pressure to the venom sac. The site of the sting should be carefully cleansed. Antihistamines may be helpful for urticaria or extensive local swelling, and application of ice to the site of the sting may help limit local swelling.

Treatment with antibiotics is necessary if superimposed infection occurs, but these are not necessary for treatment of the sterile pustule that is characteristic following fire ant stings.

Subjects who have had systemic symptoms, increasingly severe reactions to successive stings, or very large local reactions should wear medals or emblems identifying their hypersensitivity* and should observe precautions to minimize the likelihood of reexposure to the offending insect (Table 11.1). They should also be supplied with 1:1000 aqueous epinephrine for administration by a parent or for self-administration in an emergency and instructed in its use. An antihistamine and ephedrine can also be prescribed for emergency use but these do not replace the use of epinephrine. Such patients should be advised to go immediately to the nearest medical facility for further observation after instituting these emergency measures.

IMMUNOTHERAPY

Immunotherapy is indicated for patients who have had systemic reactions and positive skin tests to venom. Those with negative skin tests may have lost their sensitivity spontaneously and should not receive immunotherapy, although careful follow-up is indicated. Immunotherapy has also been recommended for patients with local reactions of increasing severity.[28] Large local reactions that have persisted for several days are sometimes associated with the development of sufficient hypersensitivity that subsequent stings may elicit systemic reactions.[29] Immunotherapy is reasonable when such local reactions are associated with positive skin tests to venom or positive RAST, but is not indicated with negative tests.[12,18]

*Medic Alert Foundation, P. O. Box 1009, Turlock, California 95380

TABLE 11.1   AVOIDANCE OF STINGING INSECTS

1. Always wear shoes when outdoors.
2. Do not wear dark clothing. White is least likely to attract bees.
3. Do not wear loose fitting clothing, which may entrap a bee.
4. Avoid hair tonics, hair spray, deodorants, perfumes, and scented soaps with strong odors which may attract bees.
5. Avoid insect feeding grounds such as flower beds, clover, garbage, picnic grounds, and orchards with ripe fruit, and do not molest wasp or hornet nests, yellow jacket burrows, or ant hills. Wasp or hornet nests or bee hives near the patient's home should be destroyed by a professional exterminator. If it is necessary to work near flowers or fruit trees wear a hat and gloves.
6. Do not leave food or garbage uncovered. It may attract ants or wasps.
7. Avoid rapid movements when near stinging insects unless being pursued.
8. Keep automobile windows closed.
9. Keep windows and doors at patient's home closed unless protected with screens.
10. Keep a fast-acting insecticide aerosol in the kitchen, glove compartment of the automobile, and someplace readily accessible from outdoors such as the garage (out of reach of small children).

Comparison of the results of immunotherapy with venom, whole body extract, and placebo has disclosed significant benefit from treatment with venom.[19] After treatment for 6-10 weeks, using a schedule which permitted attainment of maintenance dosage, participants were challenged with Hymenoptera stings. Reactions followed in 7 of the 11 treated with whole body extract, 7 of the 12 treated with placebo, and only 1 of the 18 treated with venom. After the patient for whom venom treatment had not afforded protection had been treated for 10 more weeks, he tolerated another sting without any systemic reaction. Significant increases in specific IgG antibody were found only in the patients who had received venom, and this may have been largely responsible for its protective effect. Passive administration of specific IgG antibody has been reported effective in affording protection against challenge with honeybee venom.[30] These data indicate that treatment with venom is more beneficial than treatment with whole body extract, and much of the benefit ascribed to treatment with whole body extract has probably been due to spontaneous loss of hypersensitivity or the effects of pharmacological agents administered when patients have been restung.

Treatment with venom has afforded protection to 95% of 300 patients, and reactions in the others when restung have been less severe than the reactions before treatment.[31]

The recommended treatment schedule is indicated in Table 11.2. On the days for which more than one injection is scheduled, these are administered at 30-minute intervals unless a systemic reaction or an excessive local reaction has occurred. If a systemic reaction or an excessively large local reaction with a wheal more than 10 cm in diameter occurs, no further doses are given on that day and the total dose administered at the time of the next visit is reduced to half the total dose that elicited the reaction. If a large local reaction with a wheal more than 5 cm in diameter occurs, no further doses are given on that day, and the same dose is repeated on subsequent visits until tolerated. Delayed reactions at 24-48 hours are considered to necessitate interruption in the usual schedule only if more than 10 cm in diameter. The same dose is then repeated at subsequent visits until tolerated.

The incidence of systemic reactions to venom therapy with similar treatment schedules has been reported to be 2% children, but as many as 16% adults have had systemic reactions.[32] More traditional treatment schedules, consisting of weekly administration of successively doubled doses, have also been used successfully but are reported not to decrease the frequency of reactions.[33,34]

Specific IgE concentrations in the serum usually increase during the first month of treatment and then decline, but responses are variable. After 12 months of treatment these concentrations may be either higher or lower than before treatment.[12,33]

Currently available data suggest that venom immunotherapy may be necessary indefinitely for most patients, but it has been discontinued in some after specific IgE had become undetectable in their serum, and some of these have subsequently tolerated stings without reactions.[12,18] Prospective study of beekeepers and their families has not suggested the likelihood of any substantial complications from prolonged therapy with honeybee venom.[35]

Experience with immunotherapy for fire ant hypersensitivity is much more limited than that for other Hymenoptera. Of the few reported to have been restung following immunotherapy only 1 has been reported to have had a systemic reaction.[16,36] Traditional treatment schedules have been used for treatment of fire ant hypersensitivity (see Table 14.3).

TABLE 11.2   TREATMENT SCHEDULE
             FOR HYMENOPTERA VENOM

DAY	CONCENTRATION (μg/ml)	VOLUME (ml)	VENOM INJECTED (For Single Venom) (μg protein)
1	0.01	0.1	0.001
	0.1	0.1	0.01
	1.0	0.1	0.1
8	1.0	0.1	0.1
	1.0	0.5	0.5
	10	0.1	1.0
15	10	0.1	1
	10	0.5	5
	10	1.0	10
22	100	0.1	10
	100	0.2	20
29	100	0.2	20
	100	0.3	30
36	100	0.3	30
	100	0.3	30
43	100	0.4	40
	100	0.4	40
50	100	0.5	50
	100	0.5	50
57	100	1.0	100
64	100	1.0	100
78	100	1.0	100
99	100	1.0	100
Monthly	100	1.0	100

Modification necessary if systemic or excessive local reactions
  occur.
If systemic symptoms follow a sting in a patient receiving
  maintenance therapy, increase maintenance dosage by incre-
  ments of not more than 50 μg to a new maintenance dose of
  200 μg.

REFERENCES

1. Waddell, L. A.: Egyptian civilization: Its Sumerian origin & Real Chronology and Sumerian Origin of Egyptian Hieroglyphs. Luzac & Co., London, 1930.
2. Parrish, H. M.: Analysis of 460 fatalities from venomous animals in the United States. Am J Med Sci 245:129, 1963.
3. Barnard, J. H.: Allergic and pathologic findings in fifty insect-sting fatalities. J All 40:107, 1967.
4. Barnard, J. H.: Studies of 400 Hymenoptera sting deaths in the United States. J All Clin Imm 52:259, 1973.
5. Schwartz, H. J., and Kahn, B.: Hymenoptera sensitivity. J All 45:87, 1970.
6. Insect Allergy Committee, American Academy of Allergy: Insect-sting allergy. JAMA 193:115, 1965.
7. Settipane, G. A., et al.: Frequency of Hymenoptera allergy in an atopic and normal population. J All Clin Imm 50:146, 1972.
8. Frazier, C. A.: Insect Allergy. Warren H. Green, Inc., St. Louis, 1969.
9. Barr, S. E.: Allergy to insect stings: Clinical and laboratory studies. Med Ann D C 36:395, 1967.
10. Murray, J. A.: A case of multiple bee stings. Central Africa J Med 10:249, 1964.
11. Sobotka, A. K., Franklin, R. M., Adkinson, N. F., Jr., Valentine, M., Baer, H., and Lichtenstein, L. M.: Allergy to insect stings. II. Phospholipase A: The major allergen in honeybee venom. J All Clin Immunol 57:29, 1976.
12. Lichtenstein, L. M., Valentine, M. D., and Sobotka, A. K.: Insect Allergy: The state of the art. J All Clin Immunol 64:5, 1979.
13. King, T. P., Sobotka, A. K., Alagon, A., Kochoumian, L., and Lichtenstein, L. M.: Protein allergens of white-faced hornet, yellow hornet and yellow-jacket venoms. Biochem 17:5165, 1978.
14. Smith, J. D., and Smith, E. B.: Multiple fire ant stings. A complication of alcoholism. Arch Derm 103:438, 1971.
15. Barr, S. E.: Allergy to Hymenoptera stings - review of the world literature: 1953-1970. Ann All 29:49, 1971.
16. Rhoades, R. B., et al.: Hypersensitivity to the imported fire ant. J All Clin Imm 56:84, 1975.
17. Schwartz, H. J.: Skin sensitivity in insect allergy. JAMA 194:703, 1965.
18. Reisman, R. E.: Stinging insect allergy. J All Clin Immunol 64:3, 1979.

19. Hunt, K. J., Valentine, M. D., Sobotka, A. K., Benton, A. W., Amodio, F. J., and Lichtenstein, L. M.: A controlled trial of immunotherapy in insect hypersensitivity. New Eng J Med 299:157, 1978.
20. Reisman, R. E., Arbesman, C. E., and Lazell, M.: Observations on the aetiology and natural history of stinging insect sensitivity: application of measurements of venom-specific IgE. Clin All 9:303, 1979.
21. Norman, P. S., and Marsh, D. G.: Human serum albumin and Tween 80 as stabilizers of allergen solutions. J All Clin Immunol 62:314, 1978.
22. Mueller, H. L.: Serial intracutaneous testing for bee and wasp sensitivity. J All 30:123, 1959.
23. Brown, H., and Bernton, H. S.: Studies on the Hymenoptera: VI Evolution of the skin test in Hymenoptera-sensitive patients. J All 41:92, 1968.
24. Hunt, K. J., Valentine, M. D., Sobotka, A. K., and Lichtenstein, L. M.: Diagnosis of allergy to stinging insects by skin testing with Hymenoptera venoms. Ann Int Med 85: 56, 1976.
25. Sobotka, A. K., et al.: Allergy to insect stings. I. Diagnosis of IgE-mediated Hymenoptera sensitivity by venom-induced histamine release. J All Clin Imm 53:170, 1974.
26. Conroy, M. C., Adkinson, N. F., Jr., Sobotka, A. K., and Lichtenstein, L. M.: "Releasability" of histamine from human basophils, Fed Proc 36:1216, 1977.
27. Sobotka, A. K., Adkinson, N. F., Jr., Valentine, M. D., and Lichtenstein, L. M.: Allergy to insect stings IV. Diagnosis by radioallergosorbent test (RAST). J Immunol 121: 2477, 1978.
28. Mueller, H. L.: "Insect Allergy", in Kelley, V. C. (ed): Practice of Pediatrics, Harper & Row, Hagerstown, Md., 1974, Chapter 68.
29. Green, A. W., Reisman, R. E., and Arbesman, C. E.: Clinical and immunologic studies of patients with large local reactions following insect stings. J All Clin Immunol 63:135, 1979.
30. Lessof, M. H., Sobotka, A. K., and Lichtenstein, L. M.: Effects of passive antibody in bee venom anaphylaxis. Johns Hopkins Med J 142:1, 1978.
31. Valentine, M. D., Sobotka, A. K., and Lichenstein, L. M.: Diagnosis and treatment of venom allergy: Overview. J All Clin Immunol 63:180, 1979.
32. Chipps, B. E., Valentine, M. D., Sobotka, A. K., Schuberth, K. C., and Lichenstein, L. M.: Hymenoptera hypersensitivity in children. J All Clin Immunol 63:179, 1979.

33. Reisman, R. E., Arbesman, C. E., and Lazell, M.: Clinical and immunological studies of venom immunotherapy. Clin All 9:167, 1979.
34. Golden, D., Valentine, M. D., Sobotka, A. K., and Lichtenstein, L. M.: Regimens of Hymenoptera venom immunotherapy. J All Clin Immunol 63:180, 1979.
35. Yunginger, J. W., Jones, R. T., Leiferman, K. M., Paull, B. R., Welsh, P. W., and Gleich, G. J.: Immunological and biochemical studies in beekeepers and their family members. J All Clin Immunol 61:93, 1978.
36. Triplett, R. F.: Sensitivity to the imported fire ant: Successful treatment with immunotherapy. So Med J 66: 477, 1973.

CHAPTER XII | INHALANT ALLERGENS

Inhalant allergens include pollens, molds, house dust, animal danders, dust and debris from portions of the bodies of arthropods and other environmental allergens that can be inhaled.

The importance of a particular substance as an allergen is dependent upon its capacity for acting as an antigen in the induction of formation of reaginic antibody and subsequent interaction with antibody and upon its availability in the environment in sufficient concentrations.

POLLEN

The plants responsible for atopic respiratory disease are those that are widely distributed and that produce an abundance of antigenic, airborne pollen.

Insect-pollinated plants usually produce small amounts of large, sticky pollen, which is not discharged into the air, and thus is a potential hazard only for someone in very close contact with the plant itself. Such plants have attractive, fragrant flowers which attract the insects that carry their pollen to other plants.

Wind-pollinated plants on the other hand usually have very inconspicuous flowers that discharge large amounts of light pollen into the air where it may be carried for miles by the wind. Thus, the plants responsible for pollinosis are wind-pollinated plants. Although pine, spruce, and fir produce an abundance of pollen that is carried great distances by the wind, these species rarely cause allergy, possibly because the waxy coating on the pollen prevents contact with the respiratory mucosa. [1]

The pollen grains of some insect-pollinated plants are not sticky. Limited dispersal of the pollen by wind can occur in those with open flowers, and there is some evidence of consequent sensitization to Acacia, Brassica, ligustrum, olive, Schinus (pepper tree), and others, especially in the Southern United States. [2]

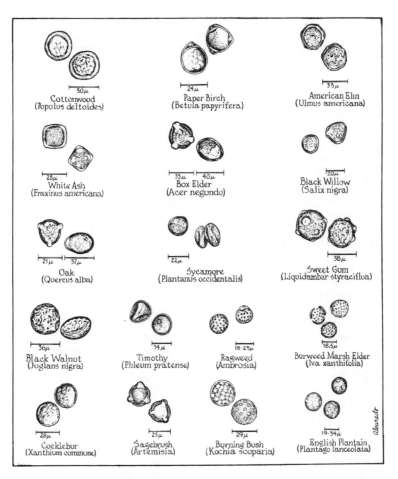

Fig. 12-1. Morphology and size of various pollen grains. Evaporation may cause some loss of size after discharge into the air. Indicated sizes are for expanded grains. [1]

Most pollen grains vary in diameter from 10-60 μ. Their size and morphology generally permit differentiation from the pollen of other plants although pollen grains of some related species may be very similar in appearance (Fig. 12.1).

Most trees pollinate for a few weeks during the spring, while the grasses pollinate for 2-10 months beginning in winter and early spring, depending upon location in the United States (Table 12.1). Most weeds pollinate between July and October

TABLE 12.1   IMPORTANT ALLERGENIC PLANTS
IN THE UNITED STATES[3,4]

REGION 1

Trees (pollinate March-May in
South and April-May in North):
Ash (Fraxinus)
Birch (Betula)
Elm (Ulmus)
Hickory (Carya)
Maple, Box Elder (Acer)
Oak (Quercus)
Poplar, Cottonwood (Populus)
Sycamore (Platanus)

Grasses (pollinate April-
June):
Bermuda (Cynodon)
Blue grass (Poa)
Meadow fescue (Festuca)
Orchard (Dactylis)
Redtop (Agrostis)
Timothy (Phleum)

Weeds (pollinate August-
October):
Cocklebur (Xanthium)
Lambs quarters (Chenopodium)
Plantain (Plantago)
Ragweed (Ambrosia)
Sorrel (Rumex)

REGION 2

Trees (pollinate February-
May):
Ash (Fraxinus)
Birch (Betula)
Cedar (Juniperus)
Elm (Ulmus)
Hackberry (Celtis)
Maple, Box elder (Acer)
Mulberry (Morus)
Oak (Quercus)

Pecan, Hickory (Carya)
Poplar, Cottonwood (Populus)
Walnut (Juglans)

Grasses (pollinate March-
July, Bermuda longer):
Bermuda (Cynodon)
Blue grass (Poa)
Johnson (Sorghum)
Orchard (Dactylis)
Redtop (Agrostis)
Rye (Lolium)
Timothy (Phleum)
Vernal (Anthoxanthum)

Weeds (pollinate August to
frost)
Cocklebur (Xanthium)
Kochia (Kochia)
Lambs quarters
(Chenopodium)
Pigweed (Amaranthus)
Plantain (Plantago)
Ragweed (Ambrosia)
Sorrel (Rumex)

REGION 3

Trees (pollinate Frbruary-
April):
Ash (Fraxinus)
Birch (Betula)
Cottonwood, Poplar (Populus)
Elm (Ulmus)
Hackberry (Celtis)
Maple (Acer)
Mesquite (Prosopis)
Red cedar (Juniperus)
Mulberry (Morus)
Oak (Quercus)
Pecan, Hickory (Carya)
Walnut (Juglans)

Table 12.1 (cont'd.)

Grasses (pollinate February-
July, Bermuda until
December):
Bermuda (Cynodon)
Blue grass (Poa)
Johnson (Sorghum)
Meadow fescue (Festuca)
Orchard (Dactylis)
Redtop (Agrostis)
Rye (Lolium)
Sweet vernal (Anthoxanthum)
Timothy (Phleum)

Weeds (pollinate August-
October)
Cocklebur (Xanthium)
Lambs quarters (Chenopodium)
Plantain (Plantago)
Ragweed (Ambrosia)
Sagewort (Artemisia)
Sorrel (Rumex)

REGION 4

Trees (pollinate February-
April):
Cottonwood, Poplar
(Populus)
Elm (Ulmus)
Maple, Box elder (Acer)
Mesquite (Prosopis)
Mountain cedar (Juniperus)
Oak (Quercus)
Palm (Palmaceae)
Pecan, Hickory (Carya)
Privet (Ligustrum)
Sycamore (Platanus)

Grasses (pollinate January-
June, Bermuda until
December):
Bahia (Paspalum)
Bermuda (Cynodon)
Blue grass (Poa)
Canary (Phalaris)

Johnson (Sorghum)
Redtop (Agrostis)
Rye (Lolium)
Salt grass (Distichlis)

Weeds (pollinate April-
December):
Lambs quarters (Chenopodium)
Marsh elder (Iva)
Pigweed (Amaranthus)
Ragweed (Ambrosia)
Sagebrush (Artemisia)
Sorrel (Rumex)

REGION 5

Trees (pollinate March-April):
Ash (Fraxinus)
Birch (Betula)
Elm (Ulmus)
Hickory, Pecan (Carya)
Maple, Box elder (Acer)
Oak (Quercus)
Poplar, Cottonwood (Populus)
Sycamore (Platanus)
Walnut (Juglans)

Grasses (pollinate March-
June):
Bermuda (Cynodon)
Blue grass (Poa)
Fescue (Festuca)
Johnson (Sorghum)
Orchard (Dactylis)
Redtop (Agrostis)
Rye (Lolium)
Timothy (Phleum)

Weeds (pollinate July-
October):
Cocklebur (Xanthium)
Lambs quarters
(Chenopodium)
Pigweed (Amaranthus)
Plantain (Plantago)

Table 12.1 (cont'd.)

Ragweed (Ambrosia)
Sagebrush (Artemisia)
Sorrel (Rumex)
Water hemp (Acnida)

REGION 6

Trees (pollinate February-
    April):
Ash (Fraxinus)
Cedar (Juniperus)
Cottonwood, Poplar (Populus)
Elm (Ulmus)
Hackberry (Celtis)
Maple, Box elder (Acer)
Mulberry (Morus)
Oak (Quercus)
Pecan, Hickory (Carya)
Sweetgum (Liquidambar)
Sycamore (Platanus)
Walnut (Juglans)
Willow (Salix)

Grasses (pollinate February-
    June, Bermuda until
    December):
Bermuda (Cynodon)
Blue grass (Poa)
Johnson (Sorghum)
Orchard (Dactylis)
Redtop (Agrostis)
Rye (Lolium)
Timothy (Phleum)

Weeds (pollinate July-
    November):
Cocklebur (Xanthium)
Lambs quarters (Chenopodium)
Marsh elder (Iva)
Pigweed (Amaranthus)
Plantain (Plantago)
Ragweed (Ambrosia)
Sagebrush (Artemisia)
Sorrel (Rumex)

REGION 7

Trees (pollinate April-June):
Alder (Alnus)
Ash (Fraxinus)
Birch (Betula)
Cottonwood, Poplar (Populus)
Elm (Ulmus)
Hickory, Pecan (Carya)
Maple, Box elder (Acer)
Oak (Quercus)
Sycamore (Platanus)
Walnut (Juglans

Grasses (pollinate April-
    June):
Blue grass (Poa)
Brome (Bromus)
Canary (Phalaris)
Fescue (Festuca)
Koelers (Koeleria)
Orchard (Dactylis)
Redtop (Agrostis)
Rye (Lolium)
Timothy (Phleum)

Weeds (pollinate July-frost):
Cocklebur (Xanthium)
Lambs quarters (Chenopodium)
Marsh elder (Iva)
Pigweed (Amaranthus)
Plantain (Plantago)
Ragweed (Ambrosia)
Russian thistle (Salsola)
Sagebrush (Artemisia)
Sorrel (Rumex)

REGION 8

Trees (pollinate March-
    May):
Ash (Fraxinus)
Birch (Betula)
Elm (Ulmus)

Table 12.1 (cont'd.)

Hickory, Pecan (Carya)
Maple, Box elder (Acer)
Mulberry (Morus)
Oak (Quercus)
Poplar, Cottonwood (Populus)
Sycamore (Platanus)
Walnut (Juglans)

Grasses (pollinate March-
    June):
Bermuda (Cynodon)
Blue grass (Poa)
Johnson (Sorghum)
Orchard (Dactylis)
Redtop (Agrostis)
Rye (Lolium)
Timothy (Phleum)

Weeds (pollinate July-October)
Kochia (Kochia)
Lambs quarters
    (Chenopodium)
Marsh elder (Iva)
Pigweed (Amaranthus)
Plantain (Plantago)
Ragweed (Ambrosia)
Russian thistle (Salsola)
Sagebrush (Artemisia)
Sorrel (Rumex)
Western water hemp (Acnida)

REGION 9

Trees (pollinate March-
    April):
Alder (Alnus)
Ash (Fraxinus)
Birch (Betula)
Elm (Ulmus)
Hazelnut (Carylus)
Hickory (Carya)
Maple, Box elder (Acer)
Oak (Quercus)
Poplar, Aspen, Cottonwood
    (Populus)
Walnut (Juglans)

Grasses (pollinate March-
    June):
Bermuda (Cynodon)
Blue grass (Poa)
Brome (Bromus)
Fescue (Festuca)
Orchard (Dactylis)
Quack (Agropyron)
Redtop (Agrostis)
Rye (Lolium)
Timothy (Phleum)

Weeds (pollinate July-October):
Cocklebur (Xanthium)
Kochia (Kochia)
Lambs quarters (Chenopodium)
Marsh elder (Iva)
Pigweed (Amaranthus)
Ragweed (Ambrosia,
    Franseria)
Russian thistle (Salsola)
Sagebrush (Artemisia)
Sorrel (Rumex)
Western water hemp (Acnida)

REGION 10

Trees (pollinate February-
    May, Mt. cedar in December-
    March):
Ash (Fraxinus)
Cottonwood (Populus)
Elm (Ulmus)
Mountain cedar, Juniper
    (Juniperus)
Maple, Box elder (Acer)
Mesquite (Prosopis)
Mulberry (Morus)
Oak (Quercus)

Grasses (pollinate March-
    November):
Bermuda (Cynodon)
Blue grass (Poa)
Fescue (Festuca)

Table 12.1 (cont'd.)

Johnson (Sorghum)
Orchard (Dactylis)
Redtop (Agrostis)
Rye (Lolium)
Timothy (Phleum)
Western wheat (Agropyron)

Weeds (pollinate July-
    October):
Cocklebur (Xanthium)
Kochia (Kochia)
Lambs quarters
    (Chenopodium)
Marsh elder (Iva)
Pigweed (Amaranthus)
Ragweed (Ambrosia)
Russian thistle (Salsola)
Sagebrush (Artemisia)
Scale (Atriplex)
Sorrel (Rumex)
Western water hemp (Acnida)

REGION 11

Trees (pollinate February-
    June, Juniper in
    December-March:
Alder (Alnus)
Ash (Fraxinus)
Birch (Betula)
Cottonwood, Poplar (Populus)
Elm (Ulmus)
Maple, Box elder (Acer)
Mountain cedar, Juniper
    (Juniperus)
Oak (Quercus)

Grasses (pollinate March-
    September):
Bermuda (Cynodon)
Blue grass (Poa)
Brome (Bromus)
Fescue (Festuca)
Koelers (Koelaria)
Orchard (Dactylis)

Redtop (Agrostis)
Rye (Lolium)
Timothy (Phleum)
Wheatgrass (Agropyron)

Weeds (pollinate July-frost
    or November):
Cocklebur (Xanthium)
Lambs quarters
    (Chenopodium)
Marsh elder (Iva)
Pigweed (Amaranthus)
Plantain (Plantago)
Ragweed (Ambrosia,
    Franseria)
Russian thistle (Salsola)
Sagebrush (Artemisia)
Scale (Atriplex)
Sugar beet (Beta)
Summer cypress (Kochia)
Western water hemp (Acnida)

REGION 12

Trees (pollinate December-
    May):
Ash (Fraxinus)
Cottonwood, Poplar (Populus)
Cypress (Cupressus)
Elm (Ulmus)
Mountain cedar (Juniperus)
Olive (Olea)
Willow (Salix)

Grasses (pollinate February-
    December):
Bermuda (Cynodon)
Blue grass (Poa)
Brome (Bromus)
Canary (Phalaris)
Rye (Lolium)
Salt grass (Distichlis)

Weeds (pollinate May-
    November):

Table 12.1 (cont'd.)

Alkaliblite (Suaeda)
Careless weed (Amaranthus)
Dicoria (Dicoria)
Hymenoclea (Hymenoclea)
Iodine bush (Allenrolfea)
Lambs quarters (Chenopodium)
Ragweed (Ambrosia,
    Franseria)
Sagebrush (Artemisia)
Scale (Atriplex)

Pigweed (Amaranthus)
Plantain (Plantago)
Ragweed (Ambrosia)
Russian thistle (Salsola)
Sagebrush (Artemisia)
Scale (Atriplex)
Sorrel (Rumex)

REGION 13

Trees (pollinate January-June;
    elm in September):
Ash (Fraxinus)
Cottonwood, Poplar (Populus)
Cypress (Cupressus)
Elm (Ulmus)
Maple, Box elder (Acer)
Mulberry (Morus)
Oak (Quercus)
Olive (Olea)
Sycamore (Platanus)
Walnut (Juglans)

Grasses (pollinate January-
    June, Bermuda until
    November):
Bermuda (Cynodon)
Blue grass (Poa)
Brome (Bromus)
Fescue (Festuca)
Johnson (Sorghum)
Oat (Avena)
Orchard (Dactylis)
Rye (Lolium)
Salt grass (Distichlis)

Weeds (pollinate July-
    November, Franseria May-
    November):
Cocklebur (Xanthium)
Lambs quarters
    (Chenopodium)

REGION 14

Trees (pollinate February-
    May):
Alder (Alnus)
Ash (Fraxinus)
Birch (Betula)
Cottonwood, Poplar (Populus)
Cypress (Cupressus)
Elm (Ulmus)
Maple, Box elder (Acer)
Oak (Quercus)
Olive (Olea)
Pecan (Carya)
Sycamore (Platanus)
Walnut (Juglans)

Grasses (pollinate February-
    June, Bermuda until
    November):
Bermuda (Cynodon)
Blue grass (Poa)
Brome (Bromus)
Canary (Phalaris)
Fescue (Festuca)
Johnson (Sorghum)
Oat (Avena)
Orchard (Dactylis)
Redtop (Agrostis)
Rye (Lolium)
Salt grass (Atriplex)
Timothy (Phleum)

Weeds (pollinate May-
    November):
Cocklebur (Xanthium)
Lambs quarters (Chenopodium)

Table 12.1 (cont'd.)

Pigweed (Amaranthus)
Plantain (Plantago)
Ragweed (Ambrosia,
    Franseria)
Russian thistle (Salsola)
Sagebrush (Artemisia)
Scale (Atriplex)
Sorrel (Rumex)
Sugar beet (Betula)

REGION 15

Trees (pollinate March-
    April):
Alder (Alnus)
Ash (Fraxinus)
Birch (Betula)
Cottonwood, Poplar
    (Populus)
Elm (Ulmus)
Juniper (Juniperus)
Maple, Box elder (Acer)
Olive (Olea)
Sycamore (Platanus)

Grasses (pollinate April-
    July, Bermuda until
    October):
Bermuda (Cynodon)
Blue grass (Poa)
Brome (Bromus)
Fescue (Festuca)
Orchard (Dactylis)
Quack, Western wheatgrass
    (Agropyron)
Redtop (Agrostis)
Rye (Lolium)
Salt grass (Distichlis)
Timothy (Phleum)

Weeds (pollinate July-
    October):
Cocklebur (Xanthium)
Iodine bush (Allenrolfea)

Kochia (Kochia)
Lambs quarters
    (Chenopodium)
Marsh elder (Iva)
Pigweed (Amaranthus)
Plantain (Plantago)
Rabbit bush (Chrysothamnus)
Ragweed (Ambrosia,
    Franseria)
Russian thistle (Salsola)
Sagebrush (Artemisia)
Scale (Atriplex)
Sorrel (Rumex)

REGION 16

Trees (pollinate April-May):
Alder (Alnus)
Aspen, Cottonwood, Poplar
    (Populus)
Birch (Betula)
Maple, Box elder (Acer)
Oak (Quercus)
Pine (Pinus)
Walnut (Juglans)
Willow (Salix)

Grasses (pollinate April-
    June):
Blue grass (Poa)
Brome (Bromus)
Koelers (Koeleria)
Orchard (Dactylis)
Quack, Western wheatgrass
    (Agropyron)
Redtop (Agrostis)
Rye (Lolium)
Timothy (Phleum)
Velvet (Holcus)
Vernal (Anthoxanthum)

Weeds (pollinate July-October):
Lambs quarters
    (Chenopodium)

Table 12.1 (cont'd.)

Marsh elder (Iva)
Pigweed (Amaranthus)
Plantain (Plantago)
Ragweed (Ambrosia,
    Franseria)
Russian thistle (Salsola)
Sagebrush (Artemisia)
Scale (Atriplex)
Sorrel (Rumex)

REGION 17

Trees (pollinate January-
    June):
Acacia (Acacia)
Alder (Alnus)
Ash (Fraxinus)
Birch (Betula)
Cottonwood, Aspen
    (Populus)
Elm (Ulmus)
Hazelnut (Carylus)
Maple, Box elder (Acer)
Oak (Quercus)
Olive (Olea)
Redwood (Sequoia)
Walnut (Juglans)
Willow (Salix)

Grasses (pollinate February-
    July):
Bermuda (Cynodon)
Blue grass (Poa)
Brome (Bromus)
Canary (Phalaris)
Fescue (Festuca)
Oat (Avena)
Orchard (Dactylis)
Redtop, Bent (Agrostis)
Rye (Lolium)
Salt grass (Distichlis)
Sudan (Andropogon)
Timothy (Phleum)
Velvet (Holcus)
Vernal (Anthoxanthum)

Weeds (pollinate June-
    October):
Cocklebur (Xanthium)
Lambs quarters (Chenopodium)
Pigweed (Amaranthus)
Plantain (Plantago)
Ragweed (Ambrosia,
    Franseria)
Russian thistle (Salsola)
Sagebrush (Artemisia)
Scale (Atriplex)
Sorrel (Rumex)

ALASKA (SOUTHWESTERN)

Trees (pollinate March-May):
Alder (Alnus)
Ash (Fraxinus)
Birch (Betula)
Cottonwood (Populus)
Maple, Box elder (Acer)
Oak (Quercus)
Willow (Salix)

Grasses (pollinate May-
    August):
Blue grass (Poa)
Brome (Bromus)
Fescue (Festuca)
Oat (Avena)
Orchard (Dactylis)
Quack (Agropyron)
Redtop (Agrostis)
Rye (Lolium)
Sweet vernal (Anthoxanthum)
Timothy (Phleum)
Velvet (Holcus)

Weeds (pollinate June-
    October):
Bitter & Yellow dock, Red
    Sorrel (Rumex)
English plantain (Plantago)
Lambs quarters
    (Chenopodium)

Table 12.1 (cont'd.)

Pickleweed (Allenrolfea)	Grasses (pollinate January-December):
Pigweed (Amaranthus)	Bermuda (Cynodon)
Sagebrush, Mugwort (Artemisia)	Blue grass (Poa)
	Johnson (Sorghum)
HAWAII	Redtop (Agrostis)
	Sugar cane (Saccharum) (pollinates November-January)
Trees (pollinate January-December):	
Algarroba, mesquite (Prosopis) (pollinates February-June)	Weeds (pollinate January-December):
Cadena de amor (Antigonon)	Cocklebur (Xanthium)
Eucalyptus (Eucalyptus)	False ragweed (Franseria)
Hibiscus (Hibiscus)	Lambs quarters (Chenopodium)
Mango (Mangifera)	Mugwort (Artemisia)
Mulberry (Morus)	Plantain (Plantago)
Olive (Olea)	Saltbush (Atriplex)
Palm (Palmaceae)	Sorrel, yellow dock (Rumex)

or November, their pollination usually ending at the time of the first frost. The specific time and duration of pollination varies somewhat from year to year depending upon variations in rainfall and temperature. Excessive rainfall before a pollen season favors plant growth, while sunshine and absence of rain during a pollen season stimulate release of pollen. High winds during a pollen season also increase its concentration in the air. Rainfall on the other hand can inhibit release of pollen and reduce its concentration in the atmosphere. Ragweed pollen and some other pollens are usually released in greatest abundance in the early morning (4:00-8:00 A.M.), but this can also vary with the species of plant producing the pollen. The continental United States has been divided into 17 botanical regions for convenience in describing the allergenic plants of importance in each area (Figure 12.2, see Table 12.1).[3]

Specific antigens have not been identified for most pollens, but antigen E, a protein with molecular weight 37,800, has been found to be the most potent allergen in ragweed pollen.[5] Other antigenically distinct allergens that are also present include antigen K, Ra3, Ra4, Ra5, and Ra6.[6-9] Antigenic and allergenic cross reactivity have been found between antigen E and antigen K, and antigenic cross reactivity has been found between antigen E and Ra4, but Ra3 and Ra5 are antigenically unique.

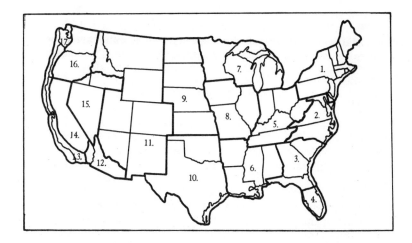

Fig. 12-2. Botanical regions of the continental United States. Within each region similar plants are of allergenic significance.

Two of three groups of antigenic proteins have been found to account for much of the allergenic activity of rye grass pollen.[10] These antigens, Group I, Group II, and Group III, are also found in fescue, orchard, and velvet grass pollens.[11] Sweet vernal pollen was found to have two Group I fractions antigenically similar to those of these other pollens, but Group I components of timothy pollen were less similar antigenically. Group II components have also been found in sweet vernal and timothy pollen extracts, and Group III components have been found in all of these pollens. None of these antigens has been found in bermuda grass pollen, however.[11]

Skin reactivity to extracts of rye, fescue, sweet vernal, blue grass, velvet, and redtop has been found to correlate well with the rye Group I allergen content of the extract.[12]

Specific antigens in most tree pollens have been studied much less extensively but considerable cross reactivity has been reported among families (poplar, alder, oak) within the order Salicales.[13] Only minor cross reactivity has been found among the orders Salicales, Saindales aceraceae (maple), and Urticales ulmaceae (elm). Thus, tree pollens representing different orders are largely antigenically distinct.

Two of ten antigenic components of birch pollen have been found to be responsible for its major allergenic activity.[14] Similar, crossreacting antigens have been detected in alder, hazel, aspen, and hazelnut pollens.

Although pine, spruce, and fir pollens rarely cause atopic hypersensitivity, Christmas trees are often responsible for exacerbations of respiratory symptoms, apparently because of other pollens and mold spores clinging to the trees or because of a nonspecific response to the pine oil fragrance.

FUNGI

Fungi include molds, smuts, rusts, and yeasts. Their growth is favored by warm temperatures (70-90°F) and high humidity. Although highest total atmospheric concentrations can be anticipated in coastal areas where such conditions prevail, fungi can be carried great distances by winds and are found throughout the United States. Those of allergenic significance are found upon plant and vegetable matter and in soil as well as in the air. In homes they are often found in mattresses and furniture, wallpaper, and old books. They often grow in damp basements, bathrooms, and in crawl spaces beneath houses. Fungi of recognized importance in atopic diseases are listed in Table 12. 2. Exposure to most fungi is possible throughout the year in most of the continental United States, but greatest total concentrations of mold spores in the atmosphere occur between June and December, largely because of Alternaria and Hormodendrum which are present in greatest concentration at those times.

Alternaria is the most important of the allergenic molds because of its antigenicity, wide distribution, and abundance.

Cladosporium is second in importance. Its spores outnumber all other airborne biologic particles.[15] Hormodendrum is considered a structural variant of Cladosporium.

TABLE 12. 2   ALLERGENIC FUNGI

Alternaria	Monilia	Smuts
Aspergillus	Mucor	barley
Botrytis	Nigrospora	corn
Cephalosporium	Penicillium	Johnson grass
Cephalothecium	Phoma	oat
Chaetomium	Pullularia	wheat
Cladosporium	Rhizopus	
(Hormodendrum)	Rusts	Spicaria
Curvularia		Sporobolomyces
Epicoccum		Stemphylium
Fusarium		Trichoderma
Geotrichum		Trichothecium
Helminthosporium		Yeast

In some parts of the United States Alternaria and Hormodendrum may be somewhat less abundant than other molds, and there
are also some regional variations in the importance of the other
allergenic fungi, but the others considered of greatest importance usually include Aspergillus, Helminthosporium, and Peni-
cillium. Many others, including some not usually reported in
atmospheric fungal surveys, can also be responsible for allergy, however. [16]
    Although clinically significant cross reactivity is very com-
mon among different species of the same genus, cross reactivity
between fungi of different orders or classes is much less frequent and often unrelated to taxonomic classification. [17]

CONTROL

    Sources of exposure to fungi include fallen leaves, mulch
piles, organic fertilizer, hay and ensilage. Industrial sources
of exposure include grain elevators and breweries as well as
farms. Common sources of mold growth in homes include foam
rubber or cotton-stuffed mattresses and furniture, kapok, wallpaper, wool carpet, house plants and the soil in which they grow,
garbage pails, refrigerator drip trays, sinks, laundry rooms,
and shower curtains.
    Exposure to airborne fungi in the home can be confirmed
by exposure to culture plates for 10-20 minutes, and specific
fungi can then be identified.
    When brief exposure is necessary for a subject with recog-
nized hypersensitivity to fungi, this can be minimized by use of
a protective mask.
    Complete eradication of fungi from the home is probably
impossible, but substantial reduction in their concentration is
possible. Obvious sources such as potted plants, old books,
and old furniture should be removed from the house. Mold
growing on shower curtains, on the walls of shower stalls, or
elsewhere should be cleaned off with a solution of sodium hypo-
chlorite. It may be necessary to use a steel brush for complete removal from some surfaces. Subsequent periodic cleaning
with a fungistatic agent, Impregon may help prevent regrowth
of molds, although there is no published proof of its effectiveness, and concentrations greater than 1 tsp./gallon of water
may be necessary for an optimal effect. [18] Impregon can also
be added to paint and to wallpaper paste to help minimize subsequent growth of fungi. Captan, a fungicide available at
garden supply houses, can be used to spray rooms, closets,
basements or crawl spaces and may eliminate fungi for several
months.

Paraformaldehyde crystals are also effective in suppressing growth of molds. Contact with the fine powder can cause local burns, and the powder is very irritating if inhaled, so all direct contact must be avoided. A flat, glass dish containing 1 tsp of the powder can be placed out of reach on a bookself or valence. A separate dish is used for each 100 sq. feet of floor space, and dishes are spaced to provide for the entire room. If suitable objects upon which the dishes can be placed are not available, the inside of a match box can be lined with aluminum foil and tacked onto the wall at an appropriate height. The room should be closed tightly for the first 24 hours after treatment is started. The powder gradually disappears over 1-4 weeks but can be replaced as it disappears. Use of a dehumidifier is also often effective in control of fungi.

HOUSE DUST

House dust is a mixture of many potential allergens, often including particles of feathers, wool, human and animal danders, arthropods, pollen, and fungi, but two components widely regarded as primary sources of an allergen specific to house dust are kapok and cotton linters.[19] As these fibers age a chemical change occurs, and they become allergenic.

House dust collected in many different parts of the world has been found to abound with mites which use keratin from feathers, hair or human skin scales as sources of food. Dermatophagoides pteronyssinus has been reported to be the commonest household mite in most of the world; D. farinae (culinae) is also found in the United States.[20] A high correlation between the results of skin testing with house dust and mite extracts led to the recognition that mites are probably the source of the allergen of primary importance in house dust.[21] Allergenic potency of house dust often correlates with its mite content,[22] and results of radioallergosorbent testing have also revealed close correlation between house dust and mite extracts.[23]

Mite allergens are not the only important allergens in house dust. Some patients have skin reactivity to house dust but not to mites[24] and quantitative histamine release from the leukocytes of patients with dust allergy has revealed greater sensitivity to house dust than to mite extract in some.[25] Antibody to human skin has been found by RAST in sera of patients with house dust allergy, and cross reactivity between human skin extract and mite extract has been demonstrated.[26] This could be due to the presence of components of the media used to culture the mites. Accordingly much of the hypersensitivity ascribed to mites could be due to human dander sensitivity, but this requires further confirmation.

CONTROL

It is most important that precautions to minimize exposure to house dust (Table 12.3) be observed in the child's bedroom because he usually spends so much more time in this room than elsewhere in the house. When outdoors or at school he is not exposed to house dust, but he is usually in his bedroom for at least 8-10 hours each night. Printed instructions should be supplied and explained to the parents. Complete compliance can be assured only by unannounced home visits.

Vacuuming the mattress has been found to reduce substantially its mite population. Mites are killed by exposure for 24 hours to a temperature of 0°F. (-17.8°C.), and exposure of mattresses, pillows, and furniture to such temperatures periodically in the winter is feasible in some parts of the world.[20] Use of an acaricide has also been found effective in killing mites.[27] Since dead mites are still allergenic they must be removed by vacuuming, whatever method of killing them has been used.

Properly installed and maintained electronic air filters can be effective in removing dust, mold, and pollen particles from the air.

Room units are less effective than central units, unless the room is isolated from the rest of the house by sealing the air vent and keeping the door closed. Unfortunately ozone is produced in small amounts by the operation of such units. Exposure of normal adults for 2 hours to ozone in concentrations of 0.37 ppm has been found to cause changes in pulmonary function consistent with small airway obstruction and increased airway resistance.[28] Although this concentration of ozone is much greater than those that manufacturers claim are produced by electronic air filters even in isolated rooms the threshold below which no adverse effect could be expected in an asthmatic is unknown.

Mechanical, high efficiency particulate air (HEPA) filters are at least as efficient as electronic air filters in cleaning air, and they produce no ozone.[29] Both room and central units are available. Air conditioning alone can substantially reduce indoor pollen and mold exposure, but the addition of a HEPA filter has been found to reduce symptoms of respiratory allergy somewhat more.[30]

Because of dust contamination of air ducts any central cleaning system is most effective if installed when the central heating and cooling system is installed. No unit for cleaning the air obviates the need for other precautions to minimize exposure to household inhalant allergens (Table 12.3).

TABLE 12.3	HOW TO PREPARE
	A DUST-FREE BEDROOM

1. Remove everything from the room and closets, including rugs, curtains, and venetian blinds.
2. Clean the room and closet thoroughly and wax the floor.
3. Hot air vents should be sealed shut or equipped with dust filters made of glass fiber or several layers of cheesecloth unless a central HEPA or electronic air filter has been installed. (Do not place flammable material in contact with metal that might become hot). Change the furnace filter at least every month when the heating or cooling system is in use -- more often if frequent inspection discloses it to be dirty. Disposable filters are preferable to permanent filters unless a HEPA filter or an electronic filter is installed. Wall or floor heating units must be thoroughly vacuumed weekly.
4. Encase the mattress and box springs in air-tight, dustproof covers. If plastic covers are used the seams should not be stitched. Seal with adhesive tape at the point where zipper ends. Handle plastic covers carefully and inspect frequently for tears. More durable covers are available from Allergen-Proof Encasings, Inc., P.O. Box 5236, 1450 E. 363rd Street, Eastlake, Ohio, 44094. All mattresses and box springs in the room must be completely encased. Because of its potential for harboring fungi, it is even best for a foam rubber mattress to be encased by such a cover. Vacuum the covered mattress at least once each week.
5. Use no mattress pads, comforters or quilts unless they are filled only with dacron, and use only dacron or polyester-filled pillows. These pillows should be replaced each year unless they are also encased in allergen-proof covers. Use blankets and bedspreads that can be washed monthly. Avoid chenille bedspreads.
6. Any stuffed toys must be filled only with synthetic stuffing such as polyester.
7. Use as little furniture as possible, none upholstered. Bare floors and windows are best, but washable curtains and throw rugs are permissible if laundered at least weekly. Clean all furniture before returning it to the room.
8. Dust the room daily and clean it at least weekly using a vacuum cleaner or a cloth or mop sprayed with Endust. Don't omit cleaning the tops of doors, window frames and sills.
9. Air the room thoroughly during and after cleaning; otherwise keep doors and windows closed.
10. Keep only clothing currently in use in the closet, and keep the closet door closed.

ANIMAL DANDERS

Dog and cat dander are potent allergens. The dander, shed epidermal cells and cell products, is easily airborne and probably contains multiple water soluble allergens. Saliva and hair are also sources of allergens. Two major allergens have been isolated from cat skin, one of which is serum albumin.[31] Cross reactivity has been found between proteins in cat saliva, serum, and skin, but there is evidence of a distinct allergen in cat saliva.[32] Albumin has also been found to be an important allergen in dog and horse epithelia.

Occasional patients may have hypersensitivity only to a single breed,[33] but the usual patient with allergy to a dog seems to be allergic to most breeds. Variability in the extent of sensitization to different breeds has been reported.[34] Some data suggest that allergy to dog or cat dander is even associated with an increased risk of allergy to other epidermoids such as cattle, horse, rabbit, goat, sheep, and squirrel.[35] It is prudent to recommend avoidance of all animal danders when allergy to one is evident. In fact it is best for anyone with an atopic disease to avoid such animals.

It is especially important that the dog or cat be eliminated completely from the house. Restriction to a kitchen or utility room at night is not adequate because dander can still be carried by others or disseminated by a forced-air heating and cooling system to the rest of the house with consequent continual exposure for the allergic child indoors.

Other possible sources of exposure to cat hair include furry toys, robes, gloves, caps, coats, and slippers, but processed furs are less antigenic than the animal itself.

Other common household pets which are allergenic include gerbils, guinea pigs, hamsters, mice, and rats.

CATTLE HAIR

Dairy farms are obvious sources of exposure to cattle hair, but it is also sometimes found in rug pads, Indian rugs, horse blankets, rope, imitation furs and toy animals, artists' brushes, and upholstered furniture as stuffing.

HORSEHAIR

Saddles, bridles, horse blankets, and the clothing worn by members of the family while riding carry horse dander and should be excluded from the house. Horsehair is also used in mattresses, furniture, brushes, and ropes, but very little dander remains.

Because serum albumin is one of the important allergens in horse epithelium, the patient with allergy to horses is likely to be allergic to horse serum. It is especially important that prophylactic active immunization against diphtheria and tetanus be maintained with toxoids in such patients. Human antitoxin rather than horse serum should be used if necessary for treatment of possible tetanus.

SHEEP WOOL

Wool can act either as an allergen or an irritant. Synthetic materials can be substituted: orlon sweaters, acrylic blankets, and nylon carpet.

GOAT HAIR

Goat hair is used in upholstered furniture, tablecloths, curtains, clothing, blankets, gloves, oriental rugs, tapestries, doll's hair, ropes, brushes, mops, and yarns. Specific types of goat hair may be identified as angora, mohair, alpaca, or cashmere, although commercial fabrics sold as cashmere may be types of sheep wool.

RABBIT FUR

Rabbit fur is found in fur coats, lining for gloves and slippers, toy animals, and stuffing for mattresses, pillows, and quilts. Felt made from rabbit fur is used in polishing pads and on the sounding hammers of pianos.

FEATHERS

Pillows are the commonest source of feathers in the home. Dacron or polyester is the best substitute, and the patient should take his dacron pillow or at least an allergen-proof cover when he travels. Pillows in many hotels are still filled with feathers.
Feathers of birds of different species are antigenically related, so there should be no pet birds in the house, but aged feathers are more highly allergenic than freshly plucked feathers, suggesting the importance of a degradation product in eliciting hypersensitivity.

OTHER INHALANT ALLERGENS

KAPOK

Kapok, a fiber from tropical trees, is used as a stuffing in sofa pillows, sleeping bags, upholstered furniture, and toys. It is also used in boat cushions and life preservers. Kapok-stuffed pillows are often misleadingly labelled "non-allergenic".

COTTONSEED

Cottonseed, a potent inhalant allergen, often clings to the cotton linters used in pads and as stuffing in pillows, mattresses, quilts, and furniture. Miniature golf courses are often covered with a mixture containing ground cottonseed. Cottonseed is also found in some cattle and poultry feeds and fertilizers. Cottonseed flour is sometimes used in making doughnuts and candy. Cottonseed oil is probably not allergenic because of the high temperatures used in its production.

FLAXSEED

Flaxseed can cause allergic reactions following ingestion, inhalation, or contact. Sources of exposure include cattle and poultry feeds, dog food, wave sets, shampoos, depilatories, insulating material, furniture polish, linseed oil, paint and varnish, putty, dust from old linoleum, Roman meal bread, breakfast cereals, flaxseed tea, laxatives, and cough medicines.

ORRIS ROOT

Orris is obtained by powdering the root of a plant of the iris family. It is used in cosmetics, scented soaps, toothpaste, mouthwashes, bath salts, perfume, sunburn lotion, shaving cream, and shaving lotions. Hypoallergenic cosmetics are free of orris root.

PYRETHRUM

Pyrethrum is obtained from a plant related to ragweed, and ragweed-sensitive subjects are often unable to tolerate exposure to pyrethrum. It is widely used in insecticides and has also been used for moth-proofing carpet, draperies, and upholstered furniture.

JUTE

Jute, a fiber from a plant grown in India, is also an inhalant allergen. It is found in rug pads, burlap bags, and rope.

GLUE

Glue is produced from animal or vegetable sources, but the glue most commonly used on labels, stickers, books, and furniture is fish glue. LePage's glue is also a fish glue. Inhalation of particles of dry glue can provoke respiratory symptoms in sensitized subjects.

SILK

Silk can elicit allergic reactions following inhalation or contact. It is still used extensively in clothing and as a stuffing material, especially in Japan.

VEGETABLE GUMS

Karaya, acacia, and tragacanth are gums that may be allergenic following either inhalation or ingestion and can also cause contact dermatitis.

Karaya gum, which is also known as Indian gum or Indian tragacanth, is used in laxatives, toothpastes, wave sets, hand lotions, certain brands of gelatin and junket, diabetic foods, fillers for commercial pies and ice cream, gum drops, jelly beans, soft centered candy, and salad dressings.

Acacia, or gum arabic, is used in medications and hair dressings and often substituted for karaya.

Tragacanth, which is antigenically closely related to acacia, is used as a filler in pharmaceuticals and is found in candy, chewing gum and salad dressing. It, too, is often substituted for karaya.

INSECTS

Mayflies and caddis flies are among the insects recognized as sources of inhalant allergens, and the cockroach has also been implicated.[36] In some communities cockroach has been found to be second only to house dust as a cause of hypersensitivity, and results of skin testing correlate well with RAST and bronchial provocation testing in asthmatics.[37, 38]

REFERENCES

1. Solomon, W. R. , et al.: "Pollens and the plants that produce them, " in Sheldon, J. M. , Lovell, R. G. , and Mathews, K. P. : A Manual of Clinical Allergy, W. B. Saunders Co. , Philadelphia, 1967, p 340.
2. Lewis, W. H. , and Vinay, P. : North American pollinosis due to insect-pollinated plants. Ann All 42:309, 1979.
3. Webb, M. E. , et al.: "The botany of allergy" in Feingold, B. F. : Introduction to Clinical Allergy. Charles C. Thomas, Springfield, 1973, p 267.
4. Chapman, J. A. : Statistical report of the pollen and mold committee of the American Academy of Allergy, 1978.
5. Lichtenstein, L. M. , et al. : In vitro assay of allergenic properties of ragweed pollen antigens. J All 38:174, 1966.
6. Goodfriend, L. , et al. : Ragweed pollen allergen Ra5: Isolation, chemical properties, and genetic basis for its cutaneous activity in man. J All Clin Imm 51:81, 1973.
7. Lichtenstein, L. , et al.: Studies of the immunological relationship of ragweed pollen antigens E and Ra3. J All Clin Imm 51:285, 1973.
8. King, T. P. , et al.: Studies on ragweed pollen allergen. Ann All 25:541, 1967.
9. Hussain, R. , and Marsh, D. G. : Allergenic activity of a rapidly released basic component of short ragweed, Ra6. J All Clin Immunol 63:193, 1979.
10. Johnson, P. , and Marsh, D. G. : The isolation and characterization of allergens from the pollen of rye grass (Lolium perenne). European Polymer J 1:63, 1965.
11. Marsh, D. G. , et al.: A new method for determining the distribution of allergenic fractions in biological materials: Its application to grass pollen extracts. J All 46:107, 1970.
12. Baer, H. , et al.: The potency and Group I antigen content of six commercially prepared grass pollen extracts. J All Clin Imm 54:157, 1974.
13. Segal, A. T. , et al.: An immunologic study of tree pollen antigens. J All 45:120, 1970.
14. Belin, L. : Immunological analyses of birch pollen antigens, with special reference to the allergenic components. Int Arch Allerg 42:300, 1972.
15. Solomon, W. R. : "Pollens and fungi" in Middleton, E. , Jr. , Reed, C. E. , and Ellis, E. F. : Allergy Principles and Practice, St. Louis, C. V. Mosby Co. , 1978, p 899.
16. Giannini, E. H. , et al.: The allergenic significance of certain fungi rarely reported as allergens. Ann All 35:372, 1975.

17. Sams, J. T., and Smith, R. E.: Cross-antigenicity of common mold antigens. Ann All 26:55, 1968.
18. Solomon, W. R., et al.: An appraisal of Impregon as a deterrent of domestic fungus growth. J All Clin Imm 57:235, 1976.
19. Deamer, W. C.: "Nonseasonal inhalant allergens", in Speer, F. (ed): The Allergic Child, Harper & Row, New York, 1963, p 92.
20. van Bronswijk, J. E. M. H., and Sinha, R. N.: Pyroglyphid mites (Acari) and house dust allergy. J All 47:31, 1971.
21. Voorhorst, R., et al.: The house-dust mite (Dermatophagoides pteronyssinus) and the allergens it produces. Identity with the house-dust allergen. J All 39:325, 1967.
22. Miyamoto, T., et al.: Allergenic potency of different house dusts in relation to contained mites. Ann All 28:405, 1970.
23. Morita, Y., et al.: Further studies in allergenic identity between house dust and the house dust mite, Dermatophagoides farinae hughes, 1961. Ann All 35:361, 1975.
24. Biliotti, G., et al.: Mites and house dust allergy. I. Comparison between house dust and mite (Dermatophagoides pteronyssinus and D. farinae) skin reactivity. Clin All 2: 109, 1972.
25. Kaiwai, T., et al.: The allergens responsible for house dust allergy. J All Clin Imm 50:117, 1972.
26. Brighton, W. D., and Topping, M. D.: Human dander in house dust allergy. Clin All 7:577, 1977.
27. Penaud, A., et al.: Methods of destroying house dust pyroglyphid mites. Clin All 5:109, 1975.
28. Hazucha, M., et al.: Pulmonary function in man after short-term exposure to ozone. Arch Environ Health 27: 183, 1973.
29. King, J. G.: Air for living. Resp Care 18:160, 1973.
30. Kooistra, J. B., Pasch, R., and Reed, C. E.: The effects of air cleaners on hay fever symptoms in air-conditioned homes. J All Clin Immunol 61:315, 1978.
31. Stokes, C. R., and Turner, M. W.: Isolation and characterization of cat allergens. Clin All 5:241, 1975.
32. Bukantz, S. C., Lockey, R. F., and Baird, I. A.: Studies with cat saliva allergen. J All Clin Immunol 63:206, 1979.
33. Hooker, S. B.: Qualitative differences among canine danders. Ann All 2:281, 1944.
34. Moore, B. S., and Hyde, J. S.: Characterization of breed-specific dog danders and serum allergens. J All Clin Immunol 63:206, 1979.

35. Crawford, L. V., and Roane, J. A.: "Miscellaneous inhalants," in Speer, F., and Dockhorn, R. J. (ed): Allergy and immunology in children. Chas. C. Thomas, Springfield, 1973, p 263.
36. Bernton, H. S., and Brown, H.: Insect allergy: The allergenic potentials of the cockroach. So Med J 62:1207, 1969.
37. Kang, B., and Sulit, N.: A comparative study of prevalence of skin hypersensitivity to cockroach and house dust antigens. Ann All 41:333, 1978.
38. Kang, B., Vellody, D., Homburger, H., and Yunginger, J. W.: Cockroach cause of allergic asthma. J All Clin Immunol 63: 80, 1979.

CHAPTER XIII | DIAGNOSTIC TESTING

Charles Blackley reported in 1873 that allegy skin testing could identify the cause of hay fever.[1] Application of grass pollen to an abrasion on his forearm was followed by whealing. Skin testing done in much the same way has continued to be the most useful method of establishing specific allergens responsible for atopic symptoms. Other methods include provocative testing, passive transfer, the radioallergosorbent test, and the leukocyte histamine release test. Whatever method is used, the significance of the results depends upon the patient's medical history and environment or diet.

SKIN TESTING

Scratch testing, prick testing, and intradermal or intracutaneous testing are the commonest methods of testing for atopic diseases.

SCRATCH TESTING

The skin over the back or volar surfaces of the forearms is suitable for scratch testing. A larger number of tests can be applied to the back, and small children may tolerate the procedure with less anxiety if they are unable to see the maneuver that produces the scratches. Their cooperation also depends upon the type of instrument used to make the scratches and upon the skill of the technician in diverting their attention from what they may have been led to expect to be a painful experience. Any sharp instrument such as a sharp needle or lancet can be used for scratching. A circular scarifier (Center Laboratories) is especially likely to appear safe to a child and can be shown to him before testing, but it may cause more nonspecific release of histamine when rotated 180° to produce a circular scratch than some instruments. Scratches should be uniform in depth. Pressure must be sufficient to interrupt the epidermis but the scratch should not be deep enough to draw blood.

If a linear scratch is made, scratches should be short and of the same length. Uniformity can be assured by using a Sterneedle apparatus.

After the skin has been cleansed with alcohol and air dried it is marked with a ball point pen to indicate sites at which scratches are to be made. These should be at least 2-3 cm apart to prevent overlapping of reactions. It is usually possible to apply 40-80 tests in rows of ten over the back.

Aqueous solutions of extracts at concentrations of 1:10-1:20 are usually used for scratch testing. House dust extracts are often used at concentrations of 1:2. The choice of allergens for testing will depend upon the medical history, environment, aeroallergens common to the particular locality, and possibly diet. Use of house dust from two or three different sources is recommended. Use of mite extract (Hollister-Stier) is also helpful. Use of a control containing diluent without allergen is essential, and a histamine control (1:1, 000 histamine acid phosphate) facilitates interpretation when there are no other positive reactions.

Excessively large reactions can often be prevented by wiping off any extract that has begun to elicit a reaction by 5 or 10 minutes after application. Reactions are read at 15-20 minutes after gentle removal of all extracts by blotting. Excessive rubbing may cause false positive reactions and should be avoided.

Advantages of scratch testing over intradermal testing include safety, the speed with which a large number of tests can be done, and the readiness with which it is accepted by most children. Scratch testing is less sensitive than intradermal testing, however. Important allergens will often remain unrecognized if scratch testing is not supplemented with intradermal testing to some of the most important inhalant allergens.

PRICK TESTING

Prick tests are done by placing the drops of aqueous extracts of allergens on the skin first and then pricking the skin through the drop with the point of a small needle such as a 26 gauge disposable needle or a sharp darning needle. Prick testing causes less discomfort than scratch testing and less nonspecific reactivity due to trauma. Consequently results of testing are read more easily with prick testing. The only disadvantage is the aversion with which most children regard needles.

INTRADERMAL
(INTRACUTANEOUS) TESTING

The skin over the outer aspect of the arm is suitable for intradermal testing. Tests should be done low enough to permit application of a tourniquet above them if necessary because of a systemic reaction, and because of this possibility the back should not be used for intradermal testing. Clothing fitting tightly enough about the arm to obstruct venous circulation, possibly lessening the intensity of skin reactions, should be loosened or removed during testing.[2]

After the skin has been cleansed with alcohol and air dried, a ball point pen is used to indicate sites at which the tests are to be applied. These should be at least 2.5-3 cm apart to minimize the possibility of overlapping reactions, which might necessitate repeating some of the tests.

Intradermal testing is much more sensitive than scratch or prick testing, and systemic reactions are more likely to follow intradermal testing. This hazard is minimized by testing initially by the scratch or prick method to obviate the need for intradermal testing with those allergens to which the patient has the most extreme hypersensitivity. Only allergens which have elicited negative or 1+ reactions with scratch or prick testing are used in intradermal testing. If this precaution is observed, 1:400-1:4,000 concentrations of aqueous extracts can safely be used for intradermal testing. Epidermoid concentrations of 1:400, or 1:500 are often used for intradermal testing, while concentrations of 1:1,000 are suitable for pollens and molds. If previous scratch or prick testing has not been done, it is safest to use only more highly dilute extracts for initial intradermal testing. Relative hypersensitivity can be estimated by testing with several different concentrations to determine the weakest dilution that elicits a significant reaction.

Disposable or glass, 1 ml. tuberculin syringes and 26 or 27 gauge disposable needles are usually used for intradermal testing. The desired small volumes can be delivered with greatest accuracy and least discomfort with a Hamilton #710 microliter syringe and 30 gauge needle, but a 25 gauge needle must be used to load the syringe.[3,4] If glass syringes are used, each should be used only for a single allergen and cleansed separately from syringes used for other allergens to prevent allergenic contamination. Glass syringes are autoclaved after cleaning.

All air must be expelled from the needle and syringe before injection to avoid a false positive reaction from intradermal injection of air. The needle is introduced into the epidermis with the bevel facing the physician or technician. The syringe is then rotated 180⁰, turning the bevel downward, and 0.01-0.02 ml. is injected to produce a very small wheal. Approximately the same volume should be injected for each test. A diluent control is necessary unless enough tests are done that the negative tests can serve as controls. A control with 1:10,000 histamine acid phosphate facilitates interpretation if all other tests are negative.

Reactions to intradermal tests are read at 10-15 minutes.

Intradermal testing is usually limited to 20-30 tests at a time to minimize the risk of systemic reactions. [5] Other disadvantages include some discomfort to the patient, although intradermal testing can be almost painless when properly done, and the greater amount of time required for applying tests. The major disadvantage is the frequent nonspecific reactions due to irritants in allergen extracts, which are more frequent with feathers, dust, and molds than with pollens. [5]

INTERPRETATION

There is no uniformly accepted method of reading allergy skin tests. One method of grading reactions as compared to the diluent control follows:

- same as control
+ erythema (with control negative)
++ wheal (3-5 mm. or twice as large as control)
+++ large wheal (8 mm. or three times as large as control)
++++ wheal with pseudopods

Distinctions based upon small differences in the sizes of wheals resulting from testing with extracts with no reliable standard of potency cannot be justified. It has been suggested that reactions could be compared to the histamine controls which might be graded as 3+ reactions, [6] but this has not gained wide acceptance.

Using this grading system and extracts of suitable composition and concentration 2+ reactions are considered significant. [7-9] Occasional 1+ reactions may be significant if correlated closely with the history, however, and 2+ reactions may lack clinical significance if not correlated with the history.

False positive reactions may be due to the presence of histamine or histamine-releasers in the extract, [10] intradermal testing with too large a volume or an extract that is too concentrated, [7] intradermal testing with extracts containing more than 5% glycerin, [7] intradermal injection of air, or mechanical trauma from too much pressure during application of the scratch. Dermographism may prevent accurate reading of tests despite comparison with controls, necessitating other methods of evaluation.

False negative reactions may be due to testing with inactive extracts. Some loss of potency of pollen extracts at concentrations of 1:1,000 stored at 4° C has been reported to occur within 4 months although horse dander extract was found to be stable over this period of time.[11] Potency has been reported to decrease more rapidly with storage in smaller volumes, an effect ascribed to adsorption of protein to glass and prevented by addition of 0.2% Tween 20. Concentrated extracts (1:20) in 50% glycerol are stable for at least 1 year and possibly much longer, and 1:10,000 Russian thistle extracts in 50% glycerosaline are stable for 1 year, but even this stabilizer cannot maintain the potency of higher dilutions for even as little as one month when stored at 17°C. or refrigerated at 4°C., except for being left at room temperature 13 hours each week to simulate conditions in some allergy clinics.[12] Glycerin, however, cannot be used in extracts for skin testing because of its irritating properties. The potency of 1:1,000 extracts was maintained for as long as 12 months by 1% human serum albumin, but was maintained for only 3 months by 0.02% or 0.2% Tween 80. The potency of 1:100 extracts, was maintained for as long as 12 months by 0.03% human serum albumin, phosphate buffer, or normal saline. Stability was poor in bicarbonate-buffered saline, and at concentrations of 1:10,000 the Russian thistle extracts lost their potency more rapidly when 0.4% phenol had been added.[12] Others have reported human serum albumin (0.03%) and Tween 80 (0.005%) equally effective in maintaining the potency of ragweed, rye, alternaria, and dust extracts for as long as 6 months, even at high dilutions.[13]

Antihistamines can have a suppressive effect upon skin reactivity for as long as 5-8 days after administration.[14] The suppressive effect of hydroxyzine is especially potent and long lasting. Neither oral aminophylline (250 mg. q.i.d.) nor ephedrine (25 mg. q.i.d.) inhibits responses to allergy skin testing in adults,[15] although inhibition has been observed in skin pretreated with isoproterenol by iontophoresis.[16] Sublingual or intravenous isoproterenol, subcutaneous or intravenous epinephrine, and intravenous aminophylline have been reported to inhibit skin reactivity to allergy testing, but terbutaline has no inhibitory effect after oral administration or following intracutaneous injection with the antigen itself.[17-20]

Although adrenal corticosteroids have definite suppressive effects upon delayed hypersensitivity, they apparently have no significant effect upon responses to allergy skin testing for immediate, Type I hypersensitivity.[15, 21]

Thus, false negative reactions due to drug therapy can be minimized by discontinuation of antihistamine therapy 1 week before testing. Small doses of theophylline or ephedrine need not be discontinued, but if large doses of theophylline are being used it may be prudent to discontinue these 6-12 hours before testing. It is probably unnecessary to modify therapy with adrenal corticosteroids, and cromolyn sodium does not affect responses to allergy skin testing.

Another cause of false negative reactions is testing during the refractory period following systemic anaphylaxis. Testing should be deferred for 2-4 weeks following such a reaction.

Reduced reactivity to allergy skin testing in children less than three years old is partly due to some decrease in the frequency of sensitization of infants and young children, but is also due to decreased reactivity of the skin itself, and the importance of intradermal testing in this age group when scratch tests have been negative has been emphasized. Response to elimination diets and precautions to minimize exposure to household inhalant allergens may obviate the need for testing in many infants and young children, however.

False negative reactions also may occur with testing for foods and certain drugs, possibly due to allergy to haptens, metabolites or digestive products of foods. Reliable, clinically significant skin reactions can also follow testing with foods, however (see Chapter IX).

Scratches that are either too superficial or too deep and intradermal tests that are too deep can also cause false negative reactions.

Testing with groups of allergens in a single extract may possibly cause a false negative reaction when allergy to only one component is present. The number of different allergens in such mixtures should be kept to a minimum and the dilutional effect of other allergens should be considered in determining the concentrations to be used in the mixture.

Positive skin tests are sometimes elicited before a particular allergen has caused clinical symptoms,[22] and skin reactivity to allergens of previous clinical significance may persist despite clinical tolerance.[23] These are not false positive reactions, but they are reactions that lack immediate clinical significance.

The size of skin reactions elicited by allergens or histamine has been found to be influenced by a circadian rhythm.[24] Maximal reactivity has been reported at 11:00 P. M. ; minimal reactivity, at 7:00-11:00 A. M.

The value of allergy skin testing has sometimes been questioned because of a possible dissociation between sensitization of mast cells in the skin and those in the shock organ. Excellent correlation has been reported between results of prick testing with pollen or mite extracts and medical history, results of provocation testing, and circulating concentrations of antigen specific IgE, however.[9, 25] Positive skin tests (scratch and intradermal) to molds have been reported to occur often in asthmatics with negative bronchial provocation tests,[26] on the other hand, and others have reported poor correlations between skin testing and provocation testing with pollens, epidermoids, and house dust as well. [8],[27] Symptoms provoked by challenge of asthmatic chlldren with ragweed pollen in a controlled environment have been reported to correlate well with results of intradermal skin testing even though pulmonary function measured a few minutes after each challenge did not generally indicate response to the challenge. [28]

Despite these discrepancies in correlation with provocation testing found by some, skin testing is still regarded as the most useful and most practical method of evaluation for most atopic subjects, although other techniques may be helpful in further evaluation of some patients.

PASSIVE TRANSFER

Passive transfer testing can be used to demonstrate the presence of reaginic antibody in serum as Prausnitz and Kustner initially did. [29] Donor serum, 0. 05 or 0. 1 ml, is injected intradermally into skin over the arm or back of a recipient with no history of atopic symptoms. Injection sites are marked, and 48 hours later each is tested with antigen, using the usual intradermal technique. Results are compared with the results of testing with a diluent control at a site that has previously received donor serum and results of testing with the diluent control and each antigen at sites that have received no serum.

Passive transfer testing is generally considered less sensitive than direct skin testing but also less subject to false positive reactions. [5] Its chief clinical applications have been for diagnosis in patients with dermographism, generalized atopic dermatitis, or such extreme hypersensitivity that direct skin testing might be dangerous.

Because of the hazard of transmission of hepatitis it is rarely used now except for experimental purposes. In vitro methods of testing are safer and more practical when direct skin testing cannot be done.

SKIN WINDOW TECHNIQUE

The skin window technique[30] utilizes the eosinophilochemotactic effect of mediator release following reaction between antigen and specific IgE antibody fixed to the surface of mast cells. A 5x5 mm area of epidermis over the arm, forearm, or thigh is shaved, cleaned with alcohol, and scraped with a razor blade or scalpel blade until fine bleeding points appear. An aqueous solution of the antigen (1:1, 000-1:10, 000) is then applied, and the abraded area is covered with a glass slide kept in place for 24 hours by cardboard, an elastic bandage, and adhesive. A control window 5-6 cm away from the test site is prepared.

Further refinements of technique have permitted continual bathing of the abrasion with the test solution.[31]

After staining with Wright stain the number of eosinophils in 200-500 cells is determined and compared with those on the control slide. If the percentage of eosinophils at the test site exceeds that at the control site by more than 3 the test is considered positive.[2]

Results of skin window testing have sometimes been found to correlate even better with clinical symptoms than have results of skin testing (scratch and intradermal).[32]

PROVOCATIVE TESTING

Provocative testing includes bronchial provocation testing, nasal testing, and conjunctival testing. Bronchial inhalation testing can be done with specific allergens or with methacholine or histamine. Ingestion of foods is a form of provocative testing that is discussed elsewhere (see Chapter IX).

BRONCHIAL
PROVOCATION TESTING

A wide variety of methods of bronchial provocation testing has been used, but an attempt has been made to standardize procedures in the United States.[33] Nebulized aqueous solutions are delivered for inhalation during an inspiration beginning at functional residual capacity and ending at inspiratory capacity. It is recommended that inhalation testing with allergens be done only after the safe initial dose for challenge has been determined by intradermal skin testing with serial dilutions of extracts. The weakest concentration that elicits a 2+ intradermal reaction is the concentration considered safe to administer by inhalation.

It is recommended that testing be done at a time when the patient is asymptomatic and FEV_1 is at least 80% of the highest previously observed value.[33] Drugs which may interfere with the response should be withheld for various periods of time before testing depending upon their anticipated duration of activity: beta adrenergic agents, theophylline, alpha adrenergic blocking agents, and anticholinergic agents for 8 hours (sustained action preparations, for 12 hours); cromolyn sodium for 24 hours; antihistamines, 48 hours; hydroxyzine, 96 hours.

Pulmonary function is measured before and 10 minutes after 5 inhalations of diluent. If FEV_1 has not decreased as much as 10% the first allergen challenge can be administered.

This consists of 5 inhalations of the weakest concentration that elicited a 2+ intradermal reaction or a weaker dilution. If a reduction in FEV_1 of less than 15% is measured 10 minutes later, 5 inhalations of the next more concentrated solution can then be administered. When a decrease of 15-19% in FEV_1 occurs an additional 5-10 minute wait is recommended. The 10 minute drop should be sustained at the 20 minute measurement. The end point is a decrease in FEV_1 of more than 20% from the value obtained following inhalation of the diluent control. [33]

The concentrations recommended for sequential use in testing are 1:500,000; 1:100,000; 1:50,000; 1:10,000; 1:5,000; 1:1,000; 1:500.

Results are expressed as the cumulative provocative dose delivered over a certain period of time to cause a 20% fall in FEV_1 ($PD_{20}-FEV_1$) with the dose expressed as antigen inhalation units. One unit is defined as one inhalation of a 1:5,000 weight by volume concentration of antigen. [33] Thus, 5 inhalations of 1:500,000 antigen would deliver a cumulative dose of 0.05 units.

There is some evidence that flow at low lung volumes may become decreased before a significant change in FEV_1 occurs, suggesting that using such a parameter might be safer than use of a significant change in FEV_1 as the end point. [34]

False positive reactions may be due to the presence of histamine or histamine-releasing agents in extracts. Use of an allergen to which a negative response is expected can serve as a control for this possibility to some extent. [35] False negative reactions can occur due to action of drugs which may affect the response or if insufficiently concentrated or inactive allergen solutions have been used. Use of solutions less concentrated than 1:20 within 7 days has been recommended. [33]

Severe asthmatic attacks have followed bronchial provocation testing when presently recommended precautions have not been observed. [36] Late asthmatic responses beginning 4-6 hours after challenge and becoming maximal at 8-12 hours have also followed bronchial provocation testing and may occur whether or not an early asthmatic response has occurred. [37] Evaluation of patients at hourly intervals for 10 hours and again at 24 hours is recommended when feasible because of this possibility and further allergen inhalation testing should be deferred for at least 24 hours after the previous test. [33]

It has also been suggested that inadvertent overdosage with antigen during inhalation testing might induce hypersensitivity or a hyperresponsive state to subsequent challenge with that antigen. [36] One study has failed to demonstrate increased sensitivity to ragweed in asthmatics following bronchial provocation testing or seasonal pollen exposure. [38]

The other drawbacks to bronchial provocation testing are that it is time consuming and only a single allergen can be tested on each day.

Reported results of bronchial provocation testing are difficult to compare because of differences in technique and interpretation. Some have found poor correlation with allergy skin testing, [8, 26, 39] while others have reported good correlation, [9, 40] and still others have found good correlation with molds, house dust, and grasses, but poor correlations with weed and tree pollens. [41] The best correlations have been reported with prick testing[9] or intradermal testing with serial dilutions to determine the weakest concentration that elicits a significant reaction. [40] Most discrepancies have consisted of negative bronchial challenge results with positive skin tests. Positive bronchial challenges only rarely have followed negative skin tests.

Bronchial provocation testing is generally recommended only for severe, chronic asthmatics who have failed to respond to therapy or when other methods have failed to identify causative agents.

METHACHOLINE
INHALATION CHALLENGE

Measurement of pulmonary function before and after inhalation of a cholinergic agent such as methacholine has been proposed as a test useful in the diagnosis of asthma. [39, 42, 43]

The technique is similar to that for inhalational challenge with allergens. [33] If FEV_1 has not decreased more than 10% following inhalation of the diluent control, 5 inhalations of the most dilute methacholine solution are administered. Pulmonary function measurements are repeated at 1 1/2 minutes, and a significant change should be sustained at 3 minutes. [33] A decrease in FEV_1 of more than 20% below the measurement obtained following inhalation of the diluent control is considered positive. If a negative response is observed, 5 inhalations of the next concentration are administered. If a borderline positive test is observed fewer than 5 inhalations of the next dose may be administered. Concentrations recommended for successive administration until a positive response is observed are 0.075, 0.15, 0.31, 0.62, 1.25, 2.5, 5.0, 10.0, 25.0 mg./ml. It is recommended that any further inhalation testing be deferred for at least 2 hours after methacholine challenge and done then only if pulmonary function has returned to the pretest baseline.

Data are expressed as PD_{20}-FEV_1 as for antigen inhalation challenge. A methacholine inhalation unit is defined as one inhalation of 1 mg/ml of methacholine in buffered diluent. Thus, 5 inhalations of 0.075 mg/ml is a dose of 0.375 cumulative units.

Positive responses to inhalation of methacholine have been reported in almost all asthmatics, most former asthmatics, and many patients with allergic rhinitis but no asthma.[39,42,43] Positive responses have usually been reported in not more than 10-15% of nonatopic subjects,[43,44] but 28% of relatives of asthmatics have been reported to have positive responses to methacholine inhalation.[44] It is possible that nonasthmatic subjects with positive responses are those destined to develop asthma later.

HISTAMINE INHALATION CHALLENGE

The recommended technique for inhalation challenge testing with histamine is identical to that for methacholine except for substitution of histamine at concentrations of 0.03, 0.06, 0.12, 0.25, 1.0, 2.5, 5.0, and 10.0 mg./ml.[33] Data are expressed as for antigen or methacholine challenge testing. A histamine inhalation unit is defined as one inhalation of 1 mg/ml of histamine base in buffered diluent.

Most asthmatics and many patients with allergic rhinitis but no asthma have been found to have positive responses to inhalation of histamine.[42,45] Although most of these respond also to methacholine inhalation, a few do not.[45] Thus, response to histamine challenge might be of assistance in establishing a diagnosis in the patient whose response to methacholine has been normal.

NASAL PROVOCATION TESTING

Nasal provocation testing consists of observation of the patient for signs and symptoms of allergic rhinitis following direct application of the allergen to the nasal mucosa. Allergen solutions can be sprayed into the nostril or powdered allergen can be sniffed from the end of a toothpick into one nostril with the other nostril closed. Talcum powder can be used as a control.

Although safer than bronchial provocation testing, nasal provocation may elicit nasal symptoms not readily controlled with topical or oral medications and can provoke asthmatic attacks.[46] Testing can be done only when the subject is relatively free of symptoms, and only one allergen can be tested at a time. Sometimes a second allergen can be tested in the other nostril 45-60 minutes after the first test.

Increased sensitivity in reactivity of the nasal mucosa has been demonstrated following allergen exposure, and such a response could cause false positive responses to testing following diagnostic and possibly even natural exposure to allergens. [47]

Good correlation with clinical histories and the results of allergy skin testing has been reported. [46]

Nasal provocation testing may occasionally be helpful when allergy skin testing results do not correlate well with the history, but results must be interpreted cautiously and precautions must be observed to avoid adverse reactions.

CONJUNCTIVAL TESTING

Conjunctival testing is accomplished by introduction of allergen extract or powder into the conjunctival sac with the patient seated and looking upward with the head tilted backward. The lower eyelid is retracted and powdered allergen dropped into the conjunctival sac from a flat toothpick or one or two drops of aqueous extract are introduced. It is prudent to use powdered extract only if skin testing with that allergen has been negative. Aqueous extracts in concentrations of 1:500-1:10,000 are suitable for conjunctival testing. The diluent control can be introduced into the conjunctival sac of the other eye.

A positive reaction consists of reddening of the caruncle with or without conjunctival injection. [5] Lacrimation, itching, and rhinorrhea may also occur. The test is read at 20 minutes or sooner if a positive reaction is evident sooner. Dry pollen is then wiped from the conjunctival sac with a cotton applicator, and the eye is washed with normal saline. One or two drops of 1:1,000 aqueous epinephrine can be instilled into the conjunctival sac if a strongly positive reaction has occurred.

Conjunctival testing has been considered more sensitive than scratch testing but less sensitive than intradermal testing. [5] It is reported sometimes helpful in assessing the clinical significance of positive skin tests to inhalant allergens. [48]

The chief drawbacks to conjunctival testing are the need for cooperation and limitation to testing a single allergen at a time.

SERUM IGE

The very small concentrations of IgE normally present in serum cannot be measured by radial immunodiffusion as serum IgG, A, and M are usually measured. Methods by which IgE can be measured include radial immunodiffusion in agarose gel containing radiolabelled anti-IgE[49] and radioimmunoassay procedures including the radioimmunosorbent test (RIST)[50] and subsequent modifications of it. [51] Measurement of serum IgE by an inhibition radioimmunoassay depends upon the capacity of the IgE in the unknown serum to inhibit reaction between iso-

tope labelled IgE and anti-IgE. In the double antibody technique
bound and unbound radiolabelled IgE are separated by precipita-
tion by a second antibody directed against the Fc portion of the
anti-IgE. [51] This method has been reported to be highly sensitive, but the direct sandwich radioimmunoassay or paper disc
radioimmunosorbent test (PRIST*), a simpler method, has been
found to be even more sensitive. [52] By this technique the IgE
to be assayed is bound to anti-IgE coupled to paper discs. After
washing, radiolabelled anti-IgE is added. Radioactivity of the
resulting complex is then measured in a gamma counter.

Serum IgE concentrations are expressed as units/ml. One
international unit is equal to approximately 2.4 ng. [53]

The initial studies greatly overestimated normal serum concentrations of IgE, apparently because of inadequacies of population selection and inaccuracy and insensitivity of techniques,
especially at low concentrations. Recent studies indicate normal geometric mean serum concentrations in adults of 36 U./
ml. or less, when those with past, present, or family histories
of allergy have been excluded from the population studied. [54, 55]

Data collected from healthy children with no history of allergy in their immediate families indicate that adult concentrations of IgE are reached by approximately 10 years of age (24
U./ml.) (Figs. 13.1, 13.2). A wide range in normal values
was observed, but these data suggest that accurate measurement
of total serum IgE may be very helpful in implicating atopic allergy when parasitic infestations and other causes of increased
concentrations can be excluded (see Chapter II). Such measurements may be especially helpful in infants and small children
where the normal range is less wide. Almost all infants whose
serum IgE concentrations exceed 20 U./ml. by 12 months of
age are reported to have developed evidence of atopic diseases. [56]

RADIOALLERGOSORBENT TEST

While the measurement of total serum IgE may be useful in
suggesting the presence of an atopic disease, the radioallergosorbent test (RAST) may be helpful in identifying the specific
allergen.

The RAST consists of incubation of the unknown serum with
allergen coupled to an insoluble polysaccharide substance such
as cellulose or filter paper discs. [57] After washing, radiolabelled anti-IgE is added and permitted to incubate. After a second
washing the radiolabelled anti-IgE-IgE-allergen complex is
counted in a gamma spectrometer to determine the amount of
specific IgE that was present in the serum. Specimens of
stored, frozen serum are suitable for analysis and even unfrozen

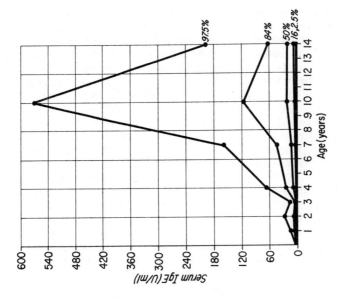

Fig. 13-2. Geometric mean serum IgE concentrations in 121 healthy infants and children with estimates of 2.5, 16, 84, and 97.5 percentiles. 55

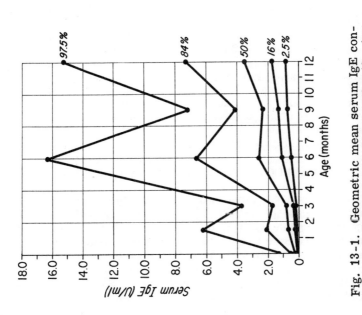

Fig. 13-1. Geometric mean serum IgE concentrations in 99 healthy infants with estimates of 2.5, 16, 84 and 97.5 percentiles. 55

specimens can be submitted to a commercial laboratory for analysis. *

Specific IgE antibodies against many inhalant allergens, a few foods, stinging insects, and ampicillin and penicillin have been measured by this technique, but it is not reported to have been used for detection of antibodies to the minor antigenic determinants of penicillin which are responsible for most acute, systemic, anaphylactic reactions to penicillin. [58]

The results of RAST have usually been reported to correlate well with the results of provocation testing, leukocyte sensitivity, symptom scores, and skin testing with serial dilutions to determine the weakest concentration that elicits a significant reaction. [9, 58, 59] Correlation with skin testing has been so good that many have concluded that the RAST and skin testing were of virtually equal accuracy. [59] When the RAST has been positive allergy skin testing has almost always been positive, but positive skin tests at higher concentrations of allergens have sometimes been associated with negative RAST. [60] Others have reported RAST more sensitive than skin testing for egg albumin, mite, and house dust. [61] Some have considered it slightly less reliable than provocation testing. [59]

The chief advantages of the RAST are lack of risk to the patient, lack of dependence upon the reactivity of the patient's skin, and stability of allergens in the solid-phase state. Present drawbacks to the RAST are expense, limited allergen selection, reduced sensitivity as compared with allergy skin testing, and the fact that results are not immediately available.

Its greatest usefulness seems to be in those patients in whom allergy skin testing may be unreliable because of severe atopic dermatitis, dermographism, or poor skin reactivity. Testing for drug hypersensitivity is an area of further potential usefulness yet to be developed. It has also been suggested that the RAST may be useful in the diagnosis of food allergy. [62]

Another important possible application of the RAST is in standardization of allergy extracts which could be accomplished indirectly by modification of the technique. [58]

LEUKOCYTE HISTAMINE RELEASE

The leukocyte histamine release test is another method of identifying antigen-specific IgE in serum. This consists of addition of increasing amounts of allergen to a standard concentration of the patient's leukocytes. [63] The percentage of total cellular histamine released (almost exclusively from basophils)

* Pharmacia Laboratories, Inc., 800 Centennial Avenue, Piscataway, New Jersey, 08854

can then be calculated. Cellular sensitivity is usually expressed as the amount of allergen required to release 50% of the total histamine. The result depends upon the IgE antibody fixed to the surface of the basophils and the sensitivity of the mediator-releasing mechanisms of the basophils. Reported modifications of the technique have included substitution of chopped human lung tissue, [64] sliced human skin, [65] and nasal polyp tissue[66] for the leukocytes.

Results of leukocyte histamine release have been reported to correlate well with clinical symptoms, bronchial provocation testing, RAST, and allergy skin testing (end point titration). [67]

The technique is limited to experimental use because of expense and the requirement of fresh blood as the source of leukocytes.

REFERENCES

1. Blackley, C. H. : Experimental Researches on the Causes and Nature of Catarrhus Aestivus (hay fever and asthma), Balliere, Tindall and Cox, London, 1873.
2. Tuft, L. , and Mueller, H. L. : Allergy in Children, W. B. Saunders Co. , Philadelphia, 1970.
3. Scherr, M. S. , et al. : Report of the committee on standardization: I. A method of evaluating skin test response. Ann All 29:30, 1971.
4. Voorhorst, R. , and van Krieken, H. : Atopic skin test reevaluated. I. Perfection of skin testing technique. Ann All 31:137, 1973.
5. Sheldon, J. M. , et al. : A Manual of Clinical Allergy, second ed. , W. B. Saunders Co. , 1967.
6. Aas, K. , and Belin, L. : Standardization of diagnostic work in allergy. Int Arch All Appl Imm 45:57, 1973.
7. Lindblad, J. H. , and Farr, R. S. : The incidence of positive intradermal reactions and the demonstration of skin sensitizing antibody to extracts of ragweed and dust in humans without history of rhinitis or asthma. J All 32:392, 1961.

8. Bronsky, E. A., and Ellis, E. F.: Inhalation bronchial challenge testing in asthmatic children. Ped Cl N A 16:85, 1969.

9. Bryant, D. H., et al.: The correlation between skin tests, bronchial provocation tests and the serum level of IgE specific for common allergens in patients with asthma. Clin All 5:145, 1975.

10. Doeglas, H. M. G., and Nater, J. P.: Histamine in foods causing false positive scratch tests. J All 42:164, 1968.

11. Foucard, T., et al.: Studies on the stability of diluted allergen extracts using the radioallergosorbent test (RAST). Clin Allergy 3:91, 1973.

12. Nelson, H. S.: The effect of preservatives and dilution on the deterioration of Russian thistle (Salsola pestifer), a pollen extract. J All Clin Immunol 63:417, 1979.

13. Norman, P. S., and Marsh, D. G.: Human serum albumin and Tween 80 as stabilizers of allergen solutions. J All Clin Immunol 62:314, 1978.

14. Cook, T. J., et al.: Degree and duration of skin test suppression and side effects with antihistamines. J All Clin Imm 51:71, 1973.

15. Galant, S. P., et al.: The inhibitory effect of antiallergy drugs on allergen and histamine induced wheal and flare response. J All Clin Imm 51:11, 1973.

16. Shereff, R. H., et al.: Effect of beta-adrenergic stimulation and blockade on immediate hypersensitivity skin test reactions. J All Clin Imm 52:328, 1973.

17. Tuft, L., and Brodsky, M. L.: The influence of various drugs upon allergic reactions. J All 7:238, 1936.

18. Sheldon, J. M., et al.: Effect of Isuprel on antigen-antibody and histamine skin reaction. Ann All 9:45, 1951.

19. Kram, J. A., et al.: Cutaneous immediate hypersensitivity in man: Effects of systemically administered adrenergic drugs. J All Clin Imm 56:387, 1975.

20. Imbeau, S. A., Harruff, R., Hirscher, M., and Reed, C. E.: Terbutaline's effects on the allergy skin test. J All Clin Immunol 62:193, 1978.

21. Slott, R. I., and Zweiman, B.: A controlled study of the effect of corticosteroids on immediate skin test reactivity. J All Clin Imm 54:229, 1974.

22. Hagy, G. W., and Settipane, G. A.: Prognosis of positive allergy skin tests in an asymptomatic population. J All Clin Imm 48:200, 1971.

23. Hill, L. W.: Food sensitivity in 100 asthmatic children. NEJM 238:657, 1948.

24. Reinberg, A., et al.: Circadian reactivity rhythms of human skin to histamine or allergen and the adrenal cycle. J All 36:273, 1965.

25. Pepys, J., et al.: RAST, skin and nasal tests and the history in grass pollen allergy. Clin All 5:431, 1975.
26. Collins-Williams, C., et al.: Provocative bronchial testing with molds. Ann All 31:401, 1973.
27. Berg, T. L. O., and Johansson, S. G. O.: Allergy diagnosis with the radioallergosorbent test. J All Clin Imm 54:209, 1974.
28. Fontana, V. J., et al.: Ragweed pollen challenges in a controlled environment. J All Clin Imm 54:235, 1974.
29. Prausnitz, C., and Kustner, H.: Studien uber die Uberempfindlichkeit. Centralbl Bakteriol 1 Abt Orig 86:160, 1921.
30. Rebuck, J. W., and Crowley, J. H.: A method of studying leukocyte functions in vivo. Ann NY Acad Sci 59:757, 1955.
31. Felarca, A. B., and Lowell, F. C.: Local effects of cortisol in the time course of eosinophilotaxis with the use of an improved technique. J All 43:114, 1969.
32. Felarca, A. B., and Lowell, F. C.: The accumulation of eosinophils and basophils at skin sites as related to intensity of skin reactivity and symptoms in atopic disease. J All Clin Imm 48:125, 1971.
33. Chai, H., et al.: Standardization of bronchial inhalation challenge procedure. J All Clin Imm 56:323, 1975.
34. Olive, J. T., Jr., and Hyatt, R. E.: Pulmonary mechanics during bronchial provocation in asthmatic subjects. J All 47:91, 1971.
35. Aas, K.: The Bronchial Provocation Test. Chas. C. Thomas, Springfield, 1975.
36. Spector, S. L., and Farr, R. S.: Comments on bronchial inhalation provocative tests. J All Clin Imm 48:120, 1971.
37. Robertson, D. G., et al.: Late asthmatic responses induced by ragweed pollen allergen. J All Clin Imm 54:244, 1974.
38. Rosenthal, R. R., et al.: Bronchoprovocation. Effect on priming and desensitization phenomenon in the lung. J All Clin Imm 56:338, 1975.
39. Spector, S. L., and Farr, R. S.: Bronchial inhalation procedures in asthmatics. Med Cl N A 58:71, 1974.
40. Bruce, C. A., et al.: Quantitative inhalation bronchial challenge in ragweed hay fever patients: a comparison with ragweed-allergic asthmatics. J All Clin Imm 56:331, 1975.
41. Holman, J. G., et al.: Bronchial challenge and skin test correlations. Ann All 30:250, 1972.
42. Itkin, I. H.: Bronchial hypersensitivity to mecholyl and histamine in asthma subjects. J All 40:245, 1967.
43. Cade, J. F., and Pain, M. C. F.: Bronchial reactivity. Its measurement and clinical significance. Austr N Z J Med 1:22, 1971.

44. Townley, R. G. , et al.: Methacholine sensitivity and atopic disease in asthmatic and nonatopic families. J All Clin Imm 53:107, 1974.
45. Spector, S. L. , and Farr, R. S.: A comparison of methacholine and histamine inhalations in asthmatics. J All Clin Imm 56:308, 1975.
46. Collins-Williams, C. , et al.: Nasal provocative testing with molds in the diagnosis of perennial allergic rhinitis. Ann All 30:557, 1972.
47. Connell, J. T.: Quantitative intranasal pollen challenges. J All 43:33, 1969.
48. Tuft, L. , et al.: Eye tests with inhalant allergens; their feasibility, indications, and clinical value. J All 30:492, 1959.
49. Arbesman, C. E. , et al.: Measurement of serum IgE by a one-step single radial radiodiffusion method. J All Clin Imm 49:72, 1972.
50. Johansson, S. G. O. , et al.: A new class of immunoglobulin in human serum. Immunol 14:265, 1968.
51. Gleich, G. J. , et al.: Measurement of IgE in normal and allergic serum by radioimmunoassay. J Lab Clin Med 77: 690, 1971.
52. Johansson, S. G. O. , et al.: Comparison of IgE values as determined with different solid phase radioimmunoassay methods. Clin All 6:91, 1976.
53. Bazaral, M. , and Hamburger, R. N.: Standardization and stability of immunoglobulin E (IgE). J All Clin Imm 49:189, 1972.
54. Nye, L. , et al.: A detailed investigation of circulating IgE levels in a normal population. Clin All 5:13, 1975.
55. Kjellman, N. -I. M. , et al.: Serum IgE levels in healthy children quantified by a sandwich technique (PRIST). Clin All 6:51, 1976.
56. Orgel, H. A. , et al.: Development of IgE and allergy in infancy. J All Clin Imm 56:296, 1975.
57. Wide, L. , et al.: Diagnosis of allergy by an in-vitro test for allergen antibodies. Lancet 2:1105, 1967.
58. Yunginger, J. W. , and Gleich, G. J.: The impact of the discovery of IgE on the practice of allergy. Ped Cl N A 22:3, 1975.
59. Berg, T. L. O. , and Johansson, S. G. O.: Allergy diagnosis with the radioallergosorbent test. J All Clin Imm 54:209, 1974.
60. Sarsfield, J. K. , and Gowland, G.: A modified radioallergosorbent test for the in vitro detection of allergen antibodies. Clin Exp Immunol 13:619, 1973.

61. Hogarth-Scott, R. S. , et al. : Diagnosis of allergy in vitro. A comparison between skin sensitivity testing and serum levels of specific IgE antibody in children. Med J Austr 1:1293, 1973.
62. Hoffman, D. R. , and Haddad, Z. H. : Diagnosis of IgE-mediated reactions to food antigens by radioimmunoassay. J All Clin Imm 54:165, 1974.
63. May, C. D. , et al. : Procedures for immunochemical study of histamine release from leukocytes with small volume of blood. J All 46:12, 1970.
64. Brocklehurst, W. E. : The release of histamine and formation of a slow-reacting substance (SRS-A) during anaphylactic shock. J Physiol 151:416, 1960.
65. Greaves, M. W. , et al. : New in vitro test for IgE-mediated hypersensitivity in man. Brit Med J 2:623, 1972.
66. Kaliner, M. , et al.: Immunologic release of chemical mediators from human nasal polyps. NEJM 289:277, 1973.
67. Bruce, C. A. , et al. : Diagnostic tests in ragweed-allergic asthma. J All Clin Imm 53:230, 1974.

CHAPTER XIV | IMMUNOTHERAPY

Immunotherapy was introduced by Noon in 1911.[1] Administration of a series of injections of boiled timothy grass pollen extract at 3-14 day intervals to 18 patients with hay fever was followed by reduced reactivity to conjunctival instillation of fresh pollen and fewer symptoms during the next pollen season in 16.[2]

By 1914 Noon's colleague, Freeman, reported improvement in 88.5% of 84 patients with hay fever treated with timothy extract.[3]

Immunotherapy has been evaluated in numerous subsequent studies with various types of extracts in patients with hay fever or asthma due to various allergens and subjects with insect sting hypersensitivity. Various doses have been administered at differing intervals for various periods of time. A lack of objective parameters of improvement has necessitated reliance upon evaluations of symptoms by the patients for assessment of response to therapy. Evidence that at least 35% of patients find treatment with a placebo effective emphasizes the importance of inclusion of placebo controls in studies seeking to establish the efficacy of any form of therapy.[4]

Despite these complexities, immunotherapy has been shown to be efficacious by many investigators (Tables 14.1, 14.2). In a few of the controlled studies little or no benefit from treatment has been evident. In one of these[19] the lack of more definite evidence of efficacy was ascribed to use of an insensitive symptom scoring system which later was improved and inclusion of treatment for a number of different allergens rather than restriction to a single allergen for which hypersensitivity could be established more definitely.[20] In another study which disclosed no benefit from immunotherapy the symptom scoring system used did not assess severity or duration of symptoms and relatively small doses of extract were used.[21] Response to therapy has been found to be related to the dose of extract administered in patients with either allergic rhinitis[22] or asthma,[12] small doses having effects similar to those of placebo.

Although immunotherapy is beneficial for most patients with allergic rhinitis, asthma, or insect sting hypersensitivity (see Chapter XI), protection is usually partial and a few patients remain unimproved. Lack of improvement is often due to exposure to allergens for which the patient is not being treated or failure to progress to high enough doses for optimal response.

TYPES OF EXTRACT

In most controlled studies of efficacy of immunotherapy aqueous extracts have been used. The chief limitations of the use of aqueous extracts have been the need for frequent injections and the occurrence of local and systemic reactions. Local reactions have consisted of painful or pruritic, erythematous swellings at the injection site subsiding within a few hours or 1-2 days. Possible systemic reactions have included generalized urticaria, angioedema, exacerbations of symptoms of allergic rhinitis or asthma, and even anaphylaxis. Other types of extract that have been studied include aqueous extracts in oil emulsions, alum-precipitated extracts, alum-precipitated pyridine extracts, and allergoids.

Repository therapy with emulsified extracts held forth the possibility that the slower release of antigen from the injection site might permit effective therapy with fewer local or systemic reactions and less frequent injections (1-4 each year), while an adjuvant effect might enhance the efficacy of therapy. Initial studies were favorable but some double blind studies indicated that repository therapy was less effective than treatment with aqueous extracts.[10] Side effects included the development of nodules and cysts or sterile abscesses at injection sites as well as immediate or delayed systemic reactions. Skin reactivity typical of Type I and Type IV hypersensitivity has been induced by administration of emulsified extracts to subjects without previous hypersensitivity, a phenomenon which has not been reported with aqueous extracts.[25] The induction of myeloma in mice by large doses of mineral oil has limited further use of repository therapy with emulsions.

Treatment with alum-precipitated pollen extracts has permitted effective therapy with fewer injections and fewer systemic reactions than occur with aqueous extracts, although severe local reactions have been somewhat more frequent.[26]

Alum-precipitated pyridine-linked extracts (Allpyral) have been reported to elicit fewer systemic and local reactions than aqueous extracts. Although its efficacy has been reported comparable to that of aqueous or repository therapy in studies without placebo controls,[27, 28] others have found the effects of alum-precipitated pyridine extracts indistinguishable from those of

TABLE 14.1 CONTROLLED STUDIES OF IMMUNOTHERAPY FOR ASTHMA

Authors	Allergens	Evaluation	Number of Patients		Patients Improved (%)	
			Placebo	Treatment	Placebo	Treatment
Bruun[5] (1949)	House dust	Symptoms	89	100	34	78
Frankland & Augustin[6] (1954)	Grass pollen	Symptoms	26	31	30	94
Johnstone[7] (1957)	Mixture	Symptoms	26	29	7	68
Citron, et al[8] (1958)	Grass pollen	Bronchial provocation	5	13	0	92
Johnstone & Crump[9] (1961)	Mixture	Symptoms	42	43	29	86
Arbesman & Reisman[10] (1964)	Ragweed pollen	Symptoms	19	21	58	76
Sanders[11] (1966)	Grass pollen (Depot)	Symptoms	16	16	50	69
Johnstone & Dutton[12] (1968)	Mixture	Absence of asthma	63	67	22	72

Table 14.1 (cont'd.)

Smith[13] (1971)	D. pteronyssinus	Symptoms	11 (human skin scales)	11	27	91
Aas[14] (1971)	House dust	Bronchial provocation	28	52	32	87
Tuchinda & Chai[15] (1973)	Alternaria, House dust, Grass, ragweed	Bronchial provocation	5 (low dose)	10	0	80
D'Souza, et al[16] (1973)*	D. pteronyssinus	Symptoms, Nasal provocation, Leukocyte histamine release	46	45		Fewer symptoms, Decreased nasal sensitivity, Decreased cell sensitivity
Pence, et al[17] (1976)*	Mountain cedar	Symptoms	15	17		Fewer symptoms
Taylor, et al[18] (1978)	Cat	Bronchial provocation Skin testing	5	5	0	100

* Some patients with allergic rhinitis included.

TABLE 14.2 CONTROLLED STUDIES OF IMMUNOTHERAPY FOR ALLERGIC RHINITIS

Authors	Allergens	Evaluation	Number of Patients		Patients Improved (%)	
			Placebo	Treatment	Placebo	Treatment
Frankland & Augustin6 (1954)	Grass Pollen	Symptoms	99	99	33	79
Lowell & Franklin19 (1963)	Mixture	Symptoms	63	59	15	32
Lowell & Franklin20 (1965)	Ragweed Pollen	Symptoms	12	12	More symptoms	Fewer symptoms
Fontana, et al21 (1966)	Ragweed Pollen †	Symptoms	26	25	50	56
Franklin & Lowell22 (1967)	Ragweed Pollen	Symptoms	13 (low dose)	12	More symptoms	Fewer symptoms
Norman, et al23 (1968)	Ragweed Pollen*	Symptoms	13	13	8	77
	Antigen E*	Symptoms	13	21	8	48

Table 14.2 (cont'd.)

			21	57	More symptoms	Fewer symptoms, Increase in blocking antibody
Lichtenstein, et al24 (1971)	Ragweed Pollen	Symptoms				
	Antigens E & K	Blocking antibody				
		Leukocyte Histamine Release				Decrease in cell sensitivity

† Treated for 3-5 seasons
* Preseasonal treatment for 3 years

placebo controls.[29,30] It has been suggested that the evident
decreased antigenicity of Allpyral may be due to inactivation
by the highly alkaline extraction with pyridine.[30,31]

Allergoids are formed by treatment of pollen extracts with
formaldehyde. Allergoids have a reduced capacity for causing
allergic reactions, but can induce formation of blocking antibody and both the skin reactivity and leukocyte sensitivity characteristic of Type I hypersensitivity.[32] Their use permits
administration of much larger doses,[33] associated with somewhat fewer symptoms than in control patients receiving treatment with the usual aqueous extracts.[34] Polymerization of
ragweed antigen by treatment with glutaraldehyde has been
found to be associated with reduced allergenicity without loss
of immunogenicity for blocking antibody.[35,36] The resulting
extract permits more rapid immunization with fewer reactions.

ANTIGENS

There is considerable evidence of the efficacy of immunotherapy with aqueous extracts for the treatment of asthma or
allergic rhinitis due to pollens and some evidence of benefit from
treatment with house dust.

Immunotherapy with fungi has also been reported effective
but controlled studies have not been reported. The only controlled evaluation of immunotherapy with animal danders reported is a study of response to immunotherapy with a cat pelt
extract that contained substantially more cat allergen 1 than
do many commercially available extracts of cat epithelium.[18]
Bronchial provocation testing disclosed a significant improvement in all five of the patients who received treatment with the
active extracts.

Treatment with antigen E, the most potent allergen isolated
from ragweed pollen, has been reported as efficacious as treatment with whole ragweed extract,[23] but it has not been more
effective and has sometimes been less effective, probably because of the presence of hypersensitivity to other components
of ragweed pollen in occasional patients.[37]

Immunotherapy has been shown to be beneficial for subjects
who have had systemic reactions to Hymenoptera stings (see
Chapter XI).

Most controlled studies of the efficacy of stock and autogenous
bacterial vaccines have demonstrated no differences from response to placebo controls.[38-40] In the single study in which
a beneficial effect of bacterial vaccine was found in children the
14 patients studied had histories of exacerbations of asthma
only with respiratory infections, no wheezing between infections,
and exacerbations always of sufficient severity to require medi-

cal consultation. [41] During the 1-2 years of treatment with stock vaccine substantial decreases in the frequency and severity of wheezing associated with respiratory infections occurred in the 9 treated patients as compared with the 5 controls. Although the numbers are few, these data suggest that bacterial vaccine may be useful in a very few, highly selected patients.

MECHANISMS

The mechanisms through which immunotherapy is beneficial are unknown, but several potentially beneficial effects have been identified.

BLOCKING ANTIBODY

Stimulation of the production of blocking antibody was first thought responsible for the clinical improvement which followed immunotherapy. [42] It was observed that blood transfusions from treated patients inhibited clinical reactions in untreated patients with hay fever. Passive transfer of mixtures of allergen and serum obtained before and after courses of immunotherapy disclosed immediate reactions only with the pretreatment sera, suggesting induction of a blocking antibody by therapy. Subsequent investigations have confirmed that increased serum concentrations of IgG blocking antibody are induced by immunotherapy[22, 43] and frequently correlate with clinical improvement. [22, 44] Serum blocking antibody concentrations usually increase within the first 4 months of treatment. [45] This antibody can react with antigen but does not sensitize the mast cell for mediator release.

IGE

In untreated atopic subjects with pollen hypersensitivity increases in specific IgE concentrations in the serum occur during their pollen seasons. Immunotherapy apparently suppresses production of specific IgE or prevents its usual seasonal increase in concentration. [45, 46] Clinical improvement has sometimes been correlated with decreased serum concentrations of reagin titers rather than increased production of blocking antibody. [47]

MAST CELL

Decreased release of histamine following challenge of peripheral leukocytes with antigen has also been reported in patients who have received immunotherapy, and such changes have also sometimes correlated with clinical improvement.[48] Decreases in cell sensitivity may occur usually only after 10-12 months of treatment.[49]

T CELL

Other changes associated with immunotherapy have included decreased lymphocyte transformation and decreased release of mitogenic factor and migration inhibition factor following challenge in vitro with specific allergen,[50,51] indicating that immunotherapy induced changes in cellular immunity as well as changes in humoral immunity. Immunotherapy has been found to decrease the proliferative response of T cells to challenge with specific allergen which otherwise can be demonstrated in atopic subjects.[52] The association of the presence of IgE specific suppressor T cells with suppression of IgE synthesis in mice treated with antigen E denatured by urea, suggests stimulation of suppressor T cells as an additional mechanism through which immunotherapy is probably beneficial.[53]

ANTIBODIES IN SECRETIONS

Increased concentrations of specific IgG and secretory IgA antibodies have been found in nasal secretions of patients receiving immunotherapy.[54] These antibodies can block histamine release.

It is likely that multiple factors are responsible for the clinical improvement associated with immunotherapy. Improvement within the first few months of treatment may be related often to increased titers of blocking antibody, while later effects may be related to decreased titers of reaginic antibody and decreased cell sensitivity. Decreases in production of IgE may be mediated by alterations in responsiveness of T cells to antigenic stimulation and stimulation of suppressor T cells as well as decreases in amounts of antigen due to blocking antibody activity.

INDICATIONS FOR IMMUNOTHERAPY

Whether or not immunotherapy is indicated depends upon the frequency and severity of symptoms as well as the ease with which they are controlled with other forms of therapy.

Immunotherapy is indicated for the treatment of asthma or allergic rhinitis only when Type I hypersensitivity is demonstrated to inhalant allergens that the patient cannot avoid, such as pollens, fungi, and house dust.

Immunotherapy is also indicated in subjects who have had

systemic reactions following Hymenoptera stings (see Chapter XI).

It is not indicated for the treatment of Type III hypersensitivity, which it might be expected to aggravate, although patients with Type I hypersensitivity to alternaria and alternaria precipitins in their sera have been reported to be able to tolerate immunotherapy usually. [55]

Specific antigens to be used in treatment should usually be those implicated by both diagnostic testing and history. If immunotherapy is indicated by these criteria, however, it is reasonable to include a few additional allergens indicated by testing only if their inclusion will not excessively dilute the allergens known to be important. Although treatment with aqueous extracts has not been reported to induce specific reaginic antibody formation in patients without prior hypersensitivity, this has been observed following treatment with emulsions and allergoids, [25, 32] so it is prudent to avoid treatment with allergens to which hypersensitivity has not been demonstrated even when aqueous extracts are used.

ANTIGEN ADMINISTRATION

Many allergists prepare their own antigen solutions for diagnosis and treatment, but antigens are also readily available commercially.

Considerable variation in potency of allergy extracts from different sources has been reported, [56] and potency of an extract from the same commercial source can vary from year to year. Neither protein nitrogen content nor weight by volume standardization accurately measures antigenic potency. Major allergenic components have been isolated and well characterized for only two important pollens (ragweed and rye grass), and only one commercial laboratory uses antigen E content for standardization of its ragweed extracts (Center Laboratories). [57, 58] The RAST inhibition technique is another method of standardization that could be applied to allergy extracts. [59]

Response to immunotherapy has been best when the highest doses tolerated have been administered. [12, 22] Treatment with large doses is most easily achieved when individual antigens are administered separately. Since multiple allergens are usually identified, it is more practical to combine these in a single extract, but each allergen added dilutes the others, and the local reaction which may follow the injection is likely to be larger than that which would have followed injection of a single allergen. Furthermore, extreme hypersensitivity to a single component of the extract may thus limit the dose of other components. Nevertheless several allergens are usually combined in a single extract because of convenience, better patient acceptance, and decreased cost.

The proportions of allergen extracts in mixtures is often varied depending upon suspected importance in the individual patient or prevalence in the local atmosphere. Such attempts to individualize mixtures are probably ineffective and unnecessary because of substantial variations in potency of extracts due to lack of accurate methods of standardization.[56]

Most children tolerate maximal doses of 0.5-1 ml of a 1:50-1:100 concentration of a pollen or mold. It has been estimated that 1 ml of a 1:100 extract approximates 6,000 protein nitrogen units, but this varies from season to season and allergen to allergen. House dust extracts are usually tolerated at concentrations of 1:100. In the treatment of hypersensitivity to Hymenoptera stings, maximal doses of 1 ml of concentrations of 100µg/ml are usually possible and adequate.

Because of the dilutional effect of additional allergens in mixtures, concentrations of individual allergens must be increased if their concentration in the final mixture is to be maintained. Thus, in both of the following prescriptions the final concentration to bermuda grass is 1:100, although each is labelled according to the concentration of the components.

Rx Equal parts: Bermuda grass,   1:20
                   Johnson grass,   1:20
                   June grass,   1:20
                   Short ragweed,   1:20
                   Marsh elder,   1:20
Mix, label 1:20, and prepare 3 additional serial ten-fold dilutions.

Rx Equal parts: Bermuda grass,   1:10
                   Johnson grass,   1:10
                   June grass,   1:10
                   Short ragweed,   1:10
                   Marsh elder,   1:10
                   Elm (Ulmus americana),   1:10
                   Maple (Acer rubrum),   1:10
                   Alternaria,   1:10
                   Helminthosporium   1:10
                   Cladosporium   1:10
Mix, label 1:10, and prepare 3 additional serial ten-fold dilutions.

Although the allergens in mixtures dilute each other all may contribute to local reactions. Thus, smaller volumes of mixtures of 10 allergens than mixtures of two or three are usually tolerated. This limitation of dosage may necessitate a modification in the treatment program with inclusion of fewer allergens in each of two mixtures. When two mixtures are used, inclusion of related allergens or allergens to which exposure will occur at the same time of year in the same mixture facilitates dosage adjustments that may be necessary because of decreased tolerance associated with seasonal exposure.

Many grass pollens are so similar antigenically that treatment with bermuda, johnson, and one other grass such as rye or timothy may sometimes afford sufficient protection when hypersensitivity to all grasses tested has been demonstrated, but some antigenic differences are found among other grasses (see Chapter XII). Treatment with timothy extract alone, however, has been reported less effective than treatment with multiple grass pollens in Sweden. [60]

TREATMENT SCHEDULE

Treatment is started with very dilute concentrations, and the dosage is gradually increased as tolerated. The initial dose for treatment of inhalant allergens is usually 0.1 ml/1:100,000. When unusually large reactions have been elicited by skin testing or systemic reactions have occurred during previous immunotherapy, treatment is started with 0.1 ml/1:1,000,000. The concentrations with which treatment of Hymenoptera sting hypersensitivity is started and the suggested progression are found in Chapter XI.

Each subsequent dose is increased by an increment of 50% if tolerated (Table 14.3), except that the dose is not increased when the first dose from the next higher concentration is administered. Loss of allergenic potency occurs more rapidly in dilute solutions and local reactions may also occur more frequently with administration of the same dose in a smaller volume because of more rapid diffusion from the injection site.

This recommended rate of progression must be modified if reactions occur. Local swelling or erythema as large as 2 cm in diameter when the injection site is examined at 20 minutes indicates that the same dose should be repeated until smaller local reactions occur before resuming the usual progression. Reactions more than 2 cm in diameter indicate a need for decreasing the next dose by at least one step. If a negligible reaction occurs then successive increases in dosage can be resumed.

If a generalized allergic reaction follows the injection, the next dose should be decreased to the same volume of the next lower concentration, a reduction to 10% of the dose that elicited the reaction. The usual progression can then again be resumed, but it is prudent to increase the dosage at a slower rate when the dose that was followed by the systemic reaction is again approached.

TABLE 14.3   IMMUNOTHERAPY TREATMENT SCHEDULE

VISIT NUMBER	DILUTION (WEIGHT BY VOLUME)	DOSE (ML)
1	1:100,000	0.1
2	1:100,000	0.15
3	1:100,000	0.22
4	1:100,000	0.33
5	1:100,000	0.50
6	1:10,000	0.05
7	1:10,000	0.07
8	1:10,000	0.10
9	1:10,000	0.15
10	1:10,000	0.22
11	1:10,000	0.33
12	1:10,000	0.50
13	1:1,000	0.05
14	1:1,000	0.07
15	1:1,000	0.10
16	1:1,000	0.15
17	1:1,000	0.22
18	1:1,000	0.33
19	1:1,000	0.50
20	1:100	0.05
21	1:100	0.07
22	1:100	0.10
23	1:100	0.15
24	1:100	0.22
25	1:100	0.33
26	1:100	0.50

If it becomes evident that the anticipated maintenance dose of 0.5-1 ml/1:100 cannot be reached because of local or systemic reactions, the maximal tolerated dose should be continued as the maintenance dose. If this dose is reached at a concentration lower than 1:100 with a mixture of allergens consideration should be given to attempting to reach higher total doses by dividing the allergens between two mixtures.

Before the maintenance dose has been reached injections are administered once or twice each week. No increase in dose is administered if more than 1 week has elapsed since the last injection, and the dose is decreased if more than 6 weeks has elapsed.

After the maintenance dose has been administered several times, the interval between injections can usually be increased gradually from 1 week to 2, 3, or 4 weeks. There is evidence that protection can be maintained by administration of maintenance doses at intervals as great as 6 weeks.[61] Occasional patients are unable to tolerate increases in the interval between injections because of increases in the size of local reactions.

Perennial treatment permits administration of larger cumulative doses and may therefore be more effective than preseasonal treatment, consisting of therapy only during the few months preceding the particular pollen season each year. When preseasonal treatment is used it is started early enough to permit maintenance doses to be reached shortly before the start of the pollen season, and therapy is discontinued during or after the season until the following year.

When perennial treatment is used a temporary reduction in dosage is sometimes necessary during the pollen season to prevent systemic reactions. If significant symptoms of allergic rhinitis or asthma are present when the child is due to receive an allergy injection, the dose should be reduced by at least 50% or omitted to minimize the possibility of a systemic reaction.

Dosage is also reduced by 50% when treatment with a fresh supply of extract is started because of the uncertainty of its relative potency. This necessitates temporary return to a weekly schedule until the proper maintenance dose with the new extract has been established.

TECHNIQUE

Allergy injections are administered with a sterile, 1 ml. tuberculin syringe and a 26 or 27 gauge, 3/8 or 1/2 inch needle. A suitable injection site is the posterior aspect of the middle third of the arm, low enough to permit use of a tourniquet above the injection site if necessary. After the skin has been cleansed with alcohol, the needle is rapidly introduced, the plunger is retracted, and if no blood has appeared in the syringe the injection is administered. Pressure is maintained for 30-60 seconds over the injection site after the needle has been withdrawn to minimize the possibility of seepage of allergen into damaged blood vessels. An injection that is too superficial may cause a large local reaction, while one which is too deep may prevent recognition of a local reaction that otherwise might have indicated a need for subsequent modification of the treatment schedule.

REACTIONS

Immunotherapy should be administered only at a physician's office, hospital, or clinic where personnel and equipment are immediately available if necessary for treatment of a systemic reaction. The patient should remain for observation for 20 minutes, and strenuous exercise should be avoided for a least one hour. The injection site should not be massaged.

Large local reactions before maintenance doses have been reached indicate a need for modification of the treatment schedule. Subsequent reductions in maintenance dosage are recommended if local reactions exceed 6 cm in diameter or persist more than 24 hours.

Antihistamines are helpful for the treatment of erythematous, pruritic local reactions. Ice packs can be applied to relieve swelling.

Local reactions occurring or persisting several hours after injections and associated with fever, malaise, or arthralgia may be due to Type III hypersensitivity and may necessitate discontinuation of therapy.[55]

Systemic reactions may consist of generalized pruritus, urticaria, coughing or wheezing, sneezing or rhinorrhea, syncope, or other symptoms of anaphylaxis (see Chapter VIII). The treatment indicated depends upon the severity of the reaction, but generally is the same as treatment for any anaphylactic reaction.

DURATION OF THERAPY

Immunotherapy is continued with maintenance doses until the patient has been free of allergic symptoms for 1-2 years or has experienced only minimal symptoms for 3 years. After discontinuation of therapy some patients remain well, but others may develop symptoms again within a few months, indicating a need for further therapy.

Some patients who show no benefit during the first year of treatment improve during the second year.[19] Initial improvement followed by an increase in symptoms during a different season suggests acquisition of hypersensitivity to additional allergens. Other causes of apparent treatment failures include inadequate dosage, inactive extracts, and an incorrect diagnosis. Food allergy or inadequate avoidance of environmental allergens may cause symptoms incorrectly ascribed to allergens for which immunotherapy has been prescribed. In some patients no explanation for a poor response to treatment is evident, and it is unreasonable to continue their therapy indefinitely if no benefit has been seen.

REFERENCES

1. Noon, L.: Prophylactic inoculation against hay fever. Lancet 1:1572, 1911.
2. Freeman, J.: Further observations on the treatment of hay fever by hypodermic inoculations of pollen vaccine. Lancet ii:814, 1911.
3. Freeman, J.: Vaccination against hay fever. Report of results during the last three years. Lancet 1:1178, 1914.
4. Shure, N.: The placebo in allergy. Ann All 23:368, 1965.
5. Bruun, E.: Control examination of the specificity of specific desensitization in asthma. Acta Allergol 2:122, 1949.
6. Frankland, A.W., and Augustin, R.: Prophylaxis of summer hay-fever and asthma. Lancet 1:1055, 1954.
7. Johnstone, D.E.: Study of the role of antigen dosage in the treatment of pollenosis and pollen asthma. Am J Dis Child 94:1, 1957.
8. Citron, K.M., et al.: Inhalation tests of bronchial hypersensitivity in pollen asthma. Thorax 13:229, 1958.
9. Johnstone, D.E., and Crump, L.: Value of hyposensitization therapy for perennial bronchial asthma in children. Ped 27:39, 1961.
10. Arbesman, C.E., and Reisman, R.E.: Hyposensitization therapy including repository: A double blind study. J All 35:12, 1964.
11. Sanders, S.: The treatment of seasonal hay fever and asthma in children. Pract 196:811, 1966.
12. Johnstone, D.E., and Dutton, A.: The value of hyposensitization therapy for bronchial asthma in children. Ped 42:793, 1968.
13. Smith, A.P.: Hyposensitization with Dermatophagoides pteronyssinus antigen. Brit Med J 4:204, 1971.
14. Aas, K.: Hyposensitization in house dust allergy asthma. Acta Paed 60:264, 1971.
15. Tuchinda, M., and Chai, H.: Effect of immunotherapy in chronic asthmatic children. J All Clin Imm 51:131, 1973.
16. D'Souza, MF.D., et al.: Hyposensitization with Dermatophagoides pteronyssinus in house dust allergy: A controlled study of clinical and immunological effects. Clin All 3:177, 1973.
17. Pence, H.L., Mitchell, D.Q., Greely, R.L., Updegraff, B.R., and Selfridge, H.A.: Immunotherapy for mountain cedar pollinosis. J All Clin Immunol 58:39, 1976.
18. Taylor, W.W., Ohman, J.L., Jr., and Lowell, F.C.: Immunotherapy in cat-induced asthma. J All Clin Immunol 61:283, 1978. (corr. Ibid, p 409).

19. Lowell, F. C., and Franklin, W.: A "double blind" study of treatment with aqueous allergenic extracts in cases of allergic rhinitis. J All 34:165, 1963.
20. Lowell, F. C., and Franklin, W.: Double-blind study of the effectiveness and specificity of injection therapy in ragweed hay fever. NEJM 273:675, 1965.
21. Fontana, V. J., et al.: Effectiveness of hyposensitization therapy in ragweed hay-fever in children. JAMA 195:985, 1966.
22. Franklin, W., and Lowell, F. C.: Comparison of two dosages of ragweed extract in the treatment of pollenosis. JA MA 201:915, 1967.
23. Norman, P. S., et al.: Immunotherapy of hay fever with ragweed antigen E: Comparisons with whole pollen extract and placebos. J All 42:93, 1968.
24. Lichtenstein, L. M., et al.: A single year of immunotherapy for ragweed hay fever. Ann Int Med 75:663, 1971.
25. Becker, R. J., et al.: Delayed and immediate skin reactivity in man after the injection of antigen in emulsion. J All 32:229, 1961.
26. Norman, P. S., et al.: Trials of alum-precipitated pollen extracts in the treatment of hay fever. J All 50:31, 1972.
27. Fuchs, A. M., and Strauss, M. B.: The clinical evaluation and the preparation and standardization of suspensions of a new water-insoluble whole ragweed pollen complex. J All 30:66, 1959.
28. Tuft, L., and Torsney, P. J.: Treatment of ragweed hay fever with Allpyral extracts. J All 36:265, 1965.
29. Reisman, R. E., and Arbesman, C. E.: Clinical studies of two ragweed preparations: "Purified" delta and Allpyral. Int Arch All 28:353, 1965.
30. Lichtenstein, L. M., et al.: Antibody response following immunotherapy in ragweed hay fever: Allpyral vs. whole ragweed extract. J All 41:49, 1968.
31. Lichtenstein, L. M., and Norman, P. S.: Letter to editor. J All 41:237, 1968.
32. Marsh, D. G., et al.: Induction of IgE-mediated immediate hypersensitivity to Group I rye grass pollen allergen and allergoids in non-allergic man. Immunol 22:1013, 1972.
33. Norman, P. S., et al.: Immunotherapy of grass pollen hay fever with grass pollen allergoid. J All Clin Imm 49:114, 1972.
34. Glovsky, M. M., Marsh, D. G., Kurata, J. H., and Ghekiere, L.: Treatment of highly grass-sensitive rhinitis patients with aqueous and formalinized grass extracts. J All Clin Immunol 63:166, 1979.

35. Metzger, W. J.: Comparison of polymerized and unpolymerized antigen E for immunotherapy of ragweed allergy. New Eng J Med 295:1160, 1976.
36. Patterson, R., Suszko, I. M., Bacal, E., Zeiss, C. R., Kelly, J. F., and Pruzansky, J. J.: Reduced allergenicity of high molecular weight ragweed polymers. J All Clin Immunol 63:47, 1979.
37. Reisman, R. E., et al.: Immunotherapy with antigen E. J All 44:82, 1969.
38. Johnstone, D. E.: Study of the value of bacterial vaccines in the treatment of bronchial asthma associated with respiratory infections. Ped 24:427, 1959.
39. Aas, K., et al.: "Bacterial allergy" in childhood asthma and the effect of vaccine treatment. Acta Paed 52:338, 1963.
40. Fontana, V. J., et al.: Bacterial vaccine and infectious asthma. JAMA 193:895, 1965.
41. Mueller, H. L., and Lang, M.: Hyposensitization with bacterial vaccine in infectious asthma. JAMA 208:1379, 1969.
42. Cooke, R. A., et al.: Serological evidence of immunity with coexisting sensitization in a type of human allergy (hay fever). J Exp Med 62:733, 1935.
43. Sadan, N., et al.: Immunotherapy of pollinosis in children. NEJM 280:623, 1969.
44. Melam, H., et al.: Clinical and immunologic studies of ragweed immunotherapy. J All 47:262, 1971.
45. Ishizaka, K., et al.: IgE and IgG antibody responses during immunotherapy. J All Clin Imm 51:79, 1973.
46. Reisman, R. E., et al.: Relationship of immunotherapy, seasonal pollen exposure and clinical response to serum concentrations of total IgE and ragweed-specific IgE. Int Arch All Appl Imm 48:721, 1975.
47. Malley, A., and Perlman, F.: Timothy pollen fractions in treatment of hay fever. J All 45:14, 1969.
48. Pruzansky, J. J., and Patterson, R.: Immunologic changes during hyposensitization therapy. JAMA 203:805, 1968.
49. Melam, H., et al.: Clinical and immunologic studies of ragweed immunotherapy. J All 47:262, 1971.
50. Malley, A., et al.: The site of action of antigen D immunotherapy. J All Clin Imm 48:267, 1971.
51. Evans, R., et al.: Effect of immunotherapy on humoral and cellular responses in ragweed hay fever. J All Clin Imm 53:114, 1974.
52. Gatien, J. G., et al.: Allergy to ragweed antigen E: Effect of specific immunotherapy on the reactivity of human T lymphocytes in vitro. Clin Imm Immunopath 4:32, 1975.

53. Ishizaka, K., Okudaira, H., and King, T. P.: Immunogenic properties of modified antigen E. II. Ability of urea-denatured antigen and α-polypeptide chain to prime cells specific for antigen E. J Immunol 114:110, 1975.
54. Platts-Mills, T. A. E., von Maur, R. K., Ishizaka, K., Norman, P. S., and Lichtenstein, L. M.: IgA and IgG anti-ragweed antibodies in nasal secretions. J Clin Invest 57: 1041, 1976.
55. Storms, W. W., et al.: A prospective look at reactions to Alternaria immunotherapy. J All Clin Imm 53:115, 1974.
56. Baer, H., et al.: The potency and antigen E content of commercially prepared ragweed extracts. J All 45:347, 1970.
57. King, T. P., et al.: Isolation and characterization of allergens from ragweed pollen. Biochemistry 3:458, 1964.
58. Johnson, P., and Marsh, D. G.: The isolation and characterization of allergens from the pollen of rye grass (Lolium perenne). European Polymer J 1:63, 1965.
59. Yunginger, J. W., and Gleich, G. J.: The impact of the discovery of IgE on the practice of allergy. Ped Clin N A 22: 3, 1975.
60. Heijer, A., and Goransson, K.: The significance of testing and hyposensitization with several grass pollens for hay fever. Acta Allergol 23:146, 1968.
61. Norman, P. S., et al.: Maintenance immunotherapy in ragweed hay fever. J All 47:273, 1971.

α-adrenergic hyperresponsiveness, 39
α-adrenergic stimulation, 25
α-1-antitrypsin deficiency, 104, 105
Absorption, gastrointestinal, 269
Acacia, 348
Acidosis, 51, 52, 87, 88, 108-110
  treatment of, 155
ACTH, 138, 139
ACTH test, 138
Adenoidectomy, 255
Adenoids, hypertrophy of, 196, 249
Adrenal corticosteroids, 133-141
  in allergic rhinitis, 202
  in anaphylaxis, 265, 266
  in atopic dermatitis, 220
  in death from asthma, 163
  effect on eosinophil counts, 72
  in exercise-induced asthma, 58
  in status asthmaticus, 156, 157
  in urticaria, 241
Adrenal suppression, 136-141
Adrenergic receptors, 110, 111, 113
Adverse drug reactions, classification, 293, 294
Ahistidinemia, 214
Air filter:
  electronic, 343
  HEPA, 343
Air pollution, 59, 60
Airway resistance, 82
Albumin, human serum, 356
Albuterol, 116, 118, 145, 162
  for exercise-induced asthma, 58
  for status asthmaticus, 156, 162
Alkalosis, 110

Allergens:
  inhalant, 328-348
  priming effect, 186
Allergic rhinitis (see Rhinitis, allergic)
Allergic toxemia (see Tension-fatigue syndrome)
Allergic vasculitis (see Anaphylactoid purpura)
Allergoids, 377
Allergy:
  classification, 2-5
  definition, 1
Allergy extracts, 377, 378
  stabilizers, 356
Allergy injection technique, 385
Alternaria, 340, 341
Alum-precipitated extracts, 377
Alum-precipitated pyridine-linked extracts, 377
Alveolitis, extrinsic allergic (see Pneumonitis, hypersensitivity)
Aminophylline, 152-154, 266
  (see also Theophylline)
Ampicillin, 304
Anaphylactoid purpura, 237, 298
Anaphylactoid reactions, 228, 260, 261
Anaphylatoxin, 227
Anaphylaxis, 1, 260-267
  due to ACTH and steroids, 139
  causes, 261, 262
  differential diagnosis, 263, 264
  due to drug allergy, 295
  in insect sting allergy, 318, 319
  local, 2
  pathogenesis, 260
  pathology, 266, 267
  prevention, 267
  signs, 263
  symptoms, 261-263
  systemic, 2, 228, 260-267
  treatment, 264-266
Anesthetics, local, 308, 309

Continuing Medical Education Program

Medical Examination Publishing Company has joined with Temple University Medical School's Continuing Medical Education Department in establishing a cooperative program for granting CME credit. Temple and MEPC have designed this program to make CME Category I credits available to practicing physicians at a reasonable cost. Formal recognition can now be given to the reading a physician does in his home or office of current books in his fields of interest.

This is how the program works. The Office for Continuing Medical Education at Temple University School of Medicine has carefully selected appropriate books for Category I CME credits. To obtain the credits, the reader must take the post-test, complete the answer sheet according to instructions, and mail to:

Albert J. Finestone, M.D.
Associate Dean, Continuing Medical Education
Office for Continuing Medical Education
Temple University School of Medicine
3400 North Broad Street
Philadelphia, PA 19140

You should also enclose your check for $10.00 (ten) dollars payable to TEMPLE POSTGRADUATE to help defray administrative costs.

In return, you will receive the correct answers, your graded answer sheet, and, if you have completed the test to the standards of the program, a certificate for the credits you have earned.

The dual objectives of updating your knowledge and securing necessary credits can now be achieved economically. We hope you find this service a valuable and rewarding one.

401

POST-TEST

Directions: Each question or incomplete statement is followed
by several suggested answers or completions. ALL, SOME,
OR NONE OF THE POSSIBLE CHOICES MAY BE CORRECT.
Correct responses will be found at the end of the examination.

CHAPTER I

1. True statements about Type I Reactions (Gell and Coombs,
   classification), include
   A. they are mediated by cytotropic antibodies
   B. signs and symptoms result from the actions of chemicals
      released from mast cells or basophils
   C. participating antibodies are usually of the IgE class
   D. reactivity can be transferred to normal subjects by serum
   E. soluble antigen-antibody complexes are formed

2. Examples of Type I Reactions include
   A. generalized, pruritic wheals that have followed ingestion
      of strawberries on three separate occasions
   B. hemolytic anemia following injection of penicillin
   C. three-week episodes of nasal congestion, sneezing, and
      rhinorrhea with nasal and conjunctival itching occurring
      in May each year
   D. acute airway obstruction with wheezing occurring shortly
      after a man had swallowed Dristan in an effort to relieve
      nasal obstruction due to nasal polyps
   E. generalized flushing and anxiety followed by dyspnea,
      wheezing, and shock after a boy had experienced a sudden,
      sharp pain over the back of the neck while enjoying a
      picnic lunch in the park beneath flowering trees

3. True statements about Type II Reactions include
   A. they are also known as cytolytic or cytotoxic reactions
   B. participation of complement is always necessary
   C. antibodies involved may include IgG or IgM
   D. chemicals are released but the target cell is not destroyed
   E. the antigen is a cell component or an antigen or hapten
      intimately associated with the cell

403

4. Examples of Type II Reactions include
   A. coughing, dyspnea, hemoptysis, and pulmonary infiltrates followed within a few weeks by hematuria in a young man with no history or other evidence of recent streptococcal infection
   B. mild hyperbilirubinemia, microspherocytosis, and slightly positive direct Coombs' test in a one-day-old, group A infant of a group O mother
   C. anemia, hyperbilirubinemia, and strongly positive direct Coombs' test in a twelve-hour-old, Rh positive infant of an Rh negative mother
   D. cough, dyspnea, chills, fever, myalgia, and malaise with fine, crepitant rales in an adolescent beginning four to six hours after he began work in a silo
   E. generalized pruritus and wheals occurring 20 minutes after the start of a whole blood transfusion in an automobile-accident victim with sex-linked hypogammaglobulinemia

5. True statements about Type III Reactions include
   A. they result from the formation of antigen-antibody complexes
   B. the inflammatory reaction consists primarily of monocytes
   C. reaction between antigen and precipitating antibody results in deposition of microprecipitates in and around small blood vessels after complement activation
   D. polymorphonuclear leukocytes phagocytize the antigen-antibody complexes
   E. neutrophils are destroyed, releasing proteolytic enzymes that cause tissue damage

6. Examples of Type III Reactions include
   A. Arthus reactions
   B. serum sickness
   C. nephritis of systemic lupus erythematosus
   D. contact dermatitis
   E. allergic rhinitis

7. True statements about Type IV Reactions include
   A. reactivity can be transferred to normal subjects by lymphoid cells
   B. the reaction is usually maximal at four to eight hours after intradermal injection of antigen
   C. lymphokines are released following interaction of sensitized lymphocytes with antigen
   D. cytolysis is dependent upon complement activity
   E. immunologic memory for Type IV Reactions is retained by B lymphocytes

8. Examples of Type IV Reactions include
   A. homograft rejection
   B. contact dermatitis
   C. generalized urticaria after injection of contrast media for intravenous pyelography
   D. tuberculin hypersensitivity
   E. psoriasis

9. Evidence for the genetic basis of atopic allergy includes
   A. pedigrees of allergic children are almost always consistent with inheritance as an autosomal recessive
   B. increased frequency of hay fever and asthma when both parents also have hay fever or asthma
   C. association of allergy to ragweed with certain HLA haplotypes in certain families
   D. identical twins are invariably concordant with respect to atopic allergy
   E. less variability in serum IgE concentrations has been found between monozygotic twins than between dizygotic twins

10. Available data on the prevalence of atopic diseases indicate that
   A. asthma is more frequent in the Northeastern U.S. than in the South
   B. atopic dermatitis has been reported to have occurred at some time in less than 1% of children
   C. asthma is more frequent in boys than in girls
   D. atopic respiratory disease may occur in more than 20% of children by 18 years of age
   E. allergic rhinitis is more frequent than asthma

CHAPTER II

11. Reaction between antigen and specific, IgE antibody fixed to the surfaces of mast cells causes the mast cell to release chemical mediators that include
   A. histamine
   B. kallikrein
   C. eosinophil chemotactic factor
   D. neutrophil chemotactic factor
   E. 5-hydroxytryptamine

12. Constriction of smooth muscle in bronchi is caused by
   A. histamine
   B. bradykinin
   C. slow reacting substance
   D. prostaglandin E
   E. heparin

13. Release of histamine from basophils is inhibited by
   A. histaminase
   B. cyclic AMP
   C. prostaglandin E
   D. arylsulfatase
   E. histamine

14. Substances that inactivate slow reacting substance and are found in eosinophils include
   A. major basic protein
   B. phospholipase D
   C. arylsulfatase
   D. 5-hydroxytryptamine
   E. prostaglandin E

15. Suppressor T cells may interfere with
   A. activation of helper T cells
   B. interaction of helper T cells with B lymphocytes
   C. differentiation of B lymphocytes to mature plasma cells producing IgE
   D. secretion of IgE antibody by plasma cells
   E. differentiation of B lymphocytes to mature memory cells

16. Antibodies for which there is evidence of fixation to the surfaces of mast cells or basophils are found in which of these classes?
   A. IgA
   B. IgD
   C. IgE
   D. IgM
   E. IgG_4

17. Immunoglobulins that have been found in secretions include
    A. IgG
    B. IgA
    C. IgM
    D. IgD
    E. IgE

18. Abnormal increases in total serum IgE are found in many children with
    A. ascariasis
    B. allergic bronchopulmonary aspergillosis
    C. Wiskott-Aldrich syndrome
    D. atopic dermatitis
    E. congenital sex-linked hypogammaglobulinemia

19. As compared with normal subjects, asthmatics are reported to have
    A. fewer beta adrenergic receptors on lymphocytes
    B. less hyperglycemia after isoproterenol infusion
    C. less vasodilation after isoproterenol infusion
    D. less eosinopenia after epinephrine injection
    E. less bronchoconstriction after administration of beta adrenergic blocking agents

CHAPTER III

20. Factors known to trigger bronchoconstriction in many asthmatics include
    A. respiratory infections with respiratory syncytial virus
    B. free range running for one minute
    C. inhalation of cold air
    D. increases in environmental temperature
    E. acute otitis media

21. Findings consistent with the diagnosis of asthma include
    A. forced expiratory volume in one second (FEV_1) 60% predicted normal, increased after inhalation of isoproterenol to 88% predicted normal
    B. digital clubbing and an increase in the antero-posterior diameter of the chest in a child who has had rectal prolapse three times. One of seven siblings died with pneumonia in infancy
    C. recurrent wheezing, improved dramatically after injection of epinephrine in a child with atelectasis of the right middle lobe

D. a history of recurrent wheezing with fever, expectoration of brown plugs, peripheral eosinophilia, serum IgE 2500 U/ml, and migrating pulmonary infiltrates
E. expiratory wheezing, inspiratory "crow", brassy cough, and recurrent pneumonia since birth in a six-month-old infant who seems to prefer the opisthotonic position. Forcible flexion of the neck is followed by apnea.

22. A six-month-old infant is examined because of wheezing said to have begun the previous day. Additional information tending to suggest possible asthma includes
A. episodes of wheezing two and four months ago improved after injections of Bronkephrine
B. both parents have allergic rhinitis
C. an epidemic of respiratory disease due to respiratory syncytial virus began four weeks ago
D. total blood eosinophil count is 800 per cubic mm
E. the family's chihuahua began to sleep in the patient's bedroom last week

23. Digital clubbing is often found in patients with
A. asthma
B. bronchiectasis
C. empyema
D. lung abscess
E. cyanotic congenital heart disease

24. A differential white blood cell count including 30% eosinophils with a total leukocyte count of 15,000 per cubic mm is consistent with
A. allergic bronchopulmonary aspergillosis
B. allergic asthma
C. trichinosis
D. hyperimmunoglobulinemia E with susceptibility to infection
E. pinworm infestation

25. Findings consistent with atelectasis of the left lower lobe include
A. reduced FEV_1 with normal vital capacity
B. reduced vital capacity
C. obliteration of the left cardiac border on PA chest roentgenogram
D. obliteration of the left hemidiaphragm on lateral chest roentgenogram
E. suppression of breath sounds posteriorly over the left lower hemithorax

26. Atelectasis of the right middle lobe
    A. occurs more often than atelectasis of any other lobe in children with asthma
    B. may be present despite normal findings on physical examination
    C. causes obliteration of the right cardiac border on the PA chest roentgenogram
    D. causes suppression of breath sounds posteriorly over the right lower hemithorax
    E. is differentiated from consolidation more easily by the lateral chest roentgenogram than by the PA view

27. Findings consistent with a foreign body forming a check valve in the right mainstem bronchus include
    A. persistent cough and wheezing after an episode of choking on peanuts
    B. expiratory wheezing more prominent over the right hemithorax than the left
    C. shift of the mediastinum to the right on expiratory chest roentgenogram
    D. equal inflation of both lungs on right lateral decubitus films
    E. widening of right intercostal spaces as compared with the left on expiration

28. True statements about pneumomediastinum as a complication of asthma include
    A. the occurrence of subcutaneous crepitus in the neck is an ominous sign indicating a need for cervical mediastinotomy
    B. it occurs more often in infants than older children
    C. it may be caused by coughing
    D. IPPB has been implicated as a cause
    E. it occurs more often than pneumothorax

29. Factors implicated as possible causes of status asthmaticus include
    A. alkalosis
    B. edema
    C. secretions
    D. overuse of nebulized isoproterenol
    E. pneumomediastinum

30. Respiratory failure in a child with status asthmaticus is suggested by
    A. arterial P_{CO_2} 50 mm mercury
    B. total "clinical score" of 4
    C. cyanosis in 40% oxygen with decreased breath sounds and maximal use of accessory muscles of respiration but no wheezing
    D. extreme wheezing with moderate use of accessory muscles of respiration and arterial P_{O_2} 75 mm mercury in air. Inspiratory breath sounds and cerebral function are normal
    E. moderate wheezing and moderate use of accessory muscles of respiration with arterial P_{O_2} in air 50 mm mercury. Inspiratory breath sounds and cerebral function are normal.

31. Limitations to the use of nebulized isoproterenol for the treatment of acute asthmatic attacks include
    A. it has a short duration of action
    B. it is inactivated by sulfatase following inhalation
    C. increased airway obstruction has followed its inhalation in some asthmatics
    D. a decrease in arterial P_{O_2} has sometimes followed its use despite improvement in ventilation
    E. IPPB is required for satisfactory administration

32. Sympathomimetics with greater activity upon beta-2 adrenergic receptors than beta-1 receptors include
    A. isoetharine (Bronkosol)
    B. terbutaline
    C. isoproterenol
    D. albuterol (salbutamol)
    E. epinephrine

33. The chief advantage offered by a micronized theophylline preparation such as Theolair tablets or Bronkodyl capsules over aminophylline tablets is
    A. micronized theophylline is absorbed as rapidly as a liquid preparation
    B. micronized theophylline affords more sustained serum concentrations
    C. Theolair and Bronkodyl are less expensive than aminophylline
    D. Theolair and Bronkodyl cause more bronchodilation at the same serum concentration
    E. Theolair and Bronkodyl are 100% anhydrous theophylline

34. Symptoms of theophylline toxicity include
    A. fever
    B. vomiting
    C. convulsions
    D. hematemesis
    E. abdominal pain

35. Optimal response to treatment with theophylline occurs in most asthmatic children without signs or symptoms of toxicity at serum concentrations of
    A. 5-15 mg/ml
    B. 2-5 μ g/ml
    C. 10-15 μ g/ml
    D. 20-25 μ g/ml
    E. 30-40 μ g/ml

36. Factors reported to prolong the plasma half-life of theophylline include
    A. heart failure
    B. hepatic cirrhosis
    C. cigarette smoking
    D. ampicillin
    E. troleandomycin

37. Serum theophylline concentrations can be determined accurately by
    A. radial immunodiffusion
    B. spectrophotometry
    C. gas chromatography
    D. high pressure liquid chromatography
    E. enzyme multiplied immunoassay

38. Rates of clearance of theophylline vary widely from patient to patient, but average doses recommended to maintain therapeutic serum concentrations are
    A. 12 mg/Kg/24 hours for a 19-year-old nonsmoker
    B. 16-18 mg/Kg/24 hours for a 14-year-old nonsmoker
    C. 20 mg/Kg/24 hours for a 10-year-old
    D. 24 mg/Kg/24 hours for a 4-year-old
    E. 28 mg/Kg/24 hours for a 10-month-old infant

39. A ten-year-old asthmatic who has been receiving Quibron, 200 mg q 6h for the past week is found to have a serum theophylline concentration of 30 μ g/ml 2 hours after his last dose. Recommendations should include
    A. omit the next two doses
    B. omit the next dose and reduce to 150 mg q 6h
    C. reduce the dose to 100 mg q 8h

D. continue same dose if wheezing is still present
E. increase the dose cautiously if there are no side effects and wheezing is still present

40. Cromolyn sodium
    A. prevents release of mediators from mast cells following antigen-antibody interaction only if administered before antigen challenge
    B. can prevent exercise-induced asthma
    C. can prevent bronchoconstriction induced by hyperventilation
    D. causes bronchodilation
    E. has antihistaminic activity

41. Appropriate recommendations for asthmatic children subject to exercise-induced asthma include
    A. nasal breathing
    B. inhalation of cromolyn shortly before exercise
    C. continual treatment with a sustained-release theophylline preparation
    D. avoidance of interscholastic sports requiring running
    E. substitution of health education for physical education class

42. True statements concerning gravity-assisted postural drainage include
    A. there is no objective evidence of any beneficial effect in asthmatics
    B. effective drainage of all bronchopulmonary segments is possible using six different positions
    C. it does not aggravate bronchoconstriction
    D. effective drainage of all segments can be accomplished within ten minutes
    E. for drainage of the right middle lobe the feet are elevated 15° and the child lies on his left side and rotated $\frac{1}{4}$ turn backwards

43. Possible complications of systemic treatment with adrenal corticosteroids include
    A. diabetes mellitus
    B. hypokalemia
    C. pseudotumor cerebri
    D. pancreatitis
    E. hirsutism

44. When treatment with corticosteroids is necessary, the risk of adrenal suppression can be reduced by administration of
   A. dexamethasone by inhalation
   B. dexamethasone PO as a single morning dose on alternate days
   C. beclomethasone dipropionate aerosol, 100 μ g qid
   D. prednisone PO as a single morning dose on alternate days
   E. the lowest dose consistent with adequate symptomatic control

45. Recommended treatment of status asthmaticus includes
   A. intravenous fluids, 2400-3000 ml/M^2/24 hours, for all patients
   B. intravenous hydrocortisone for any patient who has previously been treated for asthma with corticosteroids
   C. oxygen if hypoxemia is present
   D. intravenous aminophylline to maintain serum concentration at 10-20 μ g/ml
   E. mist to prevent inspissation of secretions

46. Treatment of status asthmaticus by administration of Bronkosol or isoproterenol, 1:200, by inhalation
   A. is unlikely to be helpful because lack of response to sympathomimetics has already been established in the patient
   B. can be given simultaneously with subcutaneous injections of epinephrine with safety
   C. is safer and more effective if given by IPPB
   D. is recommended at doses of 0.1 cc/Kg (maximum 5 cc)
   E. should be accompanied by supplemental oxygen

47. Drugs contraindicated in status asthmaticus include
   A. Morphine
   B. Thorazine
   C. hydroxyzine
   D. Benadryl
   E. penicillin

48. Beneficial effects of controlled, mechanical ventilation for the treatment of severe status asthmaticus with respiratory failure include
   A. restoration of normal acid-base balance by elimination of CO_2 through more effective ventilation
   B. reduction in the work of breathing
   C. more efficient administration of aerosol therapy
   D. a lessening of the frequency of the need for blood gas determinations
   E. facilitation of the administration of postural drainage

49. Complications of endotracheal intubation and mechanical ventilation for the treatment of status asthmaticus include
    A. hypoventilation
    B. hypotension
    C. pneumothorax
    D. hyperventilation
    E. pneumonia

50. True statements concerning intravenous administration of isoproterenol for the treatment of status asthmaticus include
    A. sudden death has been reported as a complication
    B. myocardial ischemia has occurred at relatively low doses
    C. continuous electrocardiographic monitoring is recommended
    D. the isoproterenol should be delivered by a slow infusion pump
    E. treatment for more than 12 hours is rarely necessary

51. True statements concerning death from asthma in children include
    A. a progressive decrease has been observed in the U.S. during the past 30 years
    B. occlusion of airways with thick, tenacious secretions has usually been found
    C. overtreatment with corticosteroids during the terminal episode has been implicated as a possible cause
    D. death rates in infants have usually been less than those in older children
    E. delay in treatment has been implicated as a possible cause

CHAPTER IV

52. Symptoms of allergic rhinitis include
    A. a profuse, watery nasal discharge
    B. paroxysms of repetitive sneezing
    C. frequent rubbing of the nose
    D. recurrent epistaxis
    E. fever

53. Signs of allergic rhinitis include
    A. a dark discoloration of the orbitopalpebral grooves
    B. enlargement of the inferior nasal turbinates
    C. transverse nasal crease
    D. pallor of the nasal mucosa
    E. mouth breathing

54. True statements concerning eosinophilia in the blood of patients with allergic rhinitis include
   A. peripheral eosinophilia is more likely to occur during September than June in patients with ragweed hay fever
   B. total eosinophil counts are usually greater than 800 per cubic mm in children with allergic rhinitis
   C. mild, temporary peripheral eosinophilia has been reported in normal six-week-old infants
   D. the normal mean eosinophil count in children is 150 per cubic mm

55. An absence of eosinophils in a nasal smear may be due to
   A. improper technique in collecting the specimen
   B. lack of recent exposure to allergen
   C. absence of allergic rhinitis
   D. upper respiratory infection
   E. the reduced frequency of nasal eosinophilia in young infants

56. Consultation is sought for a three-year-old boy said to have been entirely well until he suddenly developed a yellowish-green nasal discharge from the left nostril four weeks ago without sneezing or nasal itching. Physical examination is normal except for the mucopurulent discharge from the left nostril. Recommendations should include
   A. nasal smear for eosinophils
   B. serum IgE determination
   C. allergy skin testing
   D. precautions to minimize exposure to house dust
   E. otolaryngology consultation

57. Complications of allergic rhinitis include
   A. sinusitis
   B. epistaxis
   C. cor pulmonale
   D. hypertrophy of tonsils and adenoids
   E. chronic middle ear effusion

58. Symptomatic relief is sought for a 12-year-old girl with seasonal allergic rhinitis due to allergy to grass pollens. Medications that have already failed to control symptoms at doses that caused excessive drowsiness include Actifed, Chlor-Trimeton, Dimetapp, Benadryl, Phenergan, and Periactin. Her weight is 50 Kg. It would be rational to prescribe
   A. Decapryn, 25 mg qid
   B. Dimetane, 6 mg qid
   C. Pyribenzamine, 50 mg qid

D. Forhistal, 1 mg tid
E. Tripelennamine, 50 mg qid

CHAPTER V

59. True statements about children with atopic dermatitis include
    A. allergic rhinitis or asthma can be expected in fewer than 25%
    B. the extent and severity of the disease often correlates with total serum IgE concentrations
    C. peripheral eosinophilia has been reported to correlate with activity of the dermatitis
    D. an increased frequency of positive delayed skin tests to streptokinase/streptodornase has been found
    E. allergy skin testing is usually helpful in identifying allergens that can be avoided to improve the dermatitis

60. Atopic dermatitis is characterized by abnormal responses to intradermal injection of
    A. acetylcholine
    B. histamine
    C. bradykinin
    D. serotonin
    E. normal saline

61. A dermatitis similar to atopic dermatitis occurs in patients with
    A. homocystinuria
    B. phenylketonuria
    C. ahistidinemia
    D. Wiskott-Aldrich syndrome
    E. urticaria pigmentosa

62. The most common complication of atopic dermatitis is
    A. molluscum contagiosum
    B. Kaposi's varicelliform eruption
    C. cataracts
    D. keratoconus
    E. bacterial infection

CHAPTER VI

63. Urticaria may occur as a manifestation of
    A. systemic anaphylaxis
    B. cytotoxic reactions
    C. type III reactions (Gell and Coombs' classification)
    D. hepatitis
    E. complement activation

64. True statements about cold urticaria include
    A. a negative ice cube test rules it out as a possibility
    B. familial cold urticaria is inherited as an autosomal dominant
    C. acquired, idiopathic cold urticaria is more frequent in children than adults
    D. passive transfer with serum is often possible
    E. there is evidence of mediation by IgM in some patients

65. Exacerbations of cholinergic urticaria may be associated with
    A. fever
    B. exercise
    C. drinking hot coffee
    D. aspirin ingestion
    E. wheezing

66. Findings consistent with hereditary angioneurotic edema include
    A. recurrent urticaria
    B. recurrent abdominal pain with nausea and vomiting
    C. normal serum concentration of C1 esterase inhibitor, C4 decreased
    D. decreased serum concentrations of C1 esterase inhibitor and C4
    E. increased serum concentrations of C1 esterase inhibitor and C4

CHAPTER VII

67. Symptoms of chronic, secretory otitis media include
    A. "popping" in the ears
    B. fluctuating impairment of auditory acuity
    C. sensation of fullness in the ears
    D. recurrent acute otitis media
    E. itching of the external auditory canals

68. Signs of secretory otitis media include
    A. retraction of the tympanic membrane and abnormal prominence of the sort process of the malleus
    B. fluid level or bubbles behind the tympanic membrane
    C. chalky white appearance to the handle of the malleus
    D. reduced mobility to pneumatic otoscopy
    E. hyperemic, bulging tympanic membrane resembling alligator skin due to desquamation of superficial epithelium

69. Reasonable recommendations for the management of chronic, secretory otitis media may include
    A. antibiotics
    B. discontinuation of bottle-propping
    C. elimination of thumb-sucking if possible
    D. politzerization
    E. precautions to minimize exposure to household inhalant allergens

70. True statements concerning impedance audiometry include
    A. tympanometry is more sensitive than either pneumatic otoscopy or audiometry for detection of middle ear effusion or reduced pressure in the middle ear
    B. a flat, type B tympanogram may be due to impacted cerumen, improper technique, or middle ear effusion
    C. tympanometry has disclosed a much higher frequency of abnormalities among children with respiratory allergy than among unselected children
    D. middle ear abnormalities manifesed as type B or type C tympanograms often subside spontaneously without treatment within six weeks
    E. a type C tympanogram is consistent with eustachian tube dysfunction

CHAPTER VIII

71. Systemic reactions to which of the following agents are NOT usually due to anaphylaxis?
    A. Penicillin
    B. Aspirin
    C. Iodinated contrast media
    D. Honeybee venom
    E. Local anesthetics

72. Initial therapy of systemic anaphylaxis should include
    A. Benadryl
    B. Bronkephrine
    C. isoproterenol
    D. hydrocortisone
    E. epinephrine

73. Precautions useful in preventing systemic anaphylaxis or anaphylactoid reactions include
    A. wearing special emblems
    B. skin testing before administration of aspirin
    C. skin testing before administration of penicillin
    D. skin testing before administration of radiographic contrast media
    E. substitution of oral for parenteral therapy when possible

CHAPTER IX

74. Diagnostic methods of established value in identifying allergens responsible for IgE-mediated food allergy include
    A. allergy skin testing
    B. leukocytotoxic test
    C. leukopenic index
    D. intracutaneous provocative testing with provoking doses and neutralizing doses
    E. double-blind challenge

75. Effective therapy appropriate for most patients with food allergy includes
    A. cromolyn
    B. adrenal corticosteroids
    C. avoidance
    D. immunotherapy
    E. oral hyposensitization

76. A diet designed to eliminate cow's milk should also eliminate
    A. orange sherbet
    B. most brands of margarine
    C. spaghetti
    D. Vienna bread
    E. Cool Whip

77. True statements concerning disaccharidase deficiency include
    A. lactase deficiency is its commonest form
    B. it is more common in infants than in older children or adults
    C. stool pH is typically less than 6
    D. addition of a Clinitest tablet to 15 drops of a 1:1 dilution of stool in water discloses more than 0.25% reducing substance
    E. tests for stool pH and reducing substance are most reliable in breast-fed newborns

CHAPTER X

78. Patients with aspirin intolerance are often unable to tolerate
    A. acetaminophen
    B. indomethacin
    C. tartrazine
    D. antipyrine
    E. Tylenol

79. Recommended precautions before administration of radiographic contrast media to patients in whom such agents have previously elicited anaphylactoid reactions include
    A. injection of a 1 ml "test dose"
    B. treatment with prednisone beginning 18 hours before this study
    C. treatment with diphenhydramine before the study
    D. administration of the contrast media in graded doses at ten minute intervals
    E. skin testing

80. A patient who has had a systemic reaction to procaine would be likely to tolerate
    A. Xylocaine
    B. Lidocaine
    C. Carbocaine
    D. Novocaine
    E. Tetracaine

CHAPTER XI

81. The major allergen of honeybee venom is
    A. melittin
    B. antigen 5
    C. apamin
    D. phospholipase A
    E. the same as the major allergen of vespid venom

82. True statements concerning hymenoptera hypersensitivity include
    A. positive intradermal skin tests to venom, $0.1 \ \mu g/ml$, have not been found in patients without histories of hypersensitivity to insect stings
    B. life-threatening systemic anaphylaxis is unusual in patients with no previous history of systemic reactions
    C. specific IgE antibody concentrations in serum may decrease spontaneously to insignificant levels within a few weeks after a systemic reaction
    D. fatal systemic anaphylaxis has followed fire ant stings
    E. leukocytes of some patients with hymenoptera hypersensitivity do not release histamine even after challenge with anti-IgE
    F. use of RAST has elicited as many as 20% false positive reactions and 20% false negatives as compared with skin testing with hymenoptera venom

83. Immunotherapy for hymenoptera hypersensitivity is indicated for patients with
    A. large local reactions persisting several days and negative skin tests to venom
    B. histories of systemic reactions but negative skin tests to venom
    C. histories of systemic reactions and positive skin tests
    D. histories of local reactions of decreasing size with subsequent stings and positive skin tests with venom at 1 μ g/ml
    E. histories of systemic reactions followed by whole body extract injections for three to five years, but skin tests to venom that are still positive

84. True statements concerning immunotherapy with hymenoptera venom include
    A. significant increases in serum concentrations of specific IgG are elicited
    B. serum concentrations of specific IgE usually increase during the first month
    C. systemic reactions to therapy have been reported in 2% of children treated
    D. serum concentrations of specific IgE are lower than before treatment after 12 months of therapy
    E. protection against systemic reactions from hymenoptera stings can be expected within ten weeks after treatment has started in 95% of patients

85. Patients who have had systemic reactions to honeybee stings should
    A. always wear shoes outdoors
    B. wear dark clothing rather than white
    C. stop using hair tonic
    D. wear gloves while picking peaches
    E. be equipped with 1:1000 aqueous epinephrine

CHAPTER XII

86. Ragweed pollination is favored by
    A. dry weather before the pollen season
    B. dry weather during the pollen season
    C. morning rather than evening
    D. wind
    E. an early frost

87. The most potent allergen in ragweed pollen is
    A. antigen E
    B. antigen K
    C. Ra3
    D. Ra4
    E. Ra5
    F. Ra6

88. The least likely cause of an exacerbation of asthma, after
    a fir Christmas tree has been brought into a Texas home, is
    A. hypersensitivity to fir pollen
    B. hypersensitivity to mountain cedar pollen
    C. hypersensitivity to molds
    D. the fragrance

89. Common sources of exposure to fungi include
    A. mattresses
    B. upholstered furniture
    C. shower curtains
    D. wallpaper
    E. books

90. True statements concerning precautions to minimize exposure
    to house dust include
    A. they are unnecessary if an acaricide is used
    B. hot air vents in the bedroom should be sealed even if a
       central HEPA filter is used
    C. foam rubber mattresses need not be encased in air-tight
       covers
    D. synthetic carpet is acceptable
    E. regular vacuuming of the mattress substantially reduces
       its mite population

CHAPTER XIII

91. A negative skin test to a grass pollen extract may be due to
    A. lack of hypersensitivity
    B. use of an impotent extract
    C. improper technique
    D. administration of Marax 36 hours before testing
    E. administration of Tedral 12 hours before testing

92. A positive skin test may be due to
    A. intradermal testing with 1:100 dog dander rather than a
       higher dilution
    B. intradermal testing with extracts containing 20% glycerin
    C. intradermal injection of an air bubble
    D. dermographism
    E. hypersensitivity

93. Stability for at least six months has been reported for
1: 10, 000 pollen extracts containing
   A. 50% glycerosaline
   B. 0.03% human serum albumin
   C. 0.005% Tween 80
   D. bicarbonate buffered saline
   E. 0.4% phenol

94. True statements concerning total serum IgE concentrations
as determined by PRIST include
   A. a value exceeding 20 U/ml during the first year suggests
      atopic allergy
   B. adult values are normally reached by ten years of age
   C. a value of 50 U/ml is above the normal adult geometric
      mean
   D. they correlate well with determination by radial
      immunodiffusion
   E. a value of 180 U/ml is within the normal range for a
      ten-year-old child

95. Disadvantages of RAST as compared with allergy skin testing
include
   A. safety
   B. expense
   C. lack of interference of antihistamines
   D. reduced sensitivity
   E. results not immediately available

CHAPTER XIV

96. Controlled studies in patients with respiratory allergy have
established the effectiveness of immunotherapy with
   A. alternaria
   B. antigen E
   C. ragweed pollen extract
   D. mountain cedar pollen extract
   E. Dermatophagoides pteronyssinus

97. Treatment of patients with ragweed hay fever with ragweed
pollen extract is usually followed by
   A. an increase in the serum titer of specific, IgG blocking
      antibody that tends to be proportional to the dose of ex-
      tract administered
   B. an immediate decrease in the serum titer of specific,
      IgE antibody
   C. suppression of the usual seasonal increase in specific,
      IgE antibody

D. decreased release of lymphokines and a decrease in the proliferative response of T lymphocytes to challenge with ragweed antigens

E. decreased release of histamine from basophils challenged with antigen after 12 months of treatment

98. Complications of immunotherapy include
A. systemic anaphylaxis
B. swelling and erythema at the injection site persisting several hours
C. coughing and wheezing beginning eight hours after the last injection
D. pallor and diaphoresis followed by syncope without tachycardia
E. fever, malaise, and arthralgia associated with local reactions persisting several hours

99. Indications for immunotherapy include
A. severe asthma recurrent at three to ten day intervals between the months of June and October each year
B. almost continual wheezing for three months in a six-month-old boy who has cried most of the time since introduction of "mixed cereal" into his diet at two months of age
C. severe, perennial allergic rhinitis, unresponsive to antihistamines, in a three-year-old boy with cardiomegaly and large, positive reactions to skin testing with alternaria, timothy, oak, ragweed, and house dust
D. frequent, severe wheezing in a child with negative skin tests and negative RAST

100. True statements about immunotherapy with pollen extracts include
A. there is evidence that some patients who show no improvement during the first year of treatment may improve during the second year
B. most asthmatics receiving appropriate immunotherapy become completely free of symptoms within three years
C. continued treatment is recommended until the patient has been free of symptoms for one to two years or has had only minimal symptoms for three years
D. if immunotherapy is discontinued after improvement has occurred, symptoms almost never recur
E. complete retesting annually is necessary to assess the response of the patient receiving immunotherapy

ANSWER SHEET

TITLE: Pediatric Allergy, 2d Ed., Medical Outline Series
by R. Michael Sly, M.D.

INSTRUCTIONS: Blacken the box under the correct answer

	A	B	C	D	E	F		A	B	C	D	E	F
1.	☐	☐	☐	☐	☐		29.	☐	☐	☐	☐	☐	
2.	☐	☐	☐	☐	☐		30.	☐	☐	☐	☐	☐	
3.	☐	☐	☐	☐	☐		31.	☐	☐	☐	☐	☐	
4.	☐	☐	☐	☐	☐		32.	☐	☐	☐	☐	☐	
5.	☐	☐	☐	☐	☐		33.	☐	☐	☐	☐	☐	
6.	☐	☐	☐	☐	☐		34.	☐	☐	☐	☐	☐	
7.	☐	☐	☐	☐	☐		35.	☐	☐	☐	☐	☐	
8.	☐	☐	☐	☐	☐		36.	☐	☐	☐	☐	☐	
9.	☐	☐	☐	☐	☐		37.	☐	☐	☐	☐	☐	
10.	☐	☐	☐	☐	☐		38.	☐	☐	☐	☐	☐	
11.	☐	☐	☐	☐	☐		39.	☐	☐	☐	☐	☐	
12.	☐	☐	☐	☐	☐		40.	☐	☐	☐	☐	☐	
13.	☐	☐	☐	☐	☐		41.	☐	☐	☐	☐	☐	
14.	☐	☐	☐	☐	☐		42.	☐	☐	☐	☐	☐	
15.	☐	☐	☐	☐	☐		43.	☐	☐	☐	☐	☐	
16.	☐	☐	☐	☐	☐		44.	☐	☐	☐	☐	☐	
17.	☐	☐	☐	☐	☐		45.	☐	☐	☐	☐	☐	
18.	☐	☐	☐	☐	☐		46.	☐	☐	☐	☐	☐	
19.	☐	☐	☐	☐	☐		47.	☐	☐	☐	☐	☐	
20.	☐	☐	☐	☐	☐		48.	☐	☐	☐	☐	☐	
21.	☐	☐	☐	☐	☐		49.	☐	☐	☐	☐	☐	
22.	☐	☐	☐	☐	☐		50.	☐	☐	☐	☐	☐	
23.	☐	☐	☐	☐	☐		51.	☐	☐	☐	☐	☐	
24.	☐	☐	☐	☐	☐		52.	☐	☐	☐	☐	☐	
25.	☐	☐	☐	☐	☐		53.	☐	☐	☐	☐	☐	
26.	☐	☐	☐	☐	☐		54.	☐	☐	☐	☐		
27.	☐	☐	☐	☐	☐		55.	☐	☐	☐	☐	☐	
28.	☐	☐	☐	☐	☐		56.	☐	☐	☐	☐	☐	

	A	B	C	D	E	F		A	B	C	D	E	F
57.	☐	☐	☐	☐	☐		79.	☐	☐	☐	☐	☐	
58.	☐	☐	☐	☐	☐		80.	☐	☐	☐	☐	☐	
59.	☐	☐	☐	☐	☐		81.	☐	☐	☐	☐	☐	
60.	☐	☐	☐	☐	☐		82.	☐	☐	☐	☐	☐	☐
61.	☐	☐	☐	☐	☐		83.	☐	☐	☐	☐	☐	
62.	☐	☐	☐	☐	☐		84.	☐	☐	☐	☐	☐	
63.	☐	☐	☐	☐	☐		85.	☐	☐	☐	☐	☐	
64.	☐	☐	☐	☐	☐		86.	☐	☐	☐	☐	☐	
65.	☐	☐	☐	☐	☐		87.	☐	☐	☐	☐	☐	☐
66.	☐	☐	☐	☐	☐		88.	☐	☐	☐	☐		
67.	☐	☐	☐	☐	☐		89.	☐	☐	☐	☐	☐	
68.	☐	☐	☐	☐	☐		90.	☐	☐	☐	☐	☐	
69.	☐	☐	☐	☐	☐		91.	☐	☐	☐	☐	☐	
70.	☐	☐	☐	☐	☐		92.	☐	☐	☐	☐	☐	
71.	☐	☐	☐	☐	☐		93.	☐	☐	☐	☐	☐	
72.	☐	☐	☐	☐	☐		94.	☐	☐	☐	☐	☐	
73.	☐	☐	☐	☐	☐		95.	☐	☐	☐	☐	☐	
74.	☐	☐	☐	☐	☐		96.	☐	☐	☐	☐	☐	
75.	☐	☐	☐	☐	☐		97.	☐	☐	☐	☐	☐	
76.	☐	☐	☐	☐	☐		98.	☐	☐	☐	☐	☐	
77.	☐	☐	☐	☐	☐		99.	☐	☐	☐	☐		
78.	☐	☐	☐	☐	☐		100.	☐	☐	☐	☐	☐	

NAME (PRINT)_____

STREET _____

CITY _____STATE_____ZIP_____